Lawrence Charles Parish   Larry E. Millikan
with
Mohamed Amer   Robin A. C. Graham-Brown
Sidney N. Klaus   Joseph L. Pace
Editors

Global
Dermatology

Diagnosis and Management According to
Geography, Climate, and Culture

With 156 Illustrations and 37 Color Plates

Springer-Verlag
New York Berlin Heidelberg London Paris
Tokyo Hong Kong Barcelona Budapest

Lawrence Charles Parish, MD
1819 J. F. Kennedy Boulevard Suite 465
Philadelphia, Pennsylvania 19103, USA
and
Clinical Professor of Dermatology and Director
Jefferson Center for International Dermatology
Jefferson Medical College
Thomas Jefferson University
Philadelphia, PA
USA
and
Visiting Professor of Dermatology
Yonsei University College of Medicine
Seoul, Korea
and
Visiting Professor of Dermatology
and Venereology
Zagazig University
Zagazig, Egypt

Larry E. Millikan, MD
Professor and Chairman of Dermatology
Tulane University School of Medicine
1430 Tulane Avenue
New Orleans, LA 70112
USA

Library of Congress Cataloging-in-Publication Data

Global dermatology: diagnosis and management according to geography,
  climate, and culture / edited by Lawrence Charles Parish and Larry
  E. Millikan : with contributions by Mohamad Amer. . . [et al.].
      p.   cm.
    Includes bibliographical references and index.
    ISBN 0-387-94140-1
    1. Dermatology. 2. Medical geography. 3. Skin—Diseases—
  Epidemiology. 4. Dermatology—Cross-cultural studies. I. Parish,
  Lawrence Charles. II. Millikan, Larry E., 1938-, III. Amer, Mohamad.
    [DNLM: 1. Skin Diseases—diagnosis. 2. Skin Diseases—therapy,
  3. Climate. 4. Anthropology, Cultural.   WR 100 G562 1994]
  RL72.G58   1994
  616.5—dc20
  DNLM/DLC
  for Library of Congress   93-26905

Printed on acid-free paper.

Typeset by Techset Composition, Ltd., United Kingdom
Production by TechEdit Production Services; and supervised by Natalie Johnson.
Manufacturing Supervised by Jacqui Ashri
Printed and bound by Edwards Brothers, Inc. Ann Arbor, MI.
Printed in the United States of America.

9 8 7 6 5 4 3 2 1

ISBN 0-387-94140-1   Springer-Verlag New York Berlin Heidelberg
ISBN 3-540-94140-1   Springer-Verlag Berlin Heidelberg New York

To our wives:

Sheila and Jeanine
Susan, Margaret, Anne, and Mary Ann

Preface

The concept of a textbook of global dermatology grew from the forums conducted by us at the annual meetings of the American Academy of Dermatology. Initially, these sessions were titled "Tropical Dermatology," but later we selected Global Dermatology as a term seemingly more attractive to the North American participants. An equally important factor in the development of this book grew from a desire to revise and enlarge the textbook, *Manual of Tropical Dermatology*.[1]

By global, we hope to convey with this word the tenets of the International Society of Dermatology: Tropical, Geographic and Ecologic. The actual use of the term global dermatology should be attributed to Frederick Reiss, founding Secretary-General of the Society, who wrote two decades ago:

the investigation of geographic ecology of skin and venereal disease and basic research. This means *global dermatology* and venereology.[2]

We had originally thought we had coined the term, when four years ago we embarked on this project. We had previously discarded international as being too political, and racial as being too charged.

Many books are concerned with tropical dermatology,[1,3-5] tropical venereology,[6] racial differences,[7,8] the environment,[9] or with travel medicine,[10] but none to our knowledge has examined skin diseases and how they may differ in various parts of the world due to socioeconomic, ecologic, climatologic, or genetic influences. We wanted to know why the dermatologists of yesteryear always focused on national or racial origin. Were they correct in stating that some diseases were those of the poor or that ethnic background was significant?[11,12]

As we began to look into the problems of sorting out what global dermatology encompasses, we asked ourselves several questions: Does geography make a difference? Does climate really alter disease states? Do genetics significantly change the type of cutaneous affliction? Do socioeconomic factors create new problems?

We then organized the book into the various sections as listed in Contents, agonizing over the outline at the Zagazig International Conferences of Dermatology and Venereology and at other congresses. Experts from around the world were invited to discuss selected aspects. We had first thought that all chapters would fit into a proper form, but we soon discovered that many terms are not universal, comparative epide-miologic data are not available everywhere, and most important, what we might think worthy of discussion was uninteresting in another area of the world.[13,14]

Global Dermatology should be considered an adventure into uncharted areas of dermatology. We have not intended to create another major textbook in the field, but we have gathered contributions from many parts of the world about aspects of the specialty that are often not included in major review articles or even lengthy book chapters. We have not intended to cover every country of the world—too many are created everyday to include every race, with too much disagreement and variation—or to discuss every variable; rather, we are presenting a distillation of dermato-logy as it appears around the globe in the closing years of the twentieth century.

We are most appreciative of the wonderful cooperation contributed by the staff at Springer-Verlag New York, Dr. Hirak Routh, Fellow in International Dermatology, Jefferson Center for International Dermato-logy, and Ms. Carmela Ciferni, Philadelphia, provided editorial assistance during the development and production of this book.

References

1. Pettit JHS, Parish LC: Manual of Tropical Dermatology. New York: Springer-Verlag, 1984: 1–260.
2. Reiss F: International Society of Tropical Dermatology. *Arch Dermatol* 1973; **107**: 916.
3. Cañizares O: Introduction to tropical dermatology: Factors and concepts. In: Clinical Tropical Dermatology, 1st ed. London: Blackwell Scientific Publications, 1975: 1–9.
4. Cañizares O: A Manual of Dermatology for Developing Countries. New York: Oxford University Press, 1982: 1–355.
5. Cañizares O, Harman R: Introduction to tropical dermatology: Factors and concepts. In: Cañizares O, Harman, R, ed. Clinical Tropical Dermatology. London: Blackwell Scientific Publications, 1992: 1–9.
6. Arya OP, Osoba AO, Bennett FJ: Tropical Venereology, 2nd ed. London: Churchill Livingstone, 1988: 1–370.
7. Basset A: Dermatology of Black Skin. Oxford: Oxford University Press, 1986: 1–114.
8. McDonald CJ, Scott D: Dermatology in black patients. *Dermatol Clin* 1988; **6**: 343–496.
9. Marks R, Plewig G: The Environmental Threat to the Skin. London: Martin Dunitz, 1992: 1–414.
10. Steffen R, Lobel HO, Hawroth J et al: Travel Medicine. New York: Springer-Verlag, 1989: 1–596.
11. Rubin MB, Parish LC: Dermatology of the 1870's: Patterns of occurrences of cutaneous disease (1871–1874). *Int J Dermatol* 1974; **13**: 42–46.
12. Parish LC: History of tropical dermatology. *Int J Dermatol* 1985; **24**: 191–193.
13. Rook A, Savin JA, Wilkinson DS: The prevalence, incidence and ecology of diseases of the skin. In: Rook A, Wilkinson DS, Ebling FJG et al, eds. Textbook of Dermatology, 3rd ed. London: Blackwell Scientific Publications, 1979: 39–53.

14. Burton JL, Savin JA, Champion RH: Introduction, epidemiology and histor-
    ical bibliography. In: Champion RH, Burton JL, Ebling FJG, eds. Textbook
    of Dermatology, 5th ed. London: Blackwell Scientific Publications, 1992:
    1–15.
15. Goihman Yahr, M: Nehushtan: The Globality of Cutaneous Medicine. *Int J
    Dermatol* 1994; **33**: 105–106.

February 9, 1994   Lawrence Charles Parish, MD
                                                                  Philadelphia
                                                          Larry E. Millikan, MD
                                                                   New Orleans

Contents

Contributors

Sung Ku Ahn, MD Assistant Professor of Dermatology, Yonsei University, Wonju College of Medicine, Wonju, 220 Korea

Mohamed Amer, MD Professor and Chairman of Dermatology and Venereology, Zagazig University Faculty of Medicine, 86, Ahmed El Zyat Street, Dokki, Cairo, Egypt, and Visiting Professor of Dermatology, Jefferson Medical College, Thomas Jefferson University, Philadelphia, Pennsylvania 19107, USA

Anthony J. Badame, MD Clinical Instructor, Department of Dermatology, Stanford University School of Medicine, Stanford, California 94304, USA

S. Bose, MD Dermatologist, Hôpital Pasteur, 06002 Nice Cedex, France

R. Estrada Castanon, MD Physician, Centro de Investigacion de Enfermedades Tropicales, Universidad Autonoma de Guerrero, Acapulco, Mexico

G. Cauwenbergh, PhD Director, Janssen Research Foundation, B-2340 Beerse, Belgium

Barnet L. Cline, MD, PhD Professor of Tropical Medicine, Tulane University School of Public Health and Tropical Medicine, 1501 Canal Street, New Orleans, Louisiana 70112-2824, USA

J. Carl Craft, MD Director, Macrolide Venture, Abbott Laboratories, Abbott Park, Illinois 60064-3500, USA

Chérie M. Ditre, MD Assistant Professor of Medicine (Dermatology), Hahnemann University School of Medicine, Broad and Vine streets, Mail Stop 401, Philadelphia, Pennsylvania 19102, USA

Luciano Domínguez-Soto, MD Professor and Chairman of Dermatology, Hospital General Dr. Manuel Gea Gonzalez, Calz. de Tlalpan 4800, Mexico City, 14 000, Mexico

Alfred Eichmann, MD Professor of Dermatology, University of Zurich, Zurich CH-8006, Switzerland

Rafael Falabella, MD Professor of Dermatology, Universidad del Valle School of Medicine, Centro Medico Imbanaco, Carrera 38 A, No 5A-108, Cali, Colombia

Abraham Feinstein, MD (deceased) Formerly with The Chaim Sheba Medical Center, Sackler School of Medicine, Tel-Hashomer 52621, Israel

Aldo F. Finzi, MD Professor and Chairman of Dermatology II, Universitá di Milano, Via Pace 9, 20122 Milano, Italy

Alberto Fioroni, MD   Professor of Dermatology II, Universitá di Milano, Via Place 9, 20122 Milano, Italy

Miriam Friedman, PhD   Research Associate, Faculty of Health Sciences, Ben Gurion University of the Negev, Beer Sheva, Israel and Visiting Scientist, Educational Commission for Foreign Medical Graduates, 3624 Market Street, Philadelphia, Pennsylvania 19104-2685, USA

Adekunle O. George, MB, BS, FMCP   Lecturer in Dermatology, University of Ibadan, College of Medicine, Ibadan, Nigeria

Sander L. Gilman, PhD   The Goldwin Smith Professor Humane Studies, Cornell University, 194 Goldwin Smith Hall, Ithaca, New York 14853, USA

Mauricio Goihman-Yahr, MD PhD   Professor and Chairman of Dermatology, Vargas School of Dermatology, Central University of Venezuela, Consultorio 4-B, Avenue Los Proceres, San Bernadino, Caracas, 1011, Venezuela

Robin A. C. Graham-Brown, BSc, MB, FRCP   Consultant Dermatologist, Leicester Royal Infirmary, Leicester, LE1 5WW, United Kingdom

Allen C. Green, MD, BS, DTM&H, DPH, FRACMA, FACD   Private, Practice, P.O. Box 111, 28 Barker Road, Prospect, South Australia 5082

R. J. Hay, DM, FRCP, MRC Path   Professor of Cutaneous Medicine, St. John's Institute of Dermatology, Guys Hospital, London, SE1 9RT, United Kingdom

Juan F. Honeyman, MD   Professor of Dermatology, University of Chile, Faculty of Medicine, Bilbao 5540, Santiago, Chile

Peter J. Ihrke, VMD   Professor of Dermatology, University of California at Davis, School of Veterinary Medicine, Davis, California 95616, USA, and Adjunct Clinical Associate Professor of Dermatology, Stanford University School of Medicine, Stanford, California 94304, USA

Stefania Jablonska, MD   Professor of Dermatology, Warsaw School of Medicine, Koszykowa 82a, 02-008 Warsaw, Poland

A. Katsambas, MD   Lecturer in Dermatology, University of Athens, Skoufa 35 GR-10446 Athens, Greece

Y. Alyssa Kim, MD   Instructor in Dermatology, UMD-New Jersey Medical School, Newark, New Jersey 07103-2714, USA

Sidney N. Klaus, MD   Professor and Chairman of Dermatology, Hebrew University School of Medicine, P.O. Box 12000 IL-91120 Jerusalem, Israel

K. Erik Kostelnik, MD   Resident in Medicine, Pennsylvania Hospital, 800 Spruce Street, Philadelphia, Pennsylvania 19107, USA

Inga-Britt Krause, PhD   Lecturer, Academic Department of Psychiatry, University College and Middlesex School of Medicine, 38 Marlborough Place, London NW8 0PT, United Kingdom

Amal K. Kurban, MD   Professor of Dermatology and Director of Clinical Services, Boston University School of Medicine, 80 East Concord Street, Boston, Massachusetts 02118-2394, USA

Ramsay S. Kurban, MD   Clinical Associate in Pathology, Harvard Medical School, Boston, Massachusetts 02115, USA

Sungnack Lee, MD   Professor of Dermatology, Ajou University Medical College, 5 Wonchon-Dong, Suwon 441-749, Korea

Gunnar Lomholt, MD (deceased)   Dermatologist, Graesvangen 79, Tilst, DK-8381 Mundelstrup, Denmark

Larry E. Millikan, MD   Professor and Chairman of Dermatology, Tulane University School of Medicine, New Orleans, Louisiana 70112-2824, USA

Yoshiki Miyachi, MD   Head of Dermatology Tenri General Hospital 200 Mishima-Cho Tenri, Nara 632, Japan

Rebecca L. Neame, BSc (Hons)   Consultant Dermatologist, Leicester Royal Infirmary, Leicester, LE1 5WW, United Kingdom

Yetunde Mercy Olumide, MD   Associate Professor of Dermatology, University of Lagos College of Medicine, P.M.B. 12003, Lagos, Nigeria

J. P. Ortonne, MD   Chief of Dermatology, Hôpital Pasteur, 06002, Nice, France

Joseph L. Pace, MD   Lecturer in Dermatology, University of Malta Medical School, Boffa Hospital, Floriana, Malta

Lawrence Charles Parish, MD   Clinical Professor of Dermatology and Director, Jefferson Center for International Dermatology, Jefferson Medical College, Thomas Jefferson University, Philadelphia, Pennsylvania 19107, USA

D. Rigopoulos, MD   Lecturer in Dermatology, University of Athens, School of Medicine, 5 Dragoumi Street, Kesariani GR-161 21, Athens, Greece

Albrecht Scholz, MD   Professor of Dermatology, Dresden Medical Academy, Postanschrift Fetscherstrasse 74, D-01307 Dresden, Germany

E. Joy Schulz, MD   Professor and Chairman of Dermatology, University of the Witwaterstrand Medical School, Johannesburg, South Africa,

Robert A. Schwartz, MD, MPH   Professor and Head of Dermatology, UMD-New Jersey Medical School, Newark, New Jersey 07103-2714, USA

Rita Sigg-Martin, MD   Private Practice, Hergiswil, Switzerland, CH-6052

Ahmed Moh'd Abu Shareeah, MD   Head of Dermatology and Venereology, Mafraq Hospital, P.O. Box 46142, Abu Dhabi, United Arab Emirates

Robert Steffen, MD   Professor and Head of Epidemiology and Prevention of Communicable Diseases, Institute of Social and Preventive Medicine, University of Zurich, Sumatrastrasse 30, CH-8006 Zurich, Switzerland

John D. Stratigos, MD   Professor and Chairman of Dermatology and Venereology, University of Athens School of Medicine, 5 Dragoumi Street, Kesariani GR16121, Athens, Greece

Günter Stüttgen, MD   Formerly, Chairman of Dermatology, Rudolf Virchow Institute, Free University of Berlin, Kissinger Strasse 12, D-14199, Germany

Alton I. Sutnick, MD   Vice President, Educational Commission for Foreign Medical Graduates, 3624 Market Street, Philadelphia, Pennsylvania 19104-2685, USA

Eric Van Hecke, MD   Docent, University of Gent, De Pintelaan 185, B-90000 Gent, Belgium

Dennis A. Weigand, MD Professor and Vice-Head of Dermatology, University of Oklahoma Health Sciences Center, 619 Northeast 13th Street, Oklahoma City, Oklahoma 73190, USA

Luitgard G. Wiest, MD Private Practice, Residenzstrasse 7, 8000 Munchen 2, Germany

Marjorie P. Wilson, MD President, Educational Commission for Foreign Medical Graduates, 3624 Market Street, Philadelphia, Pennsylvania 19104-2685, USA

Patrick Yesudian, MB, BS, FRCP Dermatologist, Government General Hospital, P.A. Building, 869, P.H. Road, Madras 600 010, India

Atlas of Global Dermatology

The enormous variation in skin disease that can occur globally is so large that a color atlas of global dermatology can only be representative of the cutaneous maladies.

Selected photographs have been included in this section to illustrate representative and/or significant changes in the skin. The pictures have been grouped into four categories: genetic/hereditary, infections, metabolic/medical, and other/environmental.

Genetic/Hereditary

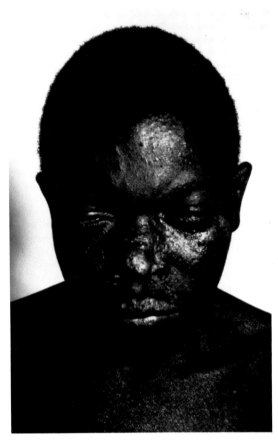

Xeroderma pigmentsoum with basal cell and squamous cell carcinoma. This Malawian man has a malignant melanoma in the right eye. (Photo courtesy of Gunnar Lomholt, M.D.)

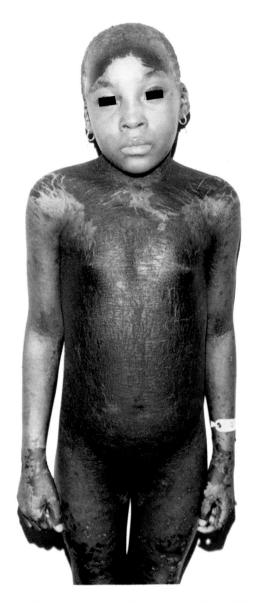

Lamellar ichthyosis in a black girl from South Africa. (Photo courtesy of E. Joy Schulz, M.D.)

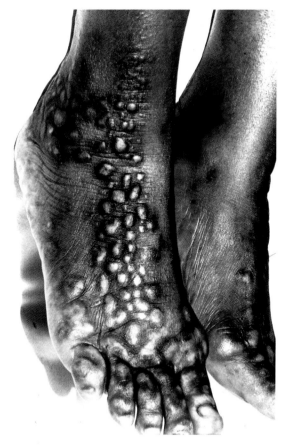

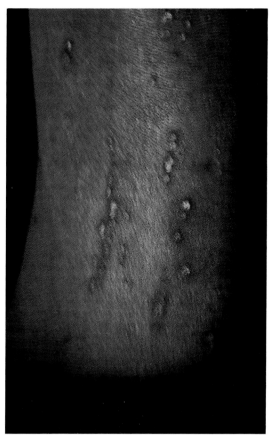

Papular keratoderma in a black man from South Africa. (Photo courtesy of E. Joy Schulz, M.D.)

Kyrle's disease in an Indian patient.

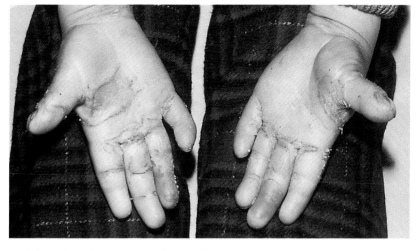

Mal de Meleda in a Greek patient. (Photo courtesy of John D. Stratigos, M.D.)

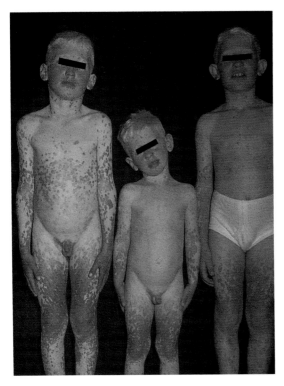

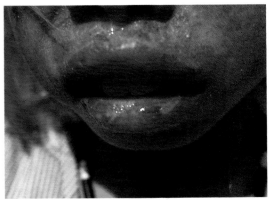

Albinism with sun damage in a 10-year-old Australian aborigine girl. (Photo courtesy of Dr. Allen C. Green.)

Albinism with deafness (Ziprkowski syndrome) in Israeli children. Three siblings of consanguineous Morrocan Sephardi Jewish origin who have piebaldism and deafness. (Photo courtesy of Abraham Feinstein, M.D.)

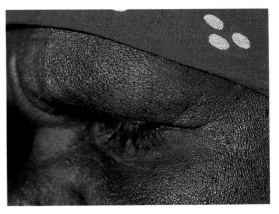

Madarosis and dermatosis papulosa nigrans in a 30-year-old Australian aborigine woman. (Photo courtesy of Dr. Allen C. Green.)

Infections

Lepromatous leprosy in an Asian immigrant to the United States. (Photo courtesy of Y. Alyssa Kim, M.D.)

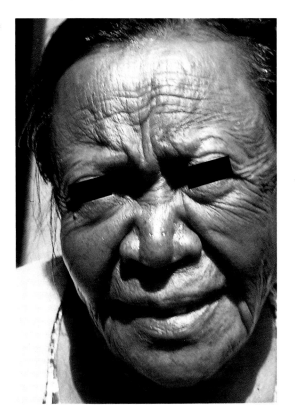

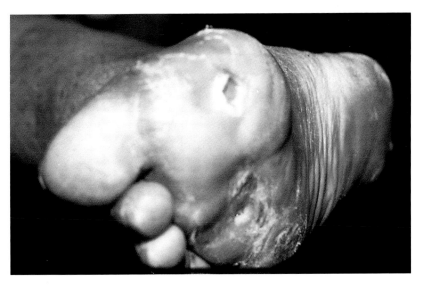

Lepromatous leprosy in an Asian immigrant to the United States. (Photo courtesy of Y. Alyssa Kim, M.D.)

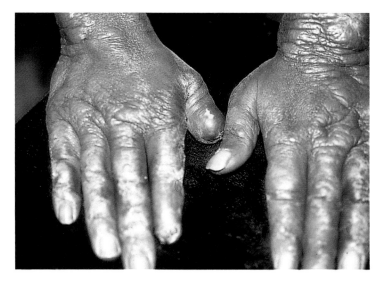

Lepromatous leprosy in an Asian immigrant to the United States. (Photo courtesy of Y. Alyssa Kim, M.D.)

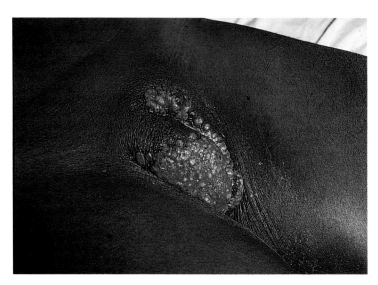

Granuloma inquinale in a 20-year-old Australian aborigine. (Photo courtesy of Dr. Allen C. Green.)

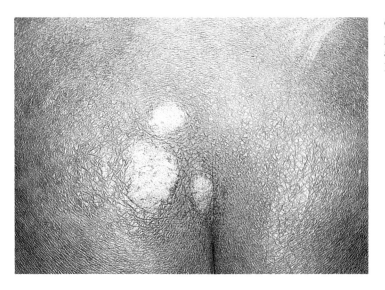

Crusted scabies in a Columbian patient who also had condyloma accuminata. (Photo courtesy of Rafael Falabella, M.D.)

Prurigo nodularis and severe pruritus in a 39-year-old Rwandese man with HIV infection. (Photo courtesy of E. Van Hecke, M.D.)

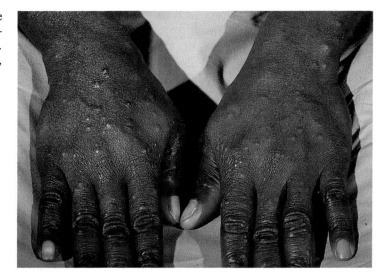

Kaposi's sarcoma in a 30-year-old Rwandese man with HIV infection. (Photo courtesy of E. Van Hecke, M.D.)

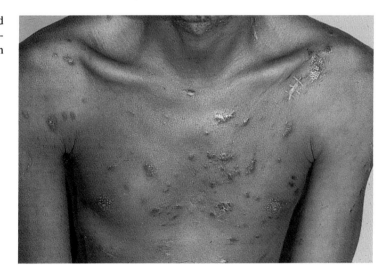

Kaposi's sarcoma not related to HIV infection (Eastern European type) in a Polish patient. (Photo courtesy of Stephania Jablonska, M.D.)

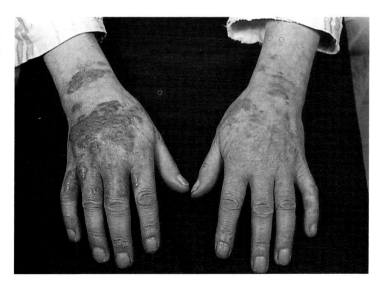

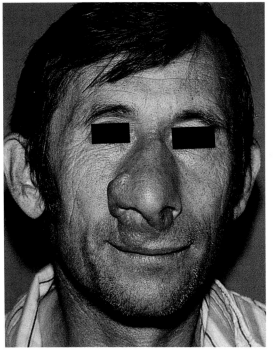

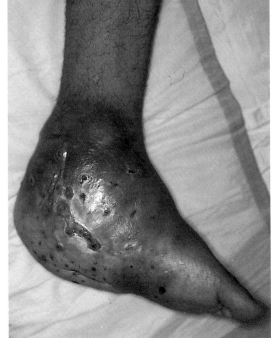

Rhinoscleroma in a Polish man. (Photo courtesy of Stephania Jablonska, M.D. and S. Chodynicki, M.D.)

Mycetoma of the foot in an American patient.

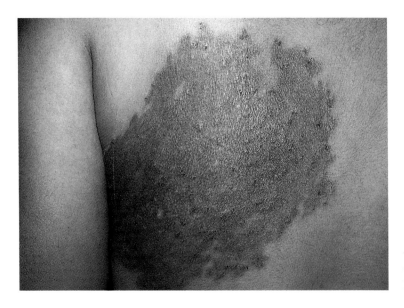

Tinea corporis in a Columbian woman. (Photo courtesy of Rafael Falabella, M.D.)

Tinea versicolor in an adolescent Australian aborigine. (Photo courtesy of Dr. Allen C. Green.)

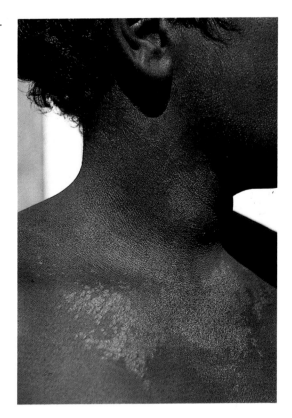

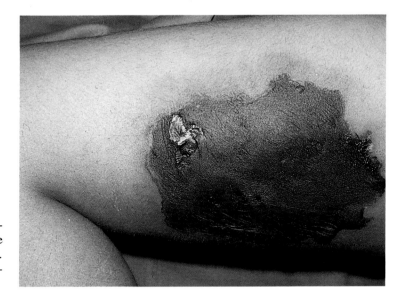

Postvaricella necrosis that developed 3 weeks after the acute
episode in a Columbian patient.
(Photo courtesy of Rafael Falabella, M.D.)

Metabolic/Medical

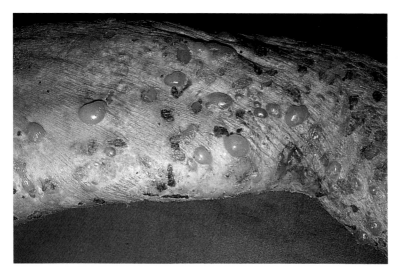

Dermatitis herpetiformis in a Columbian patient. (Photo courtesy of Dr. Rafael Falabella, M.D.)

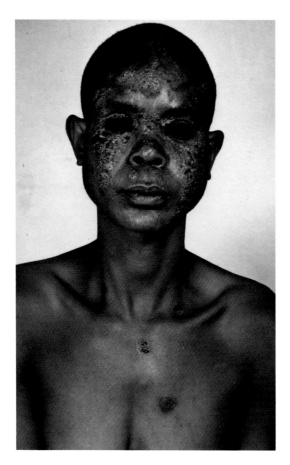

Pemphigus erythematosus in a Malawian patient. (Photo courtesy of Gunnar Lomholt, M.D.)

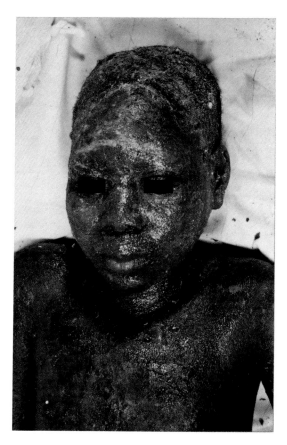

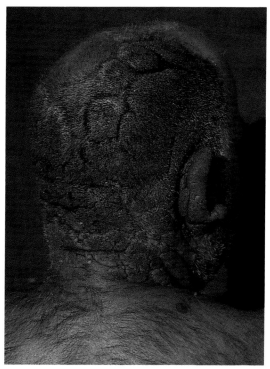

Pemphigus vegetans in an Indian patient. (Photo courtesy of Patrick Yesudian, M.D.)

Pemphigus foliaceus in a Malawian patient. (Photo courtesy of Gunnar Lomholt, M.D.)

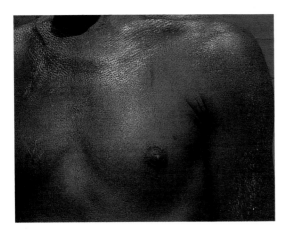

Systemic sclerosis in an Indian patient. (Photo courtesy of Patrick Yesudian, M.D.)

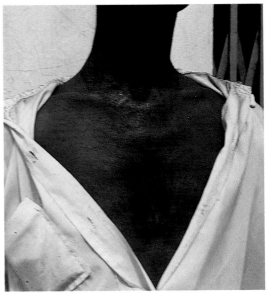

Pellagra with Casal's necklace in an Indian patient. (Photo courtesy of Patrick Yesudian, M.D.)

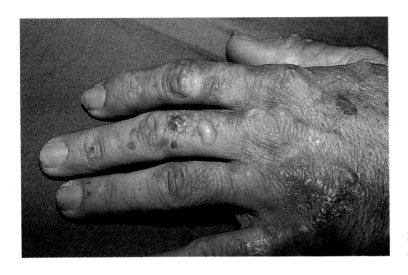

Porphyria cutanea tarda in an American patient.

Other/Environmental

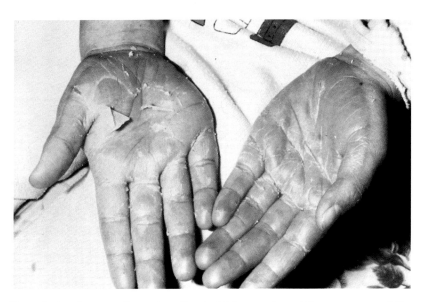

Keratolytic winter erythema in a South African patient. (Photo courtesy of Dr. J. G. L. Morrison.)

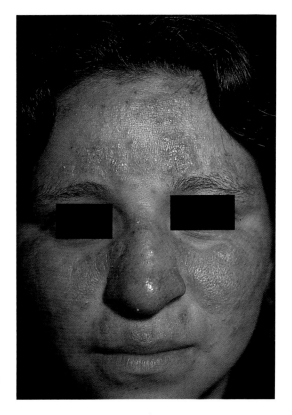

Actinic prurigo in a Mexican patient. (Photo courtesy of Luciano Domínguéz-Soto, M.D.)

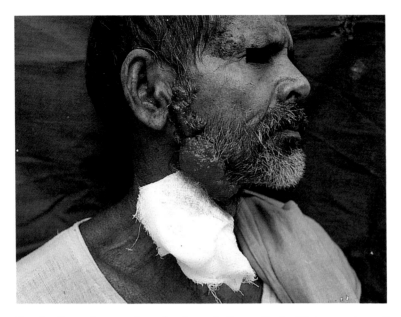

Basal cell carcinoma, ulcerating in an Indian patient. (Photo courtesy of Patrick Yesudian, M.D.)

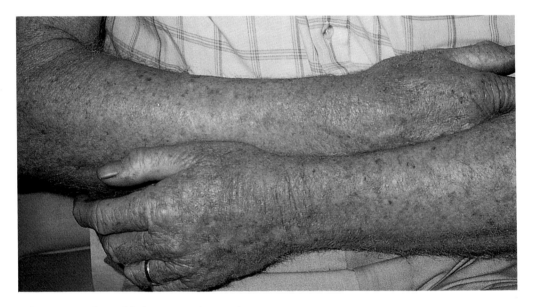

Photocontact dermatitis in an American patient.

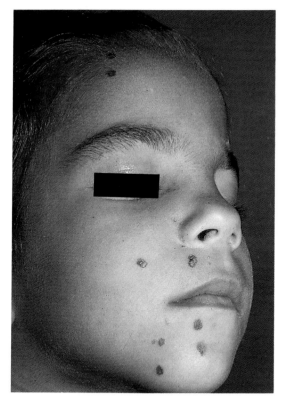

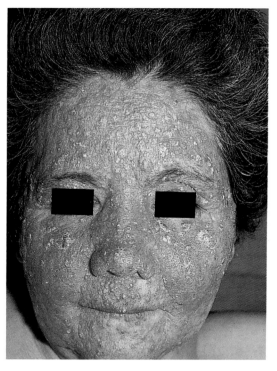

Rosacea aggravated by the chronic use of topical steroids in a Columbian woman. (Photo courtesy of Rafael Falabella, M.D.)

Mango sap irritant dermatitis in a Columbian boy. (Photo courtesy of Rafael Falabella, M.D.)

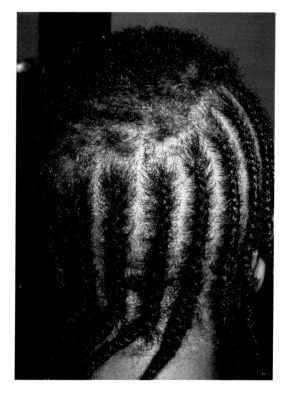

Cornrowing alopecia in an African-American woman. The hair is tightly braided in rows. (Photo courtesy of Chérie M. Ditre, M.D.)

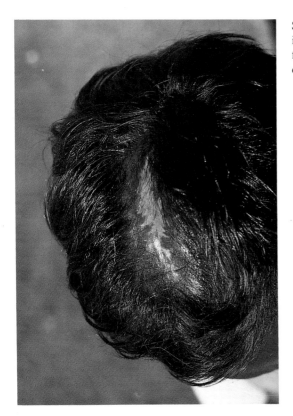

Sorry-cuts alopecia in a 43-year-old Australian aborigine woman. These scars result from injuries inflicted by a stick following the death of a baby. (Photo courtesy of Dr. Allen C. Green.)

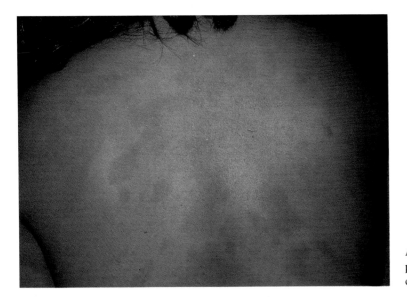

Ashy dermatosis in a Mexican patient. (Photo courtesy of Luciano Dominguéz-Soto, M.D.)

Part I
Prologue

1

Comments

Lawrence Charles Parish

The diagnosis and management of skin disease has periodically been considered sufficiently simple that dermatology was thought to be unworthy of appropriate hours in the medical school curriculum or attention by educated physicians.[1] In the mid-nineteenth century, lectures were given in America glibly proposing that all skin diseases could be divided into two categories: those responding to doses of inorganic sulfur and those that do not.

The understanding and treatment of diseases unfold and are modified with time, scientific advances, and cultural evolution. In the current era, molluscum contagiosum represents a disease in transformation. Once considered to be straightforward after it was delineated by Thomas Bateman (1778–1821) in 1817 and its infectious origin suggested in 1841,[2] in more recent times, this viral infection has been labeled a sexually transmitted disease rather than a pediatric nuisance. Treatment may be affected by the patient's pigmentation, altered by cultural taboos, or altered by public health issues, while climatic changes may create secondary pyodermas.[3]

Tropical Dermatology

Global dermatology is based on the tenets that the evaluation, treatment, and prevention of cutaneous afflictions require the understanding of many facets of medicine and the background of the patient. Aldo Castellani (1874–1971)

pioneered the modern concepts of global (i.e., tropical) dermatology in the early years of this century. By using modern scientific methods, he discovered the cause of sleeping sickness and a number of fungal infections. His carbolfuchsin paint (Castellani's paint) has been one of the first effective treatments of dermatophytosis.[4]

Attempts to understand the variations in disease have occurred over many centuries. For example, Engelbert Kaempfer (1651–1716), a German physician, traveled to the Orient and returned to the University of Leyden to present his thesis on diseases and practices he found in such countries as Japan, Persia, and Malabar. He reported on dracunculosis, filarial-induced elephantiasis, and madura foot, diseases generally unknown to seventeenth-century Europe.[5]

The colonists in North America were often confronted by diseases unrecognized in Europe. Plantation owners in the South found climates that were hotter, more humid, and sunnier than they had experienced in England or Scotland. In addition, they were responsible for the workers who had experienced forcible migration from Africa,[6] and had a different genetic background and susceptibility to previously unknown disease patterns.

Unknown diseases, new customers, and different skin color also raised many questions in North America. An eighteenth-century Virginia physician wrote in the *London Philosophical Transactions*: "An Essay upon the Causes of the Different Colors of People in Different Climates," in which he delved into the difference between white and black skin[1]

3

[The variation] does not proceed from any black humors, or fluid parts contained in their skins; for their [sic] is none such in any part of their bodies, more than in white people.

Tools of Global Dermatology

Epidemiology, climatology, cultural anthropology, and medical education all play major roles in the understanding of global dermatology. Chapters in this unit are devoted to these topics. Physical anthropology—how races differ from one another, if they do—is not addressed, as it becomes such a complex issue that the editors thought this might confuse the issues at hand.[7] Witness the absurdity of the Nurenberg laws[8] or the apartheid regulations that are now historical.

These various tools influence skin disease to a great extent. Native Alaskan peoples have lived in frigid and seemingly inhospitable environments for centuries, but "civilized" health care providers did not always comprehend their ways of adapting to the cold and the diseases found in the Arctic and Subarctic areas.[9]

Incursions into Africa also proved formidable and illustrate the need to use these tools:

Many African disease environments were extremely dangerous for outsiders. Europeans, whether traders, explorers, soldiers, missionaries, or would-be "civilizers" like the participants in the Niger expedition of 1841, generally found Africa's "fevers" and "fluxes" deadly until the beginning of tropical medicine in the late nineteenth century. With the significant exception of specific climatic regions found in extreme North and South Africa, early European activity was limited by exceedingly high death rates. The claim of a French trader that parts of the Guinea Coast were so unhealthy that the slave trade there was "an exchanged [sic] of whites for blacks" was a gross exaggeration, but the point made is understandable. The continent's epidemiological barriers also proved formidable for settlers of African descent who had lost their ancestors' immunity to tropical diseases while in North America and who found the disease environment very hazardous in Sierra Leone and Liberia. North African merchants suffered from local diseases in the Western Sudan, and visitors to the Swahili Coast no doubt had comparable problems. Africa's epidemiological

environment has played a major role in the relative isolation of the continent throughout most of its history.[10]

This unique biological environment still provides challenges. The recent augmentation of the catastrophes associated with the Marburg and HIV viruses attests to this.

Conclusions

The importance of global dermatology increases daily. With rapid travel between countries and continents and massive political upheavals, people move to foreign areas, experience different climates, and are confronted by strange cultural settings.[11] Unexpected diseases, variable treatments,[13] and new expectations[12] are created. The practitioner is constantly presented with the need for concise diagnosis and targeted therapy.

References

1. Duhring LA: The rise of American dermatology. In: Friedman R, ed. A History of Dermatology in Philadelphia. Fort Pierce Beach, FL: Froben Press, Inc., 1955:155–198.
2. Waterson AP, Wilkinson L: An Introduction to the History of Virology. New York: Cambridge University Press, 1978:42–51.
3. deWit RFE: Molluscum contagiosum. In: Parish LC, Gschnait, F, eds. Sexually Transmitted Diseases: A guide for clinicians. New York: Springer-Verlag, 1989:193–201.
4. Binazzi M: Italian memoirs of Aldo Castellani. *Int J Dermatol* 1991;**30**:741–745.
5. Bowers JZ, Carrubba RW: The doctoral thesis of Engelbert Kaempfer on tropical diseases, oriental medicine, and exotic natural phenomena. *J Hist Med* 1970;**25**:270–310.
6. Parish LC, Parish DH: Thomas Jefferson and tropical dermatology. *Int J Dermatol* 1989;**28**: 615–618.
7. Gawkroder DJ: Racial influences on skin disease. In: Champion RH, Burton JL, Ebling FJG, eds. Rook/Wilkinson/Ebling Textbook of Dermatology. London: Blackwell Scientific Publications, 1992:2859–2875.

8. Cohn W: Bearers of a common fate? The "non-aryan" Christian "Fates-Comrades" of the Paulus-Bund, 1933–1939. In: Packer A, ed. Year Book XXXIII. New York: Leo Baeck Institute, 1988:327–366.

9. Foutch RG, Mills WJ, Jr: Treatment and prevention of cold injuries by ancient peoples indigenous to Arctic and Subarctic regions. *Arctic Med Res* 1988; **47(suppl 1)**:286–289.

10. Patterson KD, Hartwig GW: The disease factor: An introductory overview. In: Hartwig GW, Patterson KD, eds. Disease in African History: An introductory survey and case studies. Durham, NC: Duke University Press, 1978:1–24.

11. Scheper–Hughes N: Social indifference to child death. *Lancet* 1991;**337**:1144–1147.

12. Fiallo P, Nunzi E, Bisighini G, Vaccari G: Leprosy in an Italian tourist visiting the tropics. *Trans Roy Soc Trop Med Hyg* 1993;**87**:675.

13. Haak H, Hardon AP: Indigenised pharmaceuticals in developing countries widely used, widely neglected. *Lancet* 1988;**i**:620–621.

14. Littlewood R: From disease to illness and back again. *Lancet* 1991;**337**:1013–1016.

2

Tropical Medicine and Tropical Public Health

Barnet L. Cline

Tropical medicine emerged as a recognized medical and scientific specialty at the beginning of the twentieth century, having evolved during European (and to a much lesser degree, American) colonialization of the tropics. The diseases encountered by newcomers to the tropics were as fascinating as they were terrifying, stimulating colonial physicians and scientists to record carefully their observations and experiments, and often to share this new information in letters to colleagues in Liverpool, London, Paris, Hamburg, Antwerp, and other European centers of learning and commerce. Thus, there evolved the first societies devoted to advances in tropical medicine; for example, the Royal Society of Tropical Medicine and Hygiene was founded in the United Kingdom in 1907, shortly after the establishment of schools of tropical medicine in Liverpool and London.

Early Tropical Medicine

Patrick Manson (1844–1922), considered by many the "father of tropical medicine," was a colonial physician in China in the 1860s and 1870s and was the first to demonstrate mosquito transmission of disease (filariasis). He wrote the first textbook of tropical medicine, published in 1898, and titled *Tropical Diseases: A Manual of the Diseases of Warm Climates.*[1] His message in the preface of the book was optimistic, though tainted by irony in retrospect: "I now firmly believe in the possibility of tropical colonization by the white races. Heat and moisture are not in themselves the direct causes of any important tropical disease. The direct causes of 99% of these diseases are germs. To kill them is simply a matter of knowledge."[2]

During a virtual explosion of new knowledge about tropical diseases during the 1890s and the 1900s, the "germs" causing many tropical diseases and their transmission cycles were discovered, including malaria, typhus, relapsing fevers, yellow fever, visceral leishmaniasis, African and American trypanosomiasis, brucellosis, bartonellosis, and others. Some of these discoveries were promptly translated into remarkable successes in disease control; for example, the elimination of yellow fever from Cuba after *Aedes aegypti* was shown to be the vector.

The new knowledge about tropical diseases rarely, however, benefitted the indigenous communities in the regions colonized. The *raison d'etre* of tropical medicine during that era was to help build and maintain empires, to make the tropics habitable by, and profitable for, Europeans. Hence, tropical medicine existed for the benefit of military troops, civil servants, merchants, and other economically productive segments of the population; women, children, and local communities were not direct beneficiaries.

Tropical Medicine and Tropical Public Health Post-World War II

The era of colonialism ended after World War II due to the weakening of European powers and growing nationalistic feelings, but the former colonies inherited a plethora of problems, including political and economic instability, few trained medical personnel, meager infrastructure, and a tradition of a more or less disease-specific approach to control of endemic diseases. It is not surprising that during the 1950s and 1960s the health status of populations in tropical and developing countries improved slowly if at all, but this was a period during which vigorous efforts were made in many countries to train indigenous medical personnel and scientists as a step toward self-sufficiency.

The past two decades have witnessed a number of milestones that helped shape the current and future direction of tropical public health, which may now be a more appropriate term than tropical medicine. The failure of malaria eradication, recognized in 1970, caused a backlash against the concept of eradication and also against targeted (vertical) disease-control programs in general.

The creation in 1975 of the WHO/UNDP-sponsored Special Programme for Tropical Diseases Research (TDR), targeting malaria, schistosomiasis, filariasis, trypanosomiasis, leishmaniasis, and leprosy, recognized that developed nations were virtually ignoring these "distant" but devastating diseases. Increased recognition of the importance of these diseases, and support for research and training in developing countries, has contributed importantly to research progress and to increasingly productive collaboration between scientists in developed and developing countries.

The first fundamental (political) shift in the relationship between developed and developing nations in the health arena has been evolving since the 1978 WHO/UNICEF Alma Ata Conference "Health for All by the Year 2000," and the concepts of primary health care were spelled out at this conference.[3] The international community recognized a broad definition of health that, in addition to traditional curative and preventive services, included concern for education, sanitation, safe water, shelter, nutrition, and other critical determinants of health and disease. Most important, however, was that at the heart of the primary health care concept was the active participation of the community, a somewhat radical concept at odds with the health services provided during the colonial and early postcolonial periods. To the surprise of some, the concept of primary health care is alive, but in many countries primary health care is struggling to become a reality rather than exist merely as a chart on the wall of an official at the ministry of health.

The eradication of smallpox in 1979 boosted the credibility of the public health sector, and the successes of the child survival initiative spearheaded by UNICEF have significantly reduced the mortality rates of infants and small children in most developing countries. These efforts have not, however, greatly enhanced the infrastructure or the ability to sustain these programs, not to mention broader primary health care efforts. The technical and financial support for the child survival programs (immunization, oral rehydration therapy, growth monitoring, breast feeding, and other "low-tech" interventions) continues to be derived from industrialized countries.

A careful examination of tropical public health today, considering recent and current trends, yields a bewildering mix of hope tempered by despair. On the positive side of the equation are dramatic advances in biotechnology offering, for example, the hope during the next decade of a "supervaccine" that could be given once shortly after birth, providing sustained protection against virtually all important infectious diseases of childhood. Polio and Guinea worm may be eradicated by the end of the century (joining smallpox as former diseases), new drugs such as praziquantel and ivermectin are powerful weapons for morbidity control of important helminthic agents, and vitamin A appears to be a valuable new intervention for child survival programs.

On the negative side, however, one must consider the HIV/AIDS pandemic, continuing rapid urbanization, staggering debt burden in the face of stagnant or declining economies, resurgence of malaria and other vector-borne diseases, rapid population growth, increased tobacco consumption, and widescale degradation of the environment.

The Challenge to Dermatology

Where do skin diseases fit into this picture? And what is the best "entry point" for dermatology on a global scale as this specialty endeavors to contribute its expertise and enormous potential to improve the health status of populations in the developing world? There are a number of potential "entry points" for dermatology into World Health Organization-sponsored and other global initiatives in health, including leprosy, sexually transmitted diseases, essential drugs, the categorical diseases of the WHO/ TDR program with prominent dermal manifestations (onchocerciasis, leishmaniasis, leprosy), and primary health care.

Appropriately, the main thrust of a new initiative of the International League of Dermatological Societies (IDLS) is to integrate care of skin disease into the primary health care system. Project UNIDERM is an important step in this direction, logical because of the great burden of skin disease in the developing world. Experience and data tell us that a large proportion of visits to health clinics in developing countries is for skin disease. In addition to providing expert skin care to patients in dermatology offices in cities worldwide (one objective of this book), an overriding concern is to encourage professionals to also contribute to the understanding of skin disease at the level of the impoverished rural or urban communities, and to develop realistic, place-specific solutions to the problems identified. An intriguing model is the "community dermatology" concept developed at the University of Guerrero, Mexico, where the Centre for the Investigation of Tropical Disease (CIET) has undertaken a comprehensive program to identify the principal skin conditions and associated risk factors, to introduce appropriate control

measures, and to train health workers to recognize and treat skin diseases using practical, low-cost approaches.[4]

Indeed, a pressing need exists to quantify more precisely the burden of skin disease in the developing world and to determine how the common, treatable conditions vary by region, season, and basic demographic factors such as race, age, sex, and urban–rural status. Carefully planned epidemiologic research is needed. Perhaps, as has been done recently for malaria (e.g., malaria of the African savannah, forest malaria, malaria associated with irrigated agriculture, highland fringe malaria, desert fringe and oasis malaria, seashore malaria, urban malaria, and so on), simple paradigms could be constructed to assist in planning more rational approaches to intervention and for training of health workers.[5]

Conclusions

Providing for prevention and care of common skin diseases in communities of the developing world can build confidence in the primary health care system, increase utilization of health services (thus improving financial sustainability), and provide a contact point for health education designed to reduce the burden of skin disease in the future. Ultimately, if developing countries are to develop self-sufficiency in the health sector, confidence must be built at the community level. Along with other "entry points" into the community, efforts to treat and prevent skin disease can contribute to the difficult challenge for developing countries and their more prosperous partners to move beyond colonial and postcolonial dependency and to create health care systems appropriate to their needs, local conditions, and resources.

References

1. Manson P: Tropical Diseases: A Manual of the Diseases of Warm Climates. London: Cassell, 1898.
2. Warren KS: Tropical medicine as tropical

health: The Heath Clark lecture. *Rev Infect Dis* 1990;**12**:142–156.

3. World Health Organization: Declaration of Alma Ata (Report on the International Conference of Primary Health Care, Alma Ata, USSR, Sept 6–12, 1978). Geneva, World Health Organization, 1978.

4. Hay R, Andersson N, Estrada R: Mexico: Community dermatology in Guerrero. *Lancet* 1991;**337**:906–907.

5. Malaria, Obstacles and Opportunities. Institute of Medicine, Washington, DC, National Academy Press, 1991;216–221.

3

Dermatological Epidemiology

R. J. Hay and R. Estrada Castanon

Epidemiology is the study of disease in populations. It encompasses the prevalence and behavior of diseases, as well as those factors that affect the clinical expression of illness. Its methods rely on a combination of clinical observation and the appropriate statistical analysis of data.[1] A particular feature of the epidemiological approach is the use of large data sets to study putative relationships and the significance of a number of different observations that are likely to affect the expression of disease. The means of deriving data from such analyses are different from those used in a scientific investigative study, more familiar to most dermatologists, where the recording or experimental manipulation of single or multiple events is the basis for determining results. In most epidemiological investigations, results are expressed as significant or nonsignificant findings depending on whether or not the coexistence of two or more events depends on chance alone.

Investigation

In this way, epidemiological investigations can throw light on key issues such as the incidence and prevalence of diseases, their mortality, and significant associations that may play a role in causation.[2] Ideally, epidemiological and scientific investigative approaches should complement one another. Surveys of the behavior of skin disease in large communities have been few despite the fact that observations can be made without recourse to complex investigational techniques; an inspection or the application of a simple questionnaire is often sufficient.

Perhaps a major obstacle to such work has been the difficulty in defining precise limits that categorize different dermatological diseases. Dermatological diagnosis requires a form of pattern recognition that is usually only acquired by a long period of training. Although there is some truth that training in the diagnosis of skin disease is important for precision, it is possible to analyze data accurately without exhaustive training. In addition to the investigators' skills in recognition, it is necessary to define in precise and comprehensible terms the disease itself in order for the results to be interpreted by others.[3] Because of the visual nature of the diagnostic features, this is a difficult task not found in other areas of medicine. For instance, the definition of hypertension can be made by specifying the normal limits of systolic and diastolic blood pressures and seeking those individuals whose blood pressure falls outside these norms.

Training in this area can be limited to acquiring the correct techniques for diagnosis, and in this area this is the main skill needed to convert the nonexpert into an expert. Definitions of visual images are more difficult to specify. Most dermatologists will be able to diagnose psoriasis with considerable accuracy. Without resorting to illustrative material showing the different clinical forms of psoriasis, it is difficult to describe verbally those features that would allow the novice to diagnose the disease because it means setting strict definitions of the disease state by nonvisual methods.

Even where it is possible to equip investigators with representative pictures of the condition under survey, the examples have to encompass a range of different morphologies that characterize the disease.[4] This task is difficult because it not only means describing the common elements of a complex visual pattern, which may vary, it also involves specifying limits of the diagnosis, that is, what is not psoriasis. This is something that even expert dermatologists find difficult. The distinction between seborrheic dermatitis and isolated psoriasis of the scalp, for instance, can be extremely difficult; the distinction between psoriasis of the palms and chronic hand dermatitis presents a similar problem.

It is small wonder, therefore, that surveys have been few,[5] and where they have been carried out they have often concentrated on the easiest diseases to describe, such as tinea versicolor, tropical ulcer, and scabies,[6] rather than those that are difficult to define such as dermatitis and pyoderma. Where such studies have been carried out, they have usually involved personnel with dermatological training[7] or, as in the large survey organized by the Institute of Dermatology in Thailand, a period of training for medical practitioners.

The problems encountered in work on the epidemiology of skin diseases are compounded by the fact that few dermatological diseases are reportable. There is, therefore, no instant source of information on the disease in the community. In the one skin disease where figures are collected in many countries, leprosy, the value of central statistics is limited because the prevalence of infection in the community is difficult to verify either because of isolation of communities or lack of resources, and often both; other problems, including manipulation of figures for political ends, are also involved in some areas. In many countries a shortage of dermatologically trained individuals is a further difficulty.[7]

Terminology

These reservations are important in understanding some of the limitations of existing epidemiological work in dermatology. The degree of occurrence of a condition in the population at any time is known as its **prevalence**. Acquiring prevalence figures is a difficult task as it involves screening large numbers of patients in the community. One of the most careful studies of prevalence rates of dermatological disease was that of Rea et al., who studied a population in South London.[8] They used a cross-sectional sample using a postal survey and backed this up by visiting and examining a cross section of this sample. Their results suggested that up to 23% of the population had at least one treatable skin disease. It is easier to obtain figures for the **incidence** of infection in hospital clinics, even though the sample sizes are often too small. Such studies describe the percentage of a hospital population with a particular disease feature within a specified period. The incidence of psoriasis, for instance, in a sample population of outpatients can be calculated. Figures for some of the main United Kingdom centers are available.[9] Published epidemiological surveys of dermatological diseases, however, all too frequently rely on small numbers of patients.

The factors affecting the distribution of skin disease in populations are complex. They encompass numerous variables from ethnic origins to climate and underlying disease. Ethnic factors, in turn, depend on a variety of different underlying variables. For instance, diet, social customs, genetic predisposition, and even exposure to disease may equally play a part in determining the manifestations of disease. Climate is often implicated in the appearance of tropical disease. The variables within climatic norms for each region need to be analyzed independently. Rainfall, mean daily temperature, and mean nocturnal temperature may all play a part and have to be analyzed independently. Exposure to infection may equally be affected by these variables, such as the presence of a suitable insect vector or intermediate host as well as the existence of appropriate soil conditions. The importance of recognizing these elements is that in order to understand the relationship between a risk factor and disease it is crucial to simplify the question into a single variable if possible: rainfall or mean nocturnal temperature rather than climate—the latter is not precise enough.

Genetic analyses are particularly difficult, although now with modern genetic techniques using, for instance, a restriction enzyme, mapping accurate identification and localization of some genetic defects is possible. The other classic approaches to identifying genetic risk in populations include HLA typing, twin studies, and the use of population genetic analyses (Hardy–Weinberg frequencies). In the latter, the frequency of occurrence of a possible genetic defect in the community is compared for significance assuming different modes of inheritance (autosomal dominant, recessive) and its occurrence in families with different sizes and where the prevalence of parental disease differs. Such analyses may be able to demonstrate that the distribution of the disease is compatible with a susceptibility trait mediated by a particular pattern of inheritance. Such an approach has been adopted to determine the genetic susceptibility to tinea imbricata.[10] The interpretation of these analyses becomes particularly difficult if the disease has a high frequency in the community and the possibility of transmission by infection rather than inherited characteristics needs to be considered.

Studying Dermatological Epidemiology

The first problem is to define the population to be studied. It is important that it be chosen for representative size and ease of handling. Sometimes it is possible to use existing data held on computer files. Generally, this is not possible, and it is then necessary to screen a large group of individuals. The size depends on availability as well as the question being asked. For instance, to find the prevalence of a disease such as psoriasis in a population, it is necessary to define the population among whom the disease, in this case psoriasis, is being studied. The size and composition of the sample is critical. Is everyone included or is this not practical? In some tropical surveys it may be possible to carry out a house-to-house enquiry, although if this is performed at certain times, the sample may show bias because, for instance, the men are all at work or the children at school. Children are often easier to screen if they are at school as this represents a common point for inspection. In a large heterogenous group, it may be necessary to take a small sample group, for instance, by using three out of every eight villages randomly distributed across the region. Prospective studies of prevalence using a group or cohort that is followed over a defined length of time is a reasonable approach to investigation.

The identification of risk factors such as age, sex, and socioeconomic group is also often a target for dermatological investigation. The approach adopted has to be carefully considered with some risk factors, for instance, sun exposure. Here, it is important to identify all potential confounding variables such as skin type, incidental versus deliberate exposure (sunbathing), and geographic location of exposure. Then it may be appropriate to try to quantify exposure; this may be simple—indoor versus outdoor work. If the limits can be identified more specifically, it may, for instance, be feasible to examine the prevalence of skin cancer in patients vacationing overseas over a specified 5-year period. Even more precise limits can be set, such as number of days on vacation per year. The main aim is to obtain some measurable difference between different individuals comprising the cohort. Incidental exposure to risk such as sun exposure is often not recorded by patients. For example, the elderly patient will often remember the few vacations spent sunbathing on a beach, but forget 4 years of military service in the tropics.

The Questionnaire

It is generally important to phrase the questions bearing in mind the sample population and the mode of acquiring information. It is nearly always a mistake to ask too many questions, which can only complicate the survey. It is also important to simplify the questions asked, for instance, to use those requiring a yes/no answer, unless a more complex answer can be analyzed. Some questions that are taken for granted may be difficult for some populations to answer. Even age may not be known to within 10 years. In these groups, age has to be related to external events such as school, going to work, or specific incidents such as a war. There is also a tendency for individuals answering surveys to give the responses they believe the questioner would like or that they believe would be most appropriate. For instance, a question on drinking habits may not be met with absolute accuracy or honesty, and questions on hygiene may be answered poorly. A question designed to find out the frequency of washing may not be accurately answered, and it may be more helpful to inquire about access to a water supply as an indicator of likely personal hygiene. The composition of families may also be difficult to chart, and in some countries, a household may harbor relatives, friends, and others belonging to a complex form of extended guardianship.

The Survey

Surveys can be planned events with specific questions, examinations, or physical measurements being carried out. Once again, it is important not to make the subject too complicated as this will inevitably result in disappointment. The survey needs to be planned so that the population is alerted to the appearance of the team and purpose of the work. Nothing is more alarming than a sudden invasion of strange doctors clutching notepads. Likewise, the population surveyed should be informed of the results. To participate in these studies is often time-consuming, and the simple task of informing the participants of some, if not all, the results in layman's terms will ease the path for further work.

Access to more specific populations such as those attending a clinic provides a more limited target, but this may be the purpose of the work and this type of population is easier to cope with. Here it is important to realize that they have usually attended for some other purpose and the

survey is generally incidental to their immediate needs.

Examination in dermatology is a key part of surveys. A good clinical examination requires total exposure and a good light. This combination is often not available. The request to remove clothes for a medical examination, often taken for granted, may be resented in many countries, particularly in the developing world, where people are naturally shy and reluctant to expose themselves to a stranger. This is a particularly difficult problem in surveys involving women, and it may not be possible to carry out an adequate examination.

In carrying out surveys in the developing world, it is important to recognize that health resources are scarce, and this may be the first time a population has seen a medical team for several months, sometimes longer. It is important to recognize that the team will have to be prepared to offer basic medical care to the population in addition to carrying out their survey.

There are many dermatological diseases, from scabies to dermatophytoses, where diagnosis of the disease can be confirmed by a simple test such as potassium hydroxide scraping, serology, or patch testing. Although these may be impracticable in a vast study, verification of the clinical diagnosis using a small cross-sectional sample is often useful. In some conditions, such as onchocerciasis, where a majority of the infected population may have no overt clinical signs, testing is of key importance;[11] in the latter example, taking skin snips from the entire study group is a routine part of a survey.

Analysis

Although analysis of a survey using a previously completed study is easier in some ways, it poses some problems, particularly in dermatology. Examinations will depend on the efforts and skills of a third party and it is not possible to validate findings. The common sources for major epidemiological data censuses and vital statistics (births, deaths, etc.) are of little use in dermatology. These generally only show gross trends, and the death certificate, useful for other medical specialties, has little value to dermatologists. There are also few reportable skin diseases apart from leprosy in some countries. Large data sources are, therefore, likely to have been specifically designed for skin disease—these are very rare—or have data of value by incidence such as cancer statistics, which may happen to have data on melanoma or other skin cancers.

Comparisons will depend on the ability to manipulate large amounts of data. The availability of good statistical packages that can be used on even small computers has eased analysis enormously. Here it is important to identify the questions or variables that need to be compared. The design of the study depends on the reliability of these sources, and it is therefore important that the means of analysis is decided on before the survey itself is finalized. In addition to helping with the comparative analysis, it may be a key factor in deciding on the numbers needed for this work. Statistical or epidemiological packages available range from the simple (such as Nanostat) to the more complex (e.g., Epi Info) where questionnaires can be designed, analyzed, and displayed visually using one program.

Conclusions

The behavior of skin disease in communities has often been ignored, although it forms a basic part of our understanding of the pathogenesis and possible means of controlling dermatoses.[12] This is of importance in all environments whether it involves the study of those variables affecting the expression of skin cancer or the risk factors and prevalence of scabies in a small village. In the developing world, in particular, knowledge of the prevalence and economic impact of disease may allow the authorities to identify those conditions that are commonest or most significant in their communities and to plan appropriate control measures where possible.[12–14] In the developing world, many of the common skin diseases are infectious, and for these, provided there are sufficient resources, effective low-cost therapy is generally available.[15]

References

1. Mausner JS, Kramer S: Epidemiology—An Introductory Text. Philadelphia: WB Saunders Company, 1985.
2. Woodall JP: Epidemiological approaches to health planning, management and evaluation. *World Health Stat Q* 1988;**41**:2–8.
3. Hay RJ, Andersson N, Estrada R: Mexico: community dermatology in Guerrero. *Lancet* 1991;**337**:906–907.
4. Perine PL, Hopkins DR, Niemel PLA, et al: Handbook of Endemic Treponematoses. Geneva: WHO, 1984.
5. Bechelli LM, Haddad N, Pimenta WPJ, et al: Epidemiological survey of skin diseases in school children living in the Purus valley. *Dermatologica* 1981;**163**:78–93.
6. Morris GE, Hay RJ, Srinavasa A, Bunat A: The diagnosis and management of tropical ulcer in East Sepik Province of Papua New Guinea. *J Trop Med Hyg* 1989;**92**:215–220.
7. George AO: Skin disease in tropical Africa. *Int J Dermatol* 1988;**29**:187–189.
8. Rea JN, Newhouse ML, Halil T: Skin disease in Lambeth. A community study of prevalence and use of medical care. *Br J Prevent Med* 1976;**30**:107–114.
9. Rook A, Savin JA, Wilkinson DS: The prevalence, incidence and ecology of disease of the skin. In: Textbook of Dermatology. Rook A, Wilkinson DS, Ebling FJG, et al, eds. Oxford: Blackwell Scientific Publications, 1991:39–53.
10. Serjeantson S, Lawrence G: Autosomal recessive inheritance of susceptibility to tinea imbricata. *Lancet* 1977;**i**:13–15.
11. Mackenzie CD, Williams JF. Variations in the clinical presentation of onchocerciasis and their relationship to host parasite interaction. *Sudan Med J* 1985;**21**:41–48.
12. Andersson N, Martinez E, Cerrato F, et al: The use of community-based data in health planning in Mexico and Central America. *Health Policy Planning* 1989;**4**(3):197–206.
13. Fordham P: Research and evaluation. In: Participation, Learning and Change. London: Commonwealth Secretariat, 1980.
14. Taplin D, Porcelain SL, Meinking TL, et al: Community control of scabies: A model based on the use of permethrin cream. *Lancet* 1991;**337**:1016–1018.
15. Caiden N, Wildavsky A: Planning and budgeting in poor countries. New York: John Wiley & Sons, 1974.

4

Climatology

Luitgard G. Wiest

Climate plays a dominant role in determining directly or indirectly the incidence of skin disease. There is no specific unit of measurement that defines climate. Climate is defined through various parameters that characterize the atmospheric conditions and processes. Different classifications and systems of climate exist; the most suitable seems to be that of Köppen.[1] Worldwide climatic and environmental factors can be divided in macroclimate, mesoclimate, and microclimate.

Background

Macroclimate, in the true geographical and meteorological sense, refers to the temperature, rainfall, humidity, clouds, winds, and wind velocity of a given area (Fig. 4.1).[2] Microclimate refers to the individual and his environment. It relates to a person's age, sex, racial background, his status in the community, and the ecological and socioeconomic conditions.[3]

Mesoclimate refers to a very localized area such as a basin of a valley or larger cities with over 100,000 inhabitants, where factors of the macroclimate and microclimate play a role. As of 1975, 24.1% of the earth's population lived in communities of such dimensions.

The best investigated local modification of climate is the so-called island of urban increased temperature in and above large cities. This phenomenon is due to decreased evaporization and anthropogenic heat production.[4]

All factors of climate are submitted to a characteristic local process that is continuously changing. The local changes are due to climate-forming processes and factors, among which the heat regulation of the surface of the earth and the atmosphere, the atmospheric circulation and the relief of such, and surface features are predominant. Temperature and rainfall are the most important climate factors that show geographical and seasonal patterns. Air temperature is the temperature of the atmosphere heated through the evaporation of the surface of the earth. With increasing geographical latitude, the temperature drops throughout the year, dropping more during the winter than during summer, and it drops with altitude, normally about 0.6°C per 100 m.[5]

The maximum temperature on earth was measured at 55°C in Arabia, Mesopotamia, the Sahara, Arizona, central California, and central Australia. The lowest temperature was measured at the cold pole of the earth with a temperature of −94.5°C near the South Pole.

Rainfalls usually have their maxima in the equatorial region and in the medium latitudes, and their minima in the extraequatorial tropics and in the polar regions. The medium yearly rainfall on the surface of the earth varies between 1 mm and over 12,000 mm.[5]

The influence of climate may be exerted more indirectly through changes induced in microorganisms, disease vectors, flora, and fauna. As a consequence, diseases of the skin in tropical regions may differ in incidence, prevalence, and appearance from identical disorders occurring in more temperate climates. Temperature,

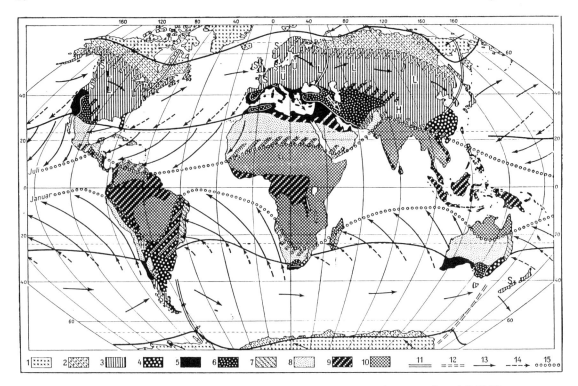

FIGURE 4.1. Generic types of climate (after E. Kupfer 1954 from "Erdkunde" 1957)

1. Polar climate
2. Subpolar climate
3. Climate of the planetary frontal zones
   S = maritime climate
   L = continental climate
   Ü = transition climate between continental and
       maritime climate
4. Humid summer east coasts
   Subtropical climates:
5. Moderate winter rain
6. Light spring rain (inland type)

Trade winds climates:
7. Damp east coasts
8. Dry west coasts and inland
   Inland tropical climates:
9. Constantly humid, evergreen virgin forests
10. Periodically humid (zenith rain)
11. Preferred sites of cold heights
12. Presumed the same
13. Winds blow all year round (trade winds very
    constant, others not constant)
14. Extended trade winds in summer
15. Site of innertropical convergence in January and July
    H = Special high altitude climate

humidity, air movement, atmospheric pressure, sunlight, electrostatic changes, and cosmic radiation may all affect the skin.

The direct effects of climate on the skin play a smaller but still significant role in determining geographical and seasonal variations in the incidence and severity of many skin functions or through long-term structural changes, cumulatively induced.

Evaluation

The first step in evaluating the effect of climate in skin diseases is to observe the relationship between disease incidence and the climatic factors during different months of the year over a sufficiently lengthy period of time. The results will provide data for the particular region, population, and period under review. Special problems emerge in comparing figures from different geographic dermatology studies in different countries and studies done at different points in time. Data are influenced by the available diagnostic competence and facilities.

Most data published are derived from hospital centers. The possibility of hospital attendance is subject to many factors and does not reflect the true incidence of a disease in large rural areas of developing countries.

Examples

A classical example for the influence of climatic factors on dermatoses is the combination of high temperature and relative humidity. The hot and humid climate of the tropical rain forest predisposes people to fungal and bacterial infection. Through increased transpiration and reduced evaporation, the acid milieu of the epidermis is altered and the barrier of the stratum corneum is reduced. The increased hydration of the horny layer promotes the colonization of the coagulase-positive staphylococcus as well as gram-negative bacteria.

Pyoderma, particularly impetigo, is more likely to occur under these conditions, and epidemics of impetigo have occurred repeatedly in tropical regions.[6] Along the coastal regions and at low altitudes in Central America,[7] fungal infections, especially tinea versicolor, and pyogenic infections account for about 19–22% of the patients in different Mexican clinics. Similar figures were obtained in Calcutta[8] and Zambia.[9] Yet, in Abu Dhabi[10] with similar climate characteristics (hot climate with a very high relative humidity) that facilitate survival and spread of fungi and bacteria producing superficial mycosis and infections, the incidence of superficial fungus infection is 8.5% and of pyoderma only 2.5%. A comparable figure of pyoderma for London is 4.6%.[11] The lower incidence in Abu Dhabi can be explained by the high standard of living, which plays a · major role in limiting the spread of infections (good hygienic measures, presence of good preventive and therapeutic measures). This emphasizes the important role of socioeconomic and environmental factors in addition to climatic factors.

Geographic location and time seem to play an important role in the prevailing causative dermatophyte. In Qatar[12] the most common pathogen found in tinea capitis was *Microsporum canis*; in the Middle East[13] and Egypt,[14] *Trichosporum violaceum*; and in Benghazi, Libya,[15] *T. rubrum*. Regional differences of the pathogen in the same country, for example, *T. violaceum* in Western Libya (Tripoli), do occur.[16] In the warm and humid microclimate of shoes, tinea pedis is promoted as an urban disease, seldom found in the barefooted peasant. Tinea pedis and toenail mycosis are rare findings in people who wear sandals most of the time.

Seasonal Changes

In most areas of hot and humid climates, there are primarily two seasons, the rainy and the dry seasons, according to the types of rainfall—the subtropical, equatorial, or monsoon type. Cyclic appearances of dermatoses have been noted in El Salvador: herpes zoster in the rainy season, and pityriasis rosea and anthrax in the dry season.[7]

In Korea,[17] the increasing number of dermatophyte infections during July and August reveals the seasonal varieties. In Panama, impetigo and fungus infections are more common during the "wet season," and insect bites and "achromia parasitaria" are more common during the dry season. The heat, combined with the low humidity of the arid and semiarid areas, favors the development of coccidioidomycosis, "desert sores."[7]

In Central America, at higher altitudes, about 3000–6000 ft, with cooler temperatures, bacterial pyoderma and superficial fungal infections are less common, whereas the soil and flora appear to favor deep fungal infections, such as sporotrichosis, chromomycosis, and mycetoma.[7] Other indirect climatic effects related to geographic factors also profoundly modify the patterns of disease incidence by influencing nutritional standards and way of life and the prevalence of parasites and their vectors.

During the rainy season, a larger number of cases of leishmaniasis, Chagas' disease, and onchocerciasis is seen due to the increase in the density of insects such as *Phlebotomus, Triatoma*, and *Simulium* that transmit disease.[7,18] Prurigo increases in the warmer months in Mexico. This is attributed to the relationship between the number of insects and the temperature.[7]

Racial Adaptation

The direct effects of climatic factors on the individual skin are influenced by racial adaptation, age, and physical state. The skin is quite sensitive to changes in the water content of the atmosphere. When the relative humidity falls, water evaporates from the stratum corneum, forming air–water interfaces that give the appearance of scaling and the texture of dryness. Thus, substantial changes in ambient conditions can influence the expression of disease in cutaneous tissue.[19]

Man is very flexible—he can adjust to environmental temperatures for a limited time between $-56°C$ and $120°C$, due to thermoregulation by transpiration, heat conduction, heat radiation, and convection.[20] During a limited time, 4 L of sweat can be produced per hour, and under extreme conditions, 14 L within 12 h.[21] Dermatoses can cause the dysfunction of thermoregulation.

Humidity

High levels of humidity in combination with a minimum dry bulb temperature favor the development of miliaria (prickly heat). These climatic conditions favor the development of miliaria due to sweat duct occlusion, hidradenitis, and acne aestivalis.[22,23] The data compiled for Central America[7] reveal that the majority of contact dermatitis was caused by plants (Anacardiacea family) of the tropical and subtropical zones.

Low atmospheric humidity and high barometric pressure can produce drying and fissuring of the horny layer—chapping.[24] Exposure to cold produces a wide range of immediate effects on the skin. Under antarctic conditions, physiological changes have been demonstra-ted,[25] such as reduction of the elastica and an increased thickness of the granular cellular layer. Cold-induced vasodilatation occurs earlier in descendants of the inhabitants of cold climates. At the colder, very high altitudes such as the altiplano on top of the Andes, with a totally different fauna and flora with low humidity, one encounters skin diseases common in temperate climates, such as xerosis, "winter itch," and even frostbites.

At higher altitudes, pigmentary disorders and light sensitivity eruptions also predominate.[7]

Ultraviolet Irradiation

The effects of shortwave ultraviolet irradiation on the skin is dependent on multiple factors, such as duration, intensity (altered by daytime), season, and geographical latitude, altitude, clouding, air pollution, ozone filter, reflection, clothing habits, wind, temperature, and humidity. These altering factors of UV irradiation determine the incidence of acute photodynamic and photoallergic dermatoses and the degree of actinic injury, reflected in the incidence of degenerative changes and of certain tumors. Races with pigmented skin are genetically adapted to the damages of solar irradiation. Precancerous actinic keratoses or basal cell carcinomas are quite uncommon in tropical areas due to the protective action of melanin in the epidermis, which decreases the damaging effect of sunlight in the more pigmented tropical races. The high incidence of epidermal malignancies in Australia[26] and in Spanish Wells, on the isolated St. George's Cay of the Bahamas, is a prime example of ill-adaptation to ultraviolet radiation in the population of British descent.

Geofactors and Socioeconomic Factors

New situations in association with geofactors and socioeconomic factors may influence the incidence and distribution of dermatoses in the future.

A very high proportion of the population living in developing countries resides in rural areas. Changes in the country's agricultural structure that are concomitant with the progress of civilization lend to new health problems arising from population movements within the country. In some large cities,[7] a shift in the pattern of dermatoses from a rural, low-economy type to a more cosmopolitan type is already evident.

Growing industrialization with increasing air pollution not only influences the local climate above larger cities but also creates health problems. Deforestation with its impact on the climate induces climatic changes and creates new breeding places for disease-transmitting vectors.[27]

With the actual rapid decrease of the protective shield of ozone above the Northern Hemisphere, the incidence of epidermal malignancies is also rising in this area.

References

1. Handbuch der Klimatologie; Köppen W, Geiger R: Stuttgart (Germany) Bornträger 1936, Vol. 1 part C.
2. Blüthgen J: Allgemeine Klimageographie. Berlin: Walter de Gruyter, 1966:519.
3. Canizares O: A Manual of Dermatology for Developing Countries. Oxford: Oxford University Press, 1982;21–22.
4. Dimitriev AA, Bessonov NP: Klimat Moskvy. Leningrad, 1969.
5. Hendl M, Marcienk J, Jäger EJ: Allgemeine Klima-, Hydro-, und Vegetationsgeographie, Gotha, Germany: VEB Hermann Haack, Geographisch-Kartographische Anstalt, 1988:12.
6. Potter EV, Ortiz JS, Sharett AR, et al: Changing types of nephritogenic streptocoocci in Trinidad. J Clin Invest 1971;50:1197–1204.
7. Canizares O: Geographic dermatology: Mexico and Central America. Arch Dermatol 1960;82:870–891.
8. Banerjee BN, Datta AK: Prevalence and incidence pattern of skin diseases in Calcutta. Int J Dermatol 1973;12:41–47.
9. Ratnam AV, Jayaraju K: Skin diseases in Zambia. Br J Dermatol 1979;101:449–455.
10. Abu Share'ah AM, Dayem HA: The incidence of skin diseases in Abu Dhabi. Int J Dermatol 1991;30:121–124.
11. Calnan CD, Meara RH: St. Johns Hospital diagnostic index. Trans St Johns Hosp Dermatol Soc London 1957;39:56–68.
12. El-Benhawi MO, Fathy S, Moubasher AH: Mycologic study of tinea capitis in Qatar. Int J Dermatol 1991;30:204–205.
13. Raubitschek F: Infectivity and family incidence of black dot tinea capitis. AMA Arch Dermatol 1959;74:477–479.
14. Amer M, Taha M, Tosson Z, et al: The frequency of causative dermatophytes in Egypt. Int J Dermatol 1981;20:431–434.
15. Kanwar AJ, Belhaj MS: Tinea capitis in Benghazi, Libya. Int J Dermatol 1987;26:371–373.
16. Bhakhtaviziam C, Shafi M, Mehta MC, et al: Tinea capitis in Tripoli. Clin Exp Dermatol 1984;9:84–88.
17. Eun HC: Dermatology in Korea. Clin Exp Dermatol 1981;6:403–406.
18. Schaller KF, Kuls W: Geomedical Monograph Series: Ethiopia. Berlin: Springer-Verlag, 1972:127.
19. Bickers DR: Skin disorders. In: Warren KS, Mahmoud AAF, eds. Tropical and Geographical Medicine. New York: McGraw–Hill, 1990:26–27.
20. Hettinger Th: In Handbuch der Arbeitsmedizin. Konietzko J, Dupius H, eds. Landsberg (Germany): Ekomed, 1989.
21. Stüttgen G, Hass N, Mittelbach F, Rudolph R: Umweltdermatosen. Wien: Springer-Verlag, 1982:116.
22. Horne GO: Climatic environmental factors in the etiology of skin diseases. J Invest Dermatol 1952;18:97–107.
23. Hjörth N, Sjölin KE, Sylvest B, et al: Akne aestivalis: Mallorca acne. Acta Derma Venereol (Stockh) 1972;52:61–63.
24. Gaul LE, Underwood GB: Relation of dewpoint and barometric pressure to chapping of normal skin. J Invest Dermatol 1952;19:9–19.
25. Bodey AS: Structural changes in skin occurring in Antarctica. Clin Exp Dermatol 1978;3:417.
26. Czarnecki MB, Meehan C, Lewis A, et al: Age and multiple basal cell carcinomas in Australia. J Int Dermatol 1991;30:713–714.
27. Dedet J-P: Cutaneous leishmaniasis in French Guiana: A review. Am J Trop Med Hyg 1990;43:25–28.

5

Culture and Socioeconomic Background: Constructing the Relationship Between the Skin, Touch, and Sexuality

Sander L. Gilman

The cultural meaning associated with the skin is the result of the skin's extreme visibility as well as its extreme invisibility. Because it is ubiquitous, covering the entire body, it is both unseen and yet always present. In Western culture, the skin becomes a *tabula rasa*, a blank slate, onto which is mapped fantasies about the interior of the body that it masks. But this fantasy interior contains both physical and moral spaces. Simultaneously, the skin is also the complex surface membrane on which realities of the function of the body—from the physical signs and symptoms of disease processes as well as dermatological pathologies— manifest themselves. In Western culture, these two aspects are hopelessly intermingled. The skin presents itself as the map of the fantasies about the body as well as the indicator of its realities.

The skin has become the place in the body, unseen and yet constantly seen, where a wide range of meanings interact. The skin is constantly being "read" in our culture. And the meanings found on the skin are shaped by the culture in which the skin is read. On one level, we inscribe culture meanings on the skin as well as reading them into the skin. We read specific antisocial meanings into the act of tattooing the skin, just as we read the emerging spots and bumps on the skin of the teenager for a clue to the psychological development of puberty. Much of this reading is undertaken as an

unconscious process—for the skin seems to be not part of the body, but the body itself. The skin's invisibility is the result of its association with the totality of the body—both the physical body as well as the psyche. The skin is the largest of all of the organs of sense and, as such, it is inherently bound to the sense of the body in its totality. The complex meaning associated with the sense of touch mirrors the complexity associated with the skin.

Touch is the most difficult of all of the senses to understand because it is at the same time the most complex and the most undifferentiated of the senses. Sight, hearing, smell, and taste all have specific, limited sensory organs, all of which have specific limited functions and are placed within gaps in the skin. The eye is placed at a specific point in the skin and the skull and it "sees" whatever we wish to understand under the act of seeing. Touch seems to be an undifferentiated quality of the entire body, but it is, in fact, a multifunctional aspect of the skin. Touch is, indeed, the complex sensory response of sensors that judge pressure, temperature, and vibration. But the receptors are not clearly differentiated by function. Ruffini's corpuscle, for example, responds to pressure and warmth, whereas Meissner's corpuscle responds to pressure and vibration. Because of this complex factor, our response to "touch," that is, to the interrelationship of all of these sensations over the entire envelope of the skin (with, of course, great concentrations of certain receptors in specific areas), is much less focused than our response to the other senses.

The skin is, thus, not only an organ of sense but it serves as the canvas on which we "see" touch and its cultural associations.[1] The skin is understood simultaneously to be such an organ, transmitting heat, cold, vibration, and pressure/pain, but it is also the blank page on which the signs associated with these sensory impressions are written. In addition, although we can "see" ourselves or "hear" ourselves, such an act is purely an act of reception; when we touch ourselves, we respond both as the object "touched" and the subject "touching."

This is especially true in terms of our touching one area of greater sensitivity, such as the genitalia, with another, such as the hand. It is not merely the genitalia that are touched and stimulated but also the hand, so that the erotic touch is double edged. No internal power is sensed to be greater than the sexual, and the skin—the ultimate organ of the sexual sensorium—is inscribed with the very cultural significance of sexual.

Thus, too, dangers that lie in the sphere of the skin have been culturally marked as sexual. The marking of the skin by syphilis (and, historically, by treatments for syphilis such as the mercury cure) was a sign of the deviancy and perversion of the individual. Here the map of the skin provides direct access to the hidden recesses of character. The sexual pathology written on the skin comes to mark the character of the individual—whether through the realities of the syphilitic lesion or the tumors of Kaposi's sarcoma. These visible signs of the bad character shine through the skin marking it, just as the marks of "good" character are associated in the popular eye with the clear, pure, shining skin of the rediscovered classical Greek sculpture or the photographic models of contemporary American advertising copy.

The blemished skin becomes the place where character is read. In classical physiognomy, the character is read not only on the face but on the skin. The example I will use to link all of these qualities ascribed to the skin—its role as a place of the link of fantasy and reality, of pathology, character, and psyche—is one taken from a long

tradition of anti-Semitic stereotypes in Western culture. It reflects many of the contradictions ascribed to the meaning of the skin and can indicate how complicated the meaning attached to the skin can be.

The "Jewish Type" and the Blackness of the Skin

The classic anti-Semitic stereotype of the Jew in the West defines the "Jewish type" within the categories of the healthy and the ill. The "Jewish type" was seen to "consist of a hooked nose, curling nasal folds (ali nasi), thick prominent lips, receding forehead and chin, large ears, curly black hair, dark skin, stooped shoulders, and piercing, cunning eyes. This is the typical Jew featured in cartoons, and these characteristics, when present in an individual, mark him as a 'Jew'"[2] It is on the skin, the "dark skin" of the Jew, that the Jew's racial difference, akin to the "black skin" of the African, is associated with the pathologically marked skin. "Blackness" of the skin has often been understood as a pathological sign.

The signs of disease had long marked the Jew as different. The earliest modern images evoked the Jews' pathology as an essential aspect of their nature. It was seen as the physical mark of their guilt for the Crucifixion. Johannes Buxtorf, writing for a fearful Christian audience about the inner nature of the Jews in an account of their nature and practices, cataloged their diseases (such as epilepsy, the plague, leprosy) in 1643.[3] Johann Jakob Schudt, the seventeenth-century Orientalist who was *the* authority on the nature of the difference of the Jews for his time, cited their physical form as diseased and repellent:

… among several hundred of their kind he had not encountered a single person without a blemish or other repulsive feature: for they are either pale and yellow or swarthy; they have in general big heads, big mouths, everted lips, protruding eyes and bristle-like eyelashes, large ears, crooked feet, hands that hang below their knees, and big shapeless warts, or are otherwise asymmetrical and malproportioned in their limbs.[4]

Schudt's view saw the diseases of the Jews as a reflex of their "Jewishness," of their stubborn refusal to acknowledge the truth of Christianity. What is striking about Schudt's early comments is the tradition of seeing the diseased Jew as "swarthy." The Jew's skin is black as a sign of the Jew's inherent illness. Here the physical signs inscribed on the skin directly reflect the flawed character of the Jew, a character ascribed to the inherent nature of the Jew.

How intensively this image of the Jew as the diseased member of society became the central means of representing the Jew can be seen in a description by the "liberal" Bavarian writer Johann Pezzl, who traveled to Vienna in the 1780s and described the typical Viennese Jew of his time:

There are about five hundred Jews in Vienna. Their sole and eternal occupation is to counterfeit (*Mauscheln*), salvage, trade in coins, and cheat Christians, Turks, heathens, indeed themselves.... This is only the beggarly filth from Canaan which can only be exceeded in filth, uncleanliness, stench, disgust, poverty, dishonesty, pushiness and other things by the trash of the twelve tribes from Galicia. Excluding the Indian fakirs, there is no category of supposed human beings which comes closer to the Orang-Utan than does a Polish Jew.... Covered from foot to head in filth, dirt and rags, covered in a type of black sack ... their necks exposed, the color of a Black, their faces covered up to the eyes with a beard, which would have given the High Priest in the Temple chills, the hair turned and knotted as if they all suffered from the *plica polonica.*[5]

The image of the Viennese Jew is of the Eastern Jew, suffering from the diseases of the East, such as the *Judenkratze*, the fabled skin and hair disease also attributed to the Poles under the designation of the *plica polonica.*[6] There had been a long tradition in Europe that held that of the skin of the Jew is marked by this disease, called "*parech*" in Yiddish.[7] In the late eighteenth century, F. L. de La Fontaine argued that the Jews were suffering an extremely disgusting form of *parech* because of their inherent nature.[8] This "disease" was a product of the social conditions in which the very poor lived. It was taken, however, to be a sign of the character of the poor rather than a sign of their circumstances.

The Jew's disease is written on the skin. It is the appearance, the skin color, the external manifestations of the Jew that marks the Jew as different. There is no question on first seeing the Jew that the Jew suffers from Jewishness. Pezzl's contemporary, Josef Rohrer, stresses the "disgusting skin diseases" of the Jew as a sign of the group's general infirmity.[9] The essential Jew for Pezzl, even worse than the Polish Jew, is the Galician Jew, the Jew from the Eastern reaches of the Hapsburg Empire.[10] This theme reappears in Arthur Schopenhauer's mid-nineteenth-century evocation of the Jews as "a sneaking dirty race afflicted with filthy diseases (scabies) that threaten to prove infectious."[11]

The Blackness of the Skin and Syphilis

But the Jew's association with the diseases of the skin reflected back to the fantasies and the realities about the sexual. In the nineteenth century, sexual questions were dealt with by the syphilologist, who, as a dermatologist, occupied the lowest rung in Viennese medicine. Indeed, when Ferdinand Hebra assumed the chair in dermatology (a field nicknamed *Judenhaut*, "Jewskin") in Vienna, he was able to recruit only Jewish assistants! It is of little surprise that the association of the low status of such a specialty and the ability of Jews to enter the medical profession through this avenue reified the view that Jews had a special relationship to diseases of the skin, especially sexually transmitted ones. When the "Syphilis Jew," the anti-Semitic rhetoric of the day, the Jewish bacteriologist August von Wassermann, discovered in 1906 the sero-diagnosis of syphilis that led to the test that bore his name, yet another association was made between the Jews and sexually transmitted disease.[12] Although ennobled in 1913, he remained in the anti-Semitic handbooks of the day as well as in public mind as the "Jew" associated with syphilis.[13]

The Jew in European science and popular thought was closely related to the spread and incidence of syphilis. Such views had two readings. The first model saw the Jews as the carriers of sexually transmitted diseases who transmitted them to the rest of the world. Syphilis had been associated with the Jews from the first appearance in Europe of the disease in the fifteenth century.[14] Indeed, it was "commonly called the Peste of the Marranos," according to the Genoese ambassador to Charles VIII in 1492.[15]

The literature on syphilis in the nineteenth century contains a substantial discussion of the special relationship of Jews to the transmission and meaning of syphilis. There is the assumption of the general risk of the Jews as the carriers of syphilis and the generalized fear that such disease would undermine the strength of the body politic. It is Jewishness that is the central category of "racial" differences for the German reader and writer of the turn of the century. The need to "see" and "label" the Jew at a time when Jews were becoming more and more "invisible" in Germany made the association with socially stigmatizing diseases that bore specific visible "signs and symptoms" especially appropriate.

Syphilis and Character

The location of the Jews and the locus of anxiety about disease in the city. Here the link between the idea of the Jew as a city dweller and the disease which lurks within the confinement of the urban environment becomes manifest. The source of the "hysteria" of the city is the diseased sexuality of the Jew. This view is to be found in Adolf Hitler's discussion of syphilis in fin-de-siècle Vienna in *Mein Kampf* (1925). There he [like his Viennese compatriot, the Jewish social worker Bertha Pappenheim[16]] links it to the Jew, the prostitute, and the power of money:

Particularly with regard to syphilis, the attitude of the nation and the state can only be designated as total capitulation.... The invention of a remedy of questionable character and its commercial exploitation can no longer help much against this plague. ... The cause lies, primarily, in our prostitution of love. ... This Jewification of our spiritual life and mammonization of our mating instinct will sooner or later destroy our entire offspring ... [17]

Hitler's view also linked Jews with prostitutes and the spread of infection. Jews were the arch-pimps; Jews ran the brothels; but Jews also

infected their prostitutes and caused the weakening of the German national fiber.[18] Jews were also associated with the false promise of a "medical" cure separate from the social "cures" that Hitler wished to see imposed: isolation and separation of the syphilitic and his/her Jewish source from the body politic. (Hitler's reference here drew upon the popular belief that particularly the specialties of dermatology and syphilology were dominated by Jews, who used their medical status to sell quack cures.)

The second model that associated Jews and syphilis seemed to postulate exactly the opposite—that Jews had a statistically lower rate for syphilitic infection—because they had become immune to it through centuries of exposure. In the medical literature of the period, reaching across all European medicine, it was assumed that Jews had a notably lower rate of infection. In a study undertaken between 1904 and 1929 of the incidence of tertiary lues (the final stage of the syphilitic infection) in the Crimea, the Jews had the lowest consistent rate of infection.[19] In an 18-year longitudinal study, H. Budel demonstrated the extraordinarily low rate of tertiary lues among Jews in Estonia during the prewar period.[20] All of these studies assumed that biological difference as well as the social difference of the Jews were at the root of their seeming "immunity."

Jewish scientists also had to explain the "statistical" fact of their immunity to syphilis. In a study of the rate of tertiary lues undertaken during World War I, the Jewish physician Max Sichel responded to the general view of the relative lower incidence of infection among Jews as resulting from the sexual difference of the Jews.[21] He uses—out of necessity—a social argument. The Jews, according to Sichel, show a lower incidence because of their early marriage and the patriarchal structure of the Jewish family, and also because of their much lower rate of alcoholism. They were, therefore, according to Sichel's implicit argument, more rarely exposed to the infection of prostitutes whose attractiveness was always associated with the greater loss of sexual control in the male attributed to inebriation. The relationship between these two "social" diseases is made into a cause for the higher incidence among other

Europeans. The Jews, because they are less likely to drink heavily, are less likely to be exposed to both the debilitating effects of alcohol (which increase the risk for tertiary lues) as well as the occasion for infection. In 1927, H. Strauß looked at the incidences of syphilitic infection in his hospital in Berlin to demonstrate whether the Jews had a lower incidence but also to see (as in the infamous Tuskegee experiments among blacks in the United States) whether they had "milder" forms of the disease because of their life-style or background.[22] He found that Jews had indeed a much lower incidence of syphilis (while having an extraordinarily higher rate of hysteria) than the non-Jewish control group. He proposed that the disease may well have a different course in Jews than in non-Jews. The marker for such a view of the heightened susceptibility or resistance to syphilis is the basic sign of difference of the Jews, the circumcised phallus.

Both of these models in the German Empire of the late-nineteenth century, then, placed the Jew in a "special" relationship to syphilis and, therefore, in a very special relationship to the "healthy" body politic that needed to make the Jew visible. (The central medical paradigm for the establishment of the healthy state was the public health program that evolved specifically to combat the "evils" of sexually transmitted disease through social control.) Western Jews had been completely acculturated by the end of the nineteenth century and thus bore no easily identifiable external signs of difference (unique clothing, group language, group-specific hair and/or beard style). These Jews had to bear the stigma of this special relationship to their diseased nature literally on the skin, where it could be seen. Their illness was not only written on the penis where (because of social practice) it could be "seen" only in the sexual act. After the gradual abandonment of circumcision, this sign of disease could not be seen at all!

Just as the hysteric is constructed out of the perceived ability to categorize and classify categories of difference visually, the syphilitic Jew has his illness written on his skin. The skin of the hysteric, like the physiognomy of the hysteric reflects the essence of the disease. Thus, the skin becomes a veritable canvas onto which

the illness of the hysteric is mapped. Seeing the hysteric means reading the signs and symptoms (the *stigmata diaboli*) of the disease and representing the disease in a manner that captures its essence. It is the reduction of the ambiguous and fleeting signs of the constructed illness of the hysteric (constructed by the very nature of the definition of the disease in the nineteenth century). If the idea of the hysteric is tied to the idea of the feminization of the healthy, Aryan male or his "Jewification" (to use one of Adolf Hitler's favorite terms), then the representation of the disease must be in terms of models of illness that are convertible into the images of the feminized male. But these images of feminization are also tied to other, salient images of a race in fin-de-siècle, for Jews bear the salient stigma the black skin of the syphilitic, the symphilitic *rupia*, "a cutaneous disease, with vesicular formation."[23]

Syphilis, Race, and Color

The Jews are black, according to nineteenth-century racial science, because they are not a pure race, because they are a race that has come from Africa. But the blackness of the African, like the blackness of the Jew, was credited to the effect of certain diseases, specifically syphilis, on the skin of the African. It is the change in the nature and color of the skin that marks the syphilitic; it is the color and quality of the skin that marks the Jew. This had been true as early as the publication in 1489 of the Spanish–Jewish physician Francisco Lopez de Villalobos's long poem on what comes to be called "syphilis":

And it makes one dark in feature and obscure in
    countenance,
Hunchback'd and indisposed, and seldom much at
    ease,
And it makes one pained and crippled in such sort as
    never was,
A scoundrel sort of thing, which also doth commence
In the rascalliest place that a man has.[24]

Beginning as a disease of the genitalia, it soon is written on the sinner's skin. In popular and scientific belief, the syphilitic *rupia* is written on the Jew's skin because of his special risk for this disease and because of his long-term exposure to it (and his increased immunity).

By the middle of the nineteenth century, *parech* had come also to be seen not as the result of God's or Nature's wrath but as the result of syphilis.[25] By the end of the nineteenth century, many Western Jews regarded it as one of the signs of difference between themselves and Eastern Jews. As late as Heinrich Singer, it was necessary to argue that "Jews show no more significant occurrence of this than other poor inhabitants of Eastern Europe."[26]

Karl Marx, writing in 1861, associated leprosy, Jews, and syphilis (with a hint of "Eastern Jewish" foreignness added in through his use of a biblical reference) in his description of his arch-rival Ferdinand Lassalle: "Lazarus the leper, is the prototype of the Jews and of Lazarus-Lassalle. But in our Lazarus, the leprosy lies in the brain. His illness was originally a badly cured case of syphilis."[27] The pathognomonic sign of the Jew is written on the skin; it is evident for all to see. Here all of the forms of disease are linked in a common symptom; all are written on the skin. It should come as no surprise in this long chain of cultural–medical associations that the blackening of the skin was also reported, in the fin de siècle, as a sign of hysteria.[28] The blackness of the Jew is written on the skin and represents the inherent difference of Jewish scientist as well as the Jewish patient.

Conclusions

This chain of association about the skin, sexuality, and color of the Jew is a classic example of how myth-making about the skin arises and is supported by cultural rhetoric. What is the cultural map that the skin provides? It is both the realities of specific forms of dermatological infections as well as the powerful myth-making that is spun about these realities.[29] The cultural significance is the need in Europe to see the Jew as different. This act had to be immediate and, thus, the usual invisibility of the skin was made visible—but only for those who were labeled as different. The realities of the body—the nature of the skin

and its pathologies—were all subsumed in this goal.

References

1. Mountcastle VB: Medical Physiology. St. Louis: C. V. Mosby, 1968;ii:1345–1675; Schiff W, Foulke E. Tactual Perception: A Source Book. Cambridge: Cambridge University Press, 1982.
2. Isaacs R: The So-Called Jewish Type. *Medical Leaves* 1940;**3**:119–122.
3. Buxtorf J: Synagoga Judaica ... Basel: Ludwig Königs selige Erben, 1643:620–622.
4. Schudt JJ: Jüdische Merkwürdigkeiten. Frankfurt am Main: S. T. Hocker, 1714–1718;ii:369. See also Haug WF: Die Faschisierung des bürgerlichen Subjekts: Die Ideologie der gesunden Normalität und die Ausrottungspolitiken im deutschen Faschismus. West Berlin: Argument Verlag, 1986.
5. Pezzl J: In: Gutitz G, Schlossar A, eds. Skizze von Wien: Ein Kultur- und Sittenbild as der josephinischen Zeit, Graz: Leykam-Verlag, 1923: 107–108.
6. See Scheiba M: Dissertatio inauguralis medica, sistens quaedam plicae pathologica: Germ. Juden–Zopff, Polon. Regiomonti: Litteris Reusnerianis [1739]; Ludolf H. Dissertatio inauguralis medica de plica, vom Juden-Zopff.... Erfordiae: Typis Groschianis [1724]; and Derblich W. De Plica Polonica. Diss, Breslau. 1848:6–9.
7. Stegmann A: De plica Judaeorum. *Miscellanea curiosa sive Ephemeridum...* 1699;**7**:57; Hamburger E: Über die Irrlehre von der Plica Polonica. Berlin: August Hirschwald, 1861:31–63.
8. de La Fontaine FL: Chirurgisch-Medicinische Abhandlungen vershiedenen [!] Inhalts Polen betreffend. Breslau, Leipzig: Wilhelm Gottlieb Korn, 1792:45–46.
9. Rohrer J: Versuch über die jüdischen Bewohner der österreichischen Monarchie. Vienna: n.p., 1804:26; Weinberg R: Zur Pathologie der Juden. *Z Demographie Statistik Juden* 1905;**1**:10–11.
10. Häusler W: Das galizische Judentum in der Habsburgermonarchie im Lichte der zeitgenössischen Publizistik und Reiseliteratur von 1772–1848. Vienna: Verlag für Geschichte und Politik, 1979.
11. Schopenhauer A: Parerga and Paralipomena, Payne EFJ trans. Oxford: Clarendon Press, 1973;**ii**:357.
12. Fleck L: Entstehung und Entwicklung einer wissenschaftlichen Tatsache. 1935; Frankfurt am Main: Suhrkamp, 1980.

13. Fritsch T: Handbuch der Judenfrage. Leipzig: Hammer, 1935:408.
14. Foa A: Il Nuova e il Vecchio: L'Insorgere della Sifilide (1494–1530). *Quaderni Storici* 1984;**55**: 11–34.
15. Cited by Friedenwald H: The Jews and Medicine: Essays. Baltimore: The Johns Hopkins University Press, 1944;**ii**:531.
16. Pappenheim B with Rabinowitsch S. Zur Lage der jüdischen Bevölkerung in Galizien: Reise-Eindrücke und Vorschläge zur Besserung der Verhältnisse. Frankfurt am Main: Neuer Frankfurter Verlag, 1904:46–51.
17. Hitler A: Mein Kampf, R Manheim trans. Boston: Houghton Mifflin Company, 1943:247.
18. Bristow EJ: Prostitution and Prejudice: The Jewish Fight against White Slavery, 1870–1939. Oxford: Clarendon, 1982.
19. Balaban N, Molotschek A: Progressive Paralyse bei den Bevölkerungen der Krim. *Allgemeine Z Psychiatrie* 1931;**94**:373–383.
20. Budul H: Beitrag zur vergleichenden Rassenpsychiatrie. *Monatsschr Psychiatrie Neurologie* 1915;**37**:199–204.
21. Sichel M: Die Paralyse der Juden in sexuologischer Beleuchtung. *Z Sexualwissensch* 1919–1920;**7**:98–104.
22. Strauß H: Erkrankungen durch Alkohol und Syphilis bei den Juden. *Z Demographie Statistik Juden* 1927;**4**:33–39.
23. Atkinson A: Clinical lecture on rupia syphilitica. *Virginian Med Monthly* 1885–1886;**12**:333–346; Muron A: Du rupia syphilitique (Gomme de la peau et du tissu cellulaire). *Gazette médicale Paris* 1872;**27**:408–410.
24. Villalobos F: The Medical Works of Francisco de Villalobos, The Celebrated Court Physician of Spain, Gaskoin G. trans. London, Churchill, 1870:94.
25. Studzieniecke F: die Cornification und die Lues Cornificative (Plica Polonica). Vienna: Carol Gerold und Sohn, 1854.
26. Singer H: Allgemeine und spezielle Krankheitslehre der Juden. Leipzig: Benno Konegen, 1904.
27. The Letters of Karl Marx. Padover SK ed. and trans. Englewood Cliffs: Prentice-Hall, 1979:459.
28. Mitchell SW: Peculiar form of rupial skin disease in an hysterical woman. *Am J Med Sci* n.s. 1893;**105**:244–246.
29. Goodman RM: Genetic Disorders among the Jewish People. Baltimore: The Johns Hopkins University Press, 1979.

6

The Cultural Construction of Illnesses of the Skin

Inga-Britt Krause

Skin is a unique part of the human body. It serves both as a physical envelope for the organism and as a boundary between the body and the external physical and social world. Because of this double significance, skin acquires social and cultural meanings intricately related to physical facts and expressed in terms of personhood. Personhood, in turn, has two aspects: that which refers to human beings as members of social groups, societies, or nations with special statuses and social roles, and that which refers to the self, namely, to a physical and mental individuality.[1,2] Both aspects are influenced by wider philosophical and cultural orientations held individually or collectively.

Dermatologists necessarily focus on the aspect of this spectrum that addresses physical individuality and pathology. Other more culturally and socially derived aspects are always at work. In contexts where cross-cultural communication between patients and doctors is difficult, culturally and socially constructed meanings are likely to cause problems and to interfere with treatment. Western medicine has made great advances in alleviating suffering from serious and stigmatizing illnesses[3-5] and in health education[6] in non-Western societies. Obstacles remain, and for dermatologists practicing in pluralist social settings where patient populations originate from a multitude of cultural backgrounds or in particular geographical areas with social and cultural contexts different from those found in Western societies, links with anthropology may prove beneficial.

What then has anthropology to offer these practitioners? In this chapter, I attempt to answer this question. Medical anthropology has received a good deal of attention recently from specialist medical audiences,[7-10] and to some extent, what anthropology has to offer medical professionals applies to cross-cultural practice whatever the specialty. Some of what I have to say, therefore, is not specifically tailored to dermatology. I also argue that as a result of the socially powerful and cross-cultural significance of skin, dermatological practice strikes deep into religious beliefs and cultural constructions of self and personhood and that this poses a particular challenge for cross-cultural dermatology. Consequently, my attention is on culturally constructed meaning rather than on biological and genetic characteristics, and I would argue that in any kind of cross-cultural medical practice, the meaning of illness and symptoms must be negotiated.

Race and Culture

Given the unique place of skin in social relationships and in social and cultural constructions of meaning, it is not surprising that physical deformities, abnormalities, and the color of the skin have been sensationalized and have served as metaphors or symbols for social difference and inequality the world over. Nor is it surprising that one of these characteristics, namely that of race, referring to differences in skin color, hair form and color, eye color, skeletal features, and predominant blood group, has served as a foundation for scientific inquiry. It is, however, now long established that racial and subracial differences in *Homo sapiens* are notoriously difficult to define and that for practical purposes, individual variations within one subgroup may be as great or greater than variations between groups.[11] Along these lines, one leading dermatologist has commented that as far as illnesses of the skin are concerned, predisposing racial factors are few and these are "mainly dependent on the amount of melanin in the skin which protects against the damaging effects of the sun."[12,22] This means that differences in the prevalence and presentation of skin symptoms between populations are more likely to be the result of differences in cultural practices and beliefs about such symptoms than of inherent differences in physical and genetic characteristics.

Nineteenth-century anthropologists were pre-occupied with another, and much more controversial, aspect, which they considered to derive from racial differences. This was the presumed differences in the mental faculties between different races and populations. This idea was in tune with the prevailing intellectual climate and theories of the day and much influenced by Darwinian thinking.[13] Subsequent anthropological work developed as a challenge to this, demonstrating that the way people think is a result not of racially inherited characteristics, but of a cultural heritage that permeates and influences both how people behave and their ideas about the world. Cultural differences could not be attributed to racial variation[14,15] and culture could be understood in its own right. In other words, this new generation of anthropologists began to consider the diversity in human thought, behavior, and beliefs not from the outside as stages on an evolutionary ladder, but from the inside and from the point of view of the individuals and the groups of individuals who share ideas and who apparently show some agreement about how they should act.[11]

This emphasis has become stronger as anthropology has come of age and, borrowing a term from linguistics, it has been referred to as the emic point of view.[16] Emic refers to that which is culturally specific, whereas etic refers to that which is universal and applicable to any number and perhaps all cultural traditions.[17] The concept of emic and its antipode, the etic, are cornerstones of medical anthropology and yet, as defined above, they also underscore the complexity of the matter. Although it is commonplace for researchers to proceed with Western medical categories and ideas as if these were etic, Western medicine is, of course, itself a result of emic processes and concepts, and as some writers have pointed out, has its own culture-bound syndromes and categories.[7,18] I do not intend to enter into a complicated philosophical debate about this here. Rather what is at issue for clinicians are the differences in the etiology, conceptualization, and classification of illnesses of the skin among different cultures, and how these differences can usefully be understood and approached.

Culture and Disease

Except for leprosy,[19] dermatological conditions have not received particular attention from anthropologists. This has largely been the case because anthropologists are more interested in the underlying principles governing concepts of health and disease in particular cultures than in specific illness behavior. Nevertheless, this general approach has provided some observations with respect to the cross-cultural study of illnesses of the skin.

Among the Gnau of New Guinea studied by Lewis,[20] who himself is a doctor, for example, the terms a person may use when he or she is ill suggests interesting differences from Western classifications. *Wola* is the term a Gnau used if he wanted to say that a part of his body, such as a leg or an organ, was ill. This term also had a wider meaning for it was used when a person was in a dangerous state such as after the performance of a ritual or for a woman during menstruation. *Wola* meant "bad" and "undesirable," but more specifically the use of the term also suggested that, although a part of the body was not right, the person was otherwise fit.

If, on the other hand, someone suffered in his or her person as a whole, the term used was *neyigeg* (to be sick) and this meant that the person was in a critical state.

On the whole, *neyigeg* referred to internal illnesses. If someone suffered from external ailments including skin diseases, limb deformities, and mental defects, he would use the term *biwola*. The prefix "bi" in Gnau language is a completed-action marker and *biwola* meant "wretched" or "ruined" and it was also the word used for "old" or "aged." It referred to a completed finite condition. Reflecting on these terms, Lewis points out that the Gnau thinking about illness and health cannot be separated from their thinking on other personal attributes, and in this sense, it can be argued, the Gnau do not have a separate medical system. Accordingly, ideas about causes and treatment of disease were also not distinguished from those applied to other misfortunes. In the case of the Gnau, these implicated spirits, sorcery, and the breaking of taboos and prohibitions. Gnau nosology and etiology was different from that of Western medicine and closely related to Gnau thinking on other matters related to physical and social existence.

The inclusion of skin conditions with other illnesses, often mental illness, is common. Ponce[21] reports on a condition in Peru referred to as *el aire*, which includes a wide range of psychological and physical symptoms ranging from eczematized dermatitis and urticaria, to epilepsy, convulsions, hysteria, and paralysis of the extremities and face, as well as other somatic symptoms and gastrointestinal complaints. All these may in varying circumstances be attributed to vapors. Prince[22] reports on two indigenous categories of illness, from the Yoruba of Nigeria, in which skin illnesses are also classified with psychological and mental distress. The two categories differ according to whether they are natural, in Yoruba terminology whether they come from God, or whether they are caused by spirits. *Inarun* is a natural condition, attributed to faulty diet and bad blood, and the symptoms are weakness, burning of the body, itching, skin rashes, dimness of vision, impotence, paralysis of the legs, and psychosis. The other category are those conditions caused by

Sopono spirits. These spirits caused smallpox as well as skin eruptions, carbuncles, boils, fevers, and psychosis, and these conditions were treated by initiation to the Sopono cult, a procedure that required the patient to become possessed. Senior women, who had themselves suffered these conditions, officiated at the initiation of new members. Possession had two functions: It revealed which Sopono spirits were responsible for the suffering and it constituted treatment. Women, in particular, were vulnerable and the treatment was expensive and often had to be repeated. A similar pattern has been observed in other African cultures where women have little power and status in the public domain, and it has been argued that such cults express not only the indigenous etiology of disease but also the social and psychological tensions experienced by powerless persons.[23]

The identification of a spirit, god, or goddess with smallpox is familiar from any parts of the world, and it is also common that smallpox is associated with rashes and skin conditions, such as measles, chickenpox, and acne. Throughout the Indo-Aryan speaking parts of India and Nepal, the smallpox goddess is Sitala. She was and is still worshipped in order to alleviate the fear of smallpox while at the same time inoculation using a cowpox vaccine was practiced by a special group of priests.[3] These practices existed alongside the ancient Ayurvedic (Hindu) and Unani (Muslim) medical traditions in which the functioning of the body was explained in terms of humoral paradigms. According to these, disease is conceptualized as an imbalance of the three humors, wind, bile, and phlegm, and treatment consists of restoring balance through correct diet and regimen.[24] Contemporary Ayurvedic practitioners largely follow these ancient ideas and operate an elaborate body of theories in the diagnosis and treatment of skin diseases.[25] Although these ideas are for the most part held and practiced by elite professionals, humoral ideas and practices are also used by lay persons. First-generation Punjabis in Britain, for example, often attribute rashes and boils to an excess of heat in their bodies and treat these conditions at home by eating and drinking cooling food substances.[26]

Personhood

These brief examples show that Western medical nosology and etiology are not universally applied and that in different cultures, medical paradigms are closely linked to more generally prevailing modes of thought that do not follow Western lines. They also show that, in some way or other, illnesses and symptoms of the skin are associated with culturally and socially constructed notions of personhood. The Gnau or the Yoruba ideas about illnesses of the skin cannot easily be separated from the social and ritual statuses and roles of the persons who suffer. The illness is not only a symptom of a physical condition afflicting the body; it is also a sign of a social state.

This is not, of course, altogether foreign to Western thinking. We also, to some extent and in some contexts, define and label persons according to the illnesses they suffer. Western biomedical paradigms, however, tend to attribute causes to naturalistic processes.[27,28] In other cultures and societies, ideas about causation of illness and misfortune may be expressed in terms of personalistic understandings, that is to say, in terms of the intentions of individual persons or of ultra-human agencies who themselves stand in cultural and social relationships to the sufferers.

Such personalistic understandings are widely applied to madness and mental illness in non-Western societies. Thus, madness may be caused by the actions of sorcerers or witches who wish the sufferer ill or by spirits who punish transgressions and violations of the moral order. These explanations are by-products of personal relationships and actions, and in a world where such a view prevails, natural and social domains overlap. Even when explanations may be offered in naturalistic terms such as those of humoral paradigms, such explanations involve individual intentions and personality. For example, individuals may themselves be seen to have caused imbalances and an excess of heat by consuming the wrong substances, and individual constitutions may be inclined toward temperaments that are particularly vulnerable to certain substances. In these modes of thought, there are,

therefore, neat distinctions between naturalistic and personalistic explanations.[28,29]

In this context of accepted personalistic understandings, the inclusion of illnesses of the skin with mental and psychological disturbances reflects the recognition of the bipolar nature of skin referred to earlier. Skin conditions, like madness, are easily detected by others and, therefore, enter interpersonal communication and interactions as socially constructed personal attributes. Their effect on the interpersonal relationships of sufferers may be as detrimental as those of madness and the explanations as incomprehensible.[30]

Leprosy

Personalistic understandings of causation and the detrimental effect of illnesses of the skin on social relationships are well illustrated by the case of leprosy. Throughout history, leprosy sufferers have been feared, shunned, and ostracized, and the disease has been considered a punishment for wrongdoings and sins.[31–34] There is hardly a more spectacular example of the effects on generations of socially constructed meanings of illness, for as we now know, leprosy is one of the least contagious of human transmissible diseases and the control of leprosy has become realistic with the availability of new drugs.

Two recent studies of leprosy in India and Pakistan illustrate the plight of contemporary leprosy victims and the way traditional medical classification and belief systems underpin that situation. Both studies were conducted as an attempt to contribute to the eradication of the disease. In one, a sample of outpatients in the dermatology clinic at King Edward's Memorial Hospital in Bombay were interviewed about their own beliefs about their conditions.[35] The patients visiting this busy city hospital were Marathi, Hindi, and Urdu speakers and most were Hindus, and a minority were Muslims and Buddhists. They presented with early or advanced stages of leprosy, with vitiligo and tinea versicolor. In the traditional Ayurvedic medical system, vitiligo is considered to be related to leprosy, whereas tinea versicolor is recognized as a less serious and less stigmatizing condition. The findings of this study show a link between stigma and personalistic understandings of disease. Thus, at initial interviews, 50% of leprosy patients, 42% of vitiligo patients, and only 17% of tinea versicolor patients attributed their conditions to magico-religious causes, such as evil eye, sorcery, possession by deities or demons, and God's will. It seems that the more stigmatizing an illness, and the more incomprehensible, the more individual and superhuman intentions are implicated. In addition, 59% of the whole sample of leprosy sufferers thought that their illness was caused by a humoral imbalance, by sexual malpractice, or by consuming harmful food substances, causes which, as I noted above, are personalistic insofar as they implicate personal action in the generation of illness.

In the second study conducted in Pakistan among leprosy victims, humoral imbalances received greater emphasis as a cause of leprosy. Here 34% of the answers given by diagnosed leprosy patients attributed the cause to religious or magical circumstances or to emotional upset, whereas 67% of the answers implicated an imbalance between hot and cold either in diet or in the physical environment.[5] These ideas agree with traditional Ayurvedic, Unani, and Greek humoral paradigms in which therapeutic intervention aims at a fit between ecological conditions and the needs of the patient. From the Indian and Pakistani point of view, however, the fit refers to appropriate action rather than to a purely biological state of affairs.[24] It is this emphasis on individual action and responsibility for health that distinguishes humoral statements about naturalistic causes from modern Western notions of empirical cause and effect.

Compliance and Explanatory Models

We have seen that the classification and explanation of both serious and less serious illnesses of the skin in different cultures is closely related to the prevailing philosophical and religious orientations in those cultures. I have also suggested that because of the very nature of skin as a socially significant aspect of personhood, explanations of illnesses of the skin tend to be personalistic, and that this personalistic emphasis is different from and perhaps even opposed to Western medical explanatory models that emphasize biomedical causes.

These differences pose problems for cross-cultural medical practice. In other cross-cultural medical fields, such as psychiatry, establishing a diagnosis in a cross-cultural encounter presents great difficulties related to the cross-cultural interpretation of symptoms, the translation of terms, and the understanding of emotions. For dermatologists, a cross-cultural context perhaps presents fewer problems for diagnosis than it does for psychiatrists. However, there are difficulties in cross-cultural dermatological practice elsewhere in the treatment process. If patient and doctor think differently about the illness, how can they communicate? When illness is so intricately related to culturally constructed notions of personhood and perhaps even involves stigmatization, how can doctors succeed in winning compliance from patients?

The research teams of the two leprosy studies referred to earlier were actively participating in leprosy eradication campaigns and became acutely aware of the cross-cultural difficulties in gaining compliance from patients. Because leprosy and other skin conditions are stigmatizing, victims who comply with medication and follow-ups also openly acknowledge the conditions and, thereby, affirm their stigmatized status.[36] In this process, the role of health professionals is but one aspect of general social processes. Thus, in India a diagnosis of leprosy is grounds for divorce, and leprosy victims may be barred from public transport unless they carry with them proof that they are receiving treatment.[4] Leprosy sufferers also frequently lose their jobs or are outcast from their families.[5] There are, therefore, good reasons to hide the disease as long as possible and to resist treatment. Once victims have become completely outcast, there is perhaps less for them to lose, but at that stage, the disease may be far advanced.

It is not entirely clear whether patients need to understand and accept Western biomedical paradigms in order to comply with Western medical treatment. Some studies have suggested that where patients have trusted those who advocated treatment, they have complied with Western medical interventions without understanding or sharing these explanations.[6,37] From the point of view of the doctor and other medical professionals, however, an understanding of patients' contexts and their thinking about illness is likely to enhance the chances of successful treatment in cross-cultural medical practice.

This point was made by Kleinman, an American psychiatrist with a cross-cultural interest. He coined the phrase "explanatory models"[38,39] to refer to the socially, culturally, and individually constructed meanings that persons place on their afflictions and on sickness. Building on the distinction between disease and illness made by Eisenberg,[40] Kleinman underlined that healing always involves not just a cure for a disease but also culturally meaningful explanations that individuals apply to their own experiences of illness. Without these, healing is not complete. Explanatory models may vary between different groups of people in the same society and they may vary between different societies, but every patient–health professional encounter in a health care system involves a negotiation between different explanatory models. When there is a fit between expectations, beliefs, behavior, and treatment, such a negotiation is relatively easily accomplished. Where no such fit exists and emic perspectives do not coincide with etic ones, the situation is more complicated. In such situations, "category fallacies" may be committed. A "category fallacy" is the application of a nosological category, developed in one cultural and social context to another such context for which its validity has not been established.[41] It is, therefore, not sufficient to establish the existence of a disease category in a particular population; the category must also make sense to the individuals in this population and it must have credibility.

Kleinman's ideas are widely referred to in cross-cultural psychiatry and their main thrust has been to caution against accepting a worldwide cross-cultural applicability of Western nosological categories and diagnoses. From an academic point of view, they have provided a focus for a cross-cultural examination and understanding of illness and have helped question the widespread practice in cross-cultural medical research of applying screening instruments and diagnoses derived from Western paradigms uncritically. From a more practical and treatment-focused point of view, however, they have also highlighted the problems inherent in cross-cultural communication about health and illness. Belief systems and culturally constructed meanings affect compliance. Weiss and his colleagues in the study quoted earlier found that patients who attributed their illness to humoral imbalances were most likely to attend the leprosy clinic and comply with treatment,[35] and in the Pakistani study, where humoral explanations were prevalent, the authors felt it necessary to widen their definition of compliance to include compliance with the treatment offered by traditional Unani practitioners.[5] This suggests that even though naturalistic humoral paradigms and Western medical models are based on different premises, the fit between these two explanatory models was good enough to facilitate a successful healing process. Patients' models, therefore, do not need to be the same as those of the healers for help to be acceptable, but there has to be some overlap. The matter may, of course, be more complex, for it is possible that patients use different models in different contexts. Referring to this type of medical pluralism, Nicholas noted about the smallpox goddess that although the treatment of a person suffering from the disease was the task of an Ayurvedic physician, an epidemic was considered a divine affliction against which a doctor was helpless.[3] For those leprosy victims who place major emphasis on magico-religious causes, a visit to a Western medical clinic must seem equally beside the point.

Ethnographic Information

Cross-cultural medical practice involves the negotiation of cultural meanings. For dermatologists, these cultural meanings are likely to be those referring to personhood, to cultural constructions of the self, and to the way social relationships are conceptualized. These are issues that directly impinge on personal experience of illness and on illness behavior. They also vary cross-culturally. What then can dermatologists do?

It is not, of course, realistic to ask dermatologists and other medical professionals to become anthropologists. Although academically interesting, this would be far too time-consuming and impractical. A cross-cultural medical practice informed by anthropology can, however, contribute to good patient–doctor communication and efficient treatment. Such a practice means that doctors show interest in personalized experiences of illness and not just in the development and treatment of disease. Along these lines, dermatologists, who practice in social and cultural settings where explanatory models are different from those of Western medicine, can ask the patient questions about causation, about indigenous terminology of sickness, and about the effect of the illness on the social status and the social relationships of the patient. Although such ethnographic data may not be comprehensible from a Western point of view, aspects of non-Western conceptualization of health and illness may overlap sufficiently with Western notions to establish a common ground. Ethnographic information and a genuine interest may thus help doctors understand the experience of the patient and tailor treatment and advice accordingly. In turn, it is also likely to reduce suffering and enhance the efficacy of medical resources.

References

 1. Mauss M: A category of the human mind: The notion of person; the notion of self. In: Carrithers M, Collins S, Lukes S, eds. The Category of the Person. Cambridge: Cambridge University Press, 1985:1–25.
 2. Carrithers M: An alternative social history of the self. In: Carrithers M, Collins S, Lukes S, eds. The Category of the Person. Cambridge: Cambridge University Press, 1985;234–256.
 3. Nicholas RW: The goddess Sitala and epidemic smallpox in Bengal. *J Asian Stud* 1981;**41**:21–44.
 4. Berreman J: Childhood leprosy and social response in South India. *Soc Sci Med* 1984;**19**:853–865.
 5. Mull JD, Wood CS, Gans LP, et al: Culture and "compliance" among leprosy patients in Pakistan. *Soc Sci Med* 1989;**29**:799–811.
 6. Mull DS, Anderson JW, Mull JD: Cow dung, rock salt, and medical innovation in the Hindu Kush of Pakistan: The cultural transformation of neonatal tenatus and iodine deficiency. *Soc Sci Med* 1990;**30**:675–691.
 7. Littlewood R: From categories to contexts: A decade of the new "cross-cultural" psychiatry. *Br J Psychiatr* 1990;**156**:308–327.
 8. Littlewood R: From disease to illness and back again. *Lancet* 1991;**337**:1013–1016.
 9. Littlewood R: DSM-IV and culture: Is the classification internationally valid? *Psychiatr Bull* 1992;**16**:257–261.
10. Helman CG: Limits of biomedical explanation. *Lancet* 1991;**337**:1080–1083.
11. Cole S: Races of Man. London: Trustees of the British Museum, 1965.
12. Canizares O: A Manual of Dermatology for Developing Countries. Oxford: Oxford University Press, 1982.
13. Ingold T: Evolution and Social Life. Cambridge: Cambridge University Press, 1986.
14. Boas F: Race, Language and Culture. New York: Free Press, 1948.
15. Kroeber AL. The Nature of Culture. Chicago: Chicago University Press, 1952.
16. Headland TN, Pike KL, Harris M: Emics and Etics: The Insider/Outsider Debate. Newbury Park, CA: Sage Publications, 1990.
17. Marsella AJ, White GM: Cultural Conceptions of Mental Health and Therapy. Dordrecht: D. Reidel, 1982.
18. Littlewood R, Lipsedge M: The butterfly and the serpent: Culture, psychopathology and medicine. *Culture Med Psychiatr* 1986;**11**:43–89.
19. Waxler NE: Learning to be a leper: A case study in the social construction of illness. In: Mishler E et al, eds. Social Contexts of Health, Illness and Patient Care. Cambridge: Cambridge University Press, 1981.
20. Lewis G: Knowledge of Illness in a Sepik Society. London: The Athlone Press, 1975.
21. Ponce OV: Historia de la psiquiatria Peruana. *Transcul Psychiat Res Rev* 1965;**2**:41–43 (in Spanish, abstracted in English).
22. Prince R: Indigenous Yoruba psychiatry. In: Kiev A, ed. Magic, Faith and Healing. New York: The Free Press, 1964.
23. Lewis I: Spirit possession and deprivation cults. *Man* 1966;**1**:307–329.

24. Zimmermann F: The Jungle & the Aroma of Meats. An Ecological Theme in Hindu Medicine. Berkeley, CA: The University of California Press, 1987.

25. Devaraj TL: Speaking of Ayurvedic Remedies for Common Diseases. New Delhi: Sterling Publishers, 1985.

26. Krause I-B: Statistics and hermeneutics: A dialogue in cross-cultural psychiatry. *J Roy Soc Med*, in press.

27. Foster GM: Disease etiologies in nonwestern medical systems. *Am Anthrop* 1976;**78**: 773–782.

28. Littlewood R: From vice to madness: The semantics of naturalistic and personalistic understandings of Trinidadian local medicine. *Soc Sci Med* 1988;**27**:129–148.

29. Krause I-B: The sinking heart: A Punjabi communication of distress. *Soc Sci Med* 1989;**29**: 563–575.

30. Horwitz AV: The Social Control of Mental Illness. New York: Academic Press, 1982.

31. Brody SN: The Disease of the Soul: Leprosy in Medieval Literature. Ithaca NY: Cornell University Press, 1974.

32. Browne SG: Some aspects of the history of leprosy: The leprosy of yesterday. *Proc Roy Soc Med* 1975;**68**:485–493.

33. Moller-Christensen V: Ten Leppers from Naestved in Denmark. Copenhagen: Danish Science Press, 1953.

34. Skinsness OK, Chang PHC: Understanding of leprosy in ancient China. *Int J Lepr* 1985;**53**: 289–307.

35. Weiss MG, Doongaji DR, Siddharth S, et al: The explanatory model interview for classification (EMIC): A method for cross-cultural research developed in a study of leprosy and mental health. *Br J Psychiatr* 1992;**160**:819–830.

36. Volinn IJ: Health professionals as stigmatizers and destigmatizers of diseases: Alcoholism and leprosy as examples. *Soc Sci Med* 1983;**17**: 385–393.

37. Henderson RH, Davies H, Eddins DL, et al: Assessment of vaccination coverage, vaccination scar rates and smallpox scarring in five areas of West Africa. *Bull World Health Org* 1983;**48**: 183–194.

38. Kleinman A: The use of "explanatory models" as a conceptual frame for comparative experiences and the basic tasks of clinical care amongst Chinese and other populations. In: Kleinman A, Kunstadter P, Alexander ER, eds. Medicine in Chinese Culture. Washington, DC: NIH Fogarty International Center, 1975: 589–657.

39. Kleinman A: Patients and Healers in the Context of Culture. Berkeley, CA: University of California Press, 1980.

40. Eisenberg L: Disease and illness: distinctions between professional and popular ideas of sickness. *Cult Med Psychiatr* 1977;**1**:9–23.

41. Kleinman A: Anthropology and psychiatry: The role of culture in cross-cultural research on illness. *Br J Psychiatr* 1987;**151**:447–454.

7

The Globalization of Medical and Dermatologic Education

Alton I. Sutnick, Miriam Friedman, and Marjorie P. Wilson

The world is rapidly becoming a global community with similar patterns of living and working and similar problems to address.[1] These changes have an impact on how medicine is practiced, with a resultant need to redefine the goals and methods of medical education. Health care needs are international, and many diseases are rapidly becoming global in distribution.[2] The universal availability of advanced technology further contributes to the globalization of health care. International collaboration in biomedical research has been long-standing, partly related to global research technology.[3] Similar comments can be made about health care delivery systems.[4]

The Global Village and Medical Education

Technology has had an impact on medical education as well. The approach of creating a competent physician, and not just providing basic medical knowledge, has led to the assessment of clinical competence and performance,[5] utilizing computers[6] and other types of simulations.[7] The development of competency tests requires the consideration, and ultimately the demonstration, of reliability, credibility, comprehensiveness, precision, validity, and feasibility. Education of the competent physician must be a continual process, spanning undergraduate, graduate, and continuing medical education, and must include an assessment of competence at all three levels. As stated by the World Medical Association,[1] the global approach to health care includes quality preventive and curative care for individual patients and the community. Internationally acceptable standard methods of assessing professional competence and performance should be developed and applied across the continuum.

It is possible to apply identical standards across educational systems in different countries. Certification by a specialty board is a performance standard that has been shown in several studies[8-10] to correlate with quality of patient care. Ramsey and colleagues[8] demonstrated a positive correlation between internists' scores on the certifying examination of the American Board of Internal Medicine and ratings of their clinical competence by professional associates. When Lightfoot[11] questioned the relationship between graduation from foreign medical schools and Board certification, Ramsey et al.[12] pointed out that there is no significant difference in examination scores between certified internists who graduated from foreign medical schools and those who graduated from U.S. medical schools. The qualifying criterion is Board certification, and the study serves as a measure of predictive validity of that process.

Selection by a committee may also serve as an international standard, as in a study comparing performances of students accepted in transfer from foreign medical schools to a U.S. medical school, to that of first-year acceptees in the same medical school.[13] The qualifying criterion in this case is acceptance by the same

Admissions Committee. By the time these students reach their senior year and first year of residency, there is no difference in performance as measured by honors awarded in year four and by first-year residency evaluations, which serve as a measure of predictive validity of that standard setting process.

Some countries have expressed an interest in administering an examination to all of their medical students to serve as an internal standard for evaluation of their curriculum and teaching effectiveness. There has even been some discussion of the development of an international credential for the purpose of physicians moving from country to country. Physicians are to be permitted to move freely from one country to another in Europe, and a legitimate international credential may serve to enhance this increase in flexibility by certifying a baseline level of competence.

The Educational Commission for Foreign Medical Graduates (ECFMG) has had numerous inquiries from many countries regarding the potential development of an examination to serve a variety of purposes to include the following functions:

1. Internal medical school monitoring for evaluation of the curriculum, and assessment of standards for teaching effectiveness of medical education programs.
2. Certification of immigrant physicians or those entering other countries for any reason.
3. Assessment of graduates of medical education programs at all levels.
4. Standard for establishment of new medical schools in a country.
5. International certifying examination as a standard for migration of physicians between countries.
6. Evaluation of educational programs across the continuum of undergraduate, graduate, and continuing medical education.

This multinational interest in some type of medical education standards has revived the potential consideration of an international medical credential based on certifying examinations in basic and clinical sciences, both in general medicine and all specialties. Such a credential might be expected to enhance medical school and residency curricula, including derma-

tology, on a global basis. Elements relating to specific local needs should be incorporated, including the training of nonphysician health care providers.

In the United States, the National Board of Medical Examiners (NBME) has already had an influence on curricula. Of the 126 accredited medical schools in the United States, 99 (79%)[16] require NBME examinations Part I and 88 (70%) Part II of all of their students, and 72 (57%) require passing Part I for promotion to the third year, and 53 (42%) Part II for graduation.[14] Furthermore, NBME makes "subject tests" of used items available to medical school departments for their use in evaluating students and determining the adequacy of departmental curricula.

Global Dermatology

Dermatologic educators have been addressing the impact of the global village in several ways. In 1985, the American Academy of Dermatology established a task force to review the tropical dermatology content of the curriculum of residency programs.[15] The intent was to encourage the view that dermatologists worldwide have a responsibility for the global management of skin disease. The International Committee of Dermatology was elected by delegates from most of the world's dermatology societies to address global dermatology concerns. The International Foundation of Dermatology was established to focus on the management of skin disease in developing countries. A 10-mission program was defined by the foundation that delineates the training needs and the establishment of model dermatologic educational programs in developing countries. The particular value of the nurse and physician assistants in such a setting is recognized, and primary care programs offer special certified training programs for physician assistants in the management of skin disease.

The global view of international dermatology education raises the question as to whether there are any national or international standards for dermatology education, in undergraduate, graduate, or continuing education. A literature review of dermatology core curricula in several countries revealed different needs for dermatology training in different countries. The following examples indicate the importance of designing appropriate curricula for dermatology education that address both local and international health needs.

Dermatology education is emphasized in the undergraduate curriculum in China as dermatology consultation is available only in large cities, and occupational dermatology accounts for 60–70% of all occupational diseases.[16] In planning undergraduate dermatology education in China, it was decided that every clinician should be able to recognize primary and secondary lesions and use correct terms to record them, and that every doctor should be able to diagnose and treat most common dermatologic disorders and to recognize skin manifestation of internal diseases. In the United States, there are no national standards of appropriate undergraduate curriculum time and content for cutaneous disease.[17] Most dermatology teaching occurs in the fourth year, constituting 0.24% of curriculum time based on the median number of required hours in the academic year reported by 91 out of 126 medical schools in 1983–1984. Because more than 7% of ambulatory patient visits in the United States relate to skin diseases, 0.24% of curriculum time seems disproportionately small. In Tanzania, skin diseases, the majority of which are infections, account for 20–60% of all medical problems encountered in various regions of the country.[18] There is a lack of adequate training programs in dermatology along with a shortage of health personnel and facilities. In the United Kingdom, a survey was conducted of registrars and senior registrars in training posts in dermatology and a large number of consultant dermatologists regarding minimum curricular requirements for certification as a consultant dermatologist.[19]

A core curriculum for Canadian physicians in dermatology outlines undergraduate, graduate, and continuing medical education programs.[20] Case subjects in dermatology are used to stress the underlying concepts of basic science in the earlier phases of learning such as structure and morphology of the skin, infectious diseases and infestations, dermatitis-eczema, vascular reactions, drug reactions, papulosquamous erup-

tions, vesiculobullous eruptions, cutaneous manifestations of systemic disease and malignancy, disease of the appendages, and benign and malignant new growths. Emphasis will be placed on clinical exposure rather than on didactic lectures. In the graduate program, it was proposed that the following be included: immunodermatology, photobiology, geriatric dermatology, dermatologic surgery, industrial dermatology, and cosmetology.

It has been argued that, rather than developing a specific body of basic science knowledge related to dermatology, a general curriculum should be designed with emphasis on principles rather than specific skills.[21] For example, in the basic science curriculum, skin can be used to teach diffusion, differentiation, cell and tissue renewal, immunologic defense, and so on. In the clinical undergraduate curriculum, a dermatologist can show students conservative use of the laboratory, such as biopsy and modern study of living tissue. Lessons in pharmacology could include topical versus systemic therapy and the immunology of transplantation. These subjects may become invaluable learning principles that do not force students to master specific knowledge, but rather to understand how the dermatologist incorporates those principles in patient management.

The establishment of a core curriculum in dermatology is essential for improving the quality of dermatology education around the world, but it is only one step. Scarce resources in developing and other countries must be upgraded. The establishment of graduate medical education programs in developed countries for dermatologists in developing countries will enhance global integration, but only if the dermatologists return to their countries to apply their new skills[22] and if the training program has addressed the issues they will face when they return.

International Aspects of Graduate Medical Education

Foreign medical graduates from developing countries who wish to receive additional training in developed countries may come with different educational agendas. Some may be interested in upgrading the quality of care in their respective countries through their own personal training; others may be interested in the organization of health care including the training of health personnel and disease control programs. To integrate the medical knowledge acquired in developed countries, foreign medical graduates from developing countries need to acquire additional tools during their training that will allow them to adequately apply their knowledge to the specific contextual needs of their countries.

In some countries, there are no graduate medical education programs, or an inadequate number of opportunities, and their graduates must be sent to other countries for this purpose. Those who come to the United States, of course, require ECFMG certification. For many years, the United States has been receptive to graduates of foreign medical schools who wish to obtain graduate medical education in a U.S. educational institution. In fact, concern was expressed and efforts were introduced to encourage this exchange and to maximize its value. There was a sympathetic approach to the problems faced by these "medical ambassadors," and the first national symposium to address these issues was held in Philadelphia in 1969.[23] Efforts were introduced to provide a practical orientation to the hospital, the community, and the nation in which they were obtaining this advanced level of medical education.[24] These programs included an approach to English language instruction,[25,26] particularly commonly used colloquial terminology. Even with an organized orientation program, the education is commonly not geared to specific needs outside of the country in which the training is offered.

The end result of medical education is an ability to provide health care, and the level of the standard is reflected in the quality of that care. Just as a medical school admissions committee determines the level of qualification of an applicant for undergraduate medical education, so the selection process for graduate medical education sets standards for that level of the continuum. Such is the case with the International Medical Scholars Program

(IMSP) of the ECFMG,[27] which provides individually designed educational programs in the United States for physicians and other health care leaders from other countries to meet the specific needs of their nations or institutions. Candidates must be sponsored by their governments, agencies, or institutions and must agree to return to a designated position in their home countries upon completion of the program. Eligible candidates include faculty of medical schools, practitioners, physicians already participating in graduate medical education programs, research scientists, administrators of health care and educational institutions, and other scholars. Candidates are considered on the basis of their demonstrated professional accomplishments and on their potential for growth and leadership in their fields. The IMSP has the potential of markedly enhancing international dermatology programs[27] or other international health care programs if appropriate candidates are recommended by the Ministries of Health or other agencies in the countries expressing the need.

Another existing program is the Foreign Faculty Fellowship Program in the Basic Medical Sciences, which is intended to provide foreign medical academicians with an opportunity to expand their knowledge and increase their teaching skills in these sciences, to support the international exchange of information in science and technology, and to enhance cultural understanding among medical educators. The fellowships are not intended to support research or a formal curriculum leading to a degree.

The scholarships are intended for full-time teachers in the basic medical sciences in medical schools outside the United States. In reviewing applications and making awards, ECFMG gives consideration to (1) the demonstrated need to strengthen teaching the basic medical sciences in the school and (2) the extent to which the school serves the medical needs of the nation or region in which the school is located.

ECFMG expects that recipients of these awards, upon completion of their period of study in the United States, will contribute to the advancement of education in the basic medical sciences in their home institutions and countries.

According to current law, the J1 visa permits

physicians to enter the United States as exchange visitors in graduate medical education programs. ECFMG is the only organization authorized by the United States Information Agency to sponsor foreign national physicians as exchange visitors to participate in program under which they will receive graduate medical education or training. The regulations state that this graduate medical education program must be accredited, there must be a written contract with the physician entering the graduate medical education program, and the physician must pass an examination equivalent to Parts I and II of the National Board of Medical Examiners, possess English language competency, and have pursued an adequate prior medical education program. These requirements are incorporated into ECFMG certification. The physician must make a written commitment to return to his or her country and the government of that country must provide written assurance that there is need for the specialty in which the physician seeks further education. The duration of stay permitted is limited to the time "typically required to complete such a program." In no event may this extend beyond 7 years. The physician may change specialty departments one time, provided the appropriate written commitments are made by the physician and the home government. This must be within the first 2 years of the physician's stay in the United States. The duration of stay is generally defined as the time required to meet the eligibility for a specialty board certification, which may be extended to include the time required to take the certification examination. There are some exceptions permitted for those specialties whose requirements are not published in the Directory of Medical Specialists. With special permission, 1 year of clinical training may be repeated. The physician must annually submit a form indicating his/her continued good standing in the program and reaffirmation of the commitment to return to the home country.

The program in select opportunities in advanced short-term training (SOAST) allows a physician to come to the United States for a program for the purpose of observation, consultation, teaching, or research that includes no element of patient care or only incidental patient contact. The dean of the accredited medical school in the United States must specifically certify those points in a clearly structured letter. Physicians in this program are not required to meet the previously described requirements for ECFMG certification and participation in an accredited graduate medical education program. ECFMG is authorized to process visa applications for such positions, as are certain educational institutions designated as exchange visitor programs by the Director of the USIA.

Exchange visitors who are designated as research scholars when they enter the United States may not as a matter of course transfer to programs of graduate medical education. Requests for such transfers will be denied by the USIA unless very unusual extenuating circumstances exist.

Conclusions

The process of medical education in the United States is, in many ways, influenced by the legislative actions of federal and state governments. The perception that the United States would soon have, or perhaps was already experiencing, an oversupply of physicians now appears to be fading. It has become clear, however, that there should be an improvement in the distribution of specialties, particularly an increase in those related to direct primary patient care, distributed appropriately geographically around the country. Residencies in these primary care specialties are generally less competitive and more accessible to foreign medical graduates.

The results of the National Residency Matching Program for 1991[28] revealed a slight increase in the number of active applicants among non-U.S. citizens who are graduates of medical schools outside of the U.S. and an increase in the percentage who matched successfully from 59.7% to 63.4%. A review of the specialties that have less success in filling provides suggestions for recommendations to FMGs for the avoidance of stiff competition for the first-year residency programs. Dermatology ranks among the highest in competitiveness as

92.9% of the positions offered were filled in the match. The U.S. dermatology educators should consider developing special programs if they desire to create an international aspect to graduate medical education in dermatology and to contribute to advances in dermatology education and care in the boundaries of the expanding global village.

References

1. Global Perspectives for Medical Education in the 21st Century. Health and Sciences Communications, Washington. The World Medical Association's Fifth World Conference on Medical Education, October 24–28 1990. 1991: Chap. 1:3–5.
2. Sullivan LW: Presidential mission to Africa. *Med Educ* 1991;**25**:283–286.
3. Nuclear Medicine and Related Radionuclide Applications in Developing Countries. Vienna: International Atomic Energy Agency, 1978.
4. Streefland P: The frontier of modern western medicine in Nepal. *Soc Sci Med* 1985;**20**: 1151–1159.
5. Neufeld VR, Norman GR, eds: Assessing Clinical Competence. Heidelberg: Springer-Verlag, 1987.
6. Swanson DB, Norcini JJ, Grosso LJ: Assessment of clinical competence: written and computer-based simulation. *Assess Eval Higher Educ* 1987;**13**:220–246.
7. Stillman PC, Mina AG: Clinical performance evaluation in medicine and law. In: Berk RA, ed. Performance Assessment, Baltimore: The Johns Hopkins University Press, 1986:393–440.
8. Ramsey PG, Carline JD, Inui TS, et al: Predictive validity of certification by the American Board of Internal Medicine. *Ann Intern Med* 1989;**110**: 719–726.
9. Hartz AJ, Krakauer H, Kuhn EM, et al: Hospital characteristics and mortality rates. *N Engl J Med* 1989;**321**:1720–1725.
10. Kelley JV, Hellinger FJ: Physician and hospital factors associated with mortality of surgical patients. *Med Care* 1986;**24**:785–800.
11. Lightfoot RW: Foreign medical graduates and Board certification. *Ann Intern Med* 1989; **111**:345.
12. Ramsey PG, Carline JD, Inui TS, et al: "In response." Letter to the Editor. *Ann Intern Med* 1989;**111**:345.
13. Hartman ME, Sutnick AI, Hartman DG, et al: Comparison of performances of transfer students and first year acceptees. *J Med Educ* 1986;**61**: 151–156.
14. AAMC Curriculum Director 1991–1992. Anderson MB, ed. Washington, DC: Association of American Medical Colleges, 1990–1991.
15. Ryan TJ: A fresh look at the management of skin diseases in the tropics. *Int J Dermatol* 1990;**29**: 413–416.
16. Li HC: Dermatology training in the Republic of China. *Int J Dermatol* 1985;**24**:129–130.
17. Ramsay DL: National survey of undergraduate dermatologic medical education. *Arch Dermatol* 1985;**121**:1529–1530.
18. Masawe A, Samitz MH: Dermatology in Tanzania: a model for other developing countries. *Int J Dermatol* 1976;**15**:630–687.
19. Dawd PM, Lovell CR: Training in dermatology in the United Kingdom. *Br J Dermatol* 1983;**109**: 235–237.
20. DesGroseilliers JP: The teaching of dermatology in Canada. *Int J Dermatol* 1985;**24**:458–460.
21. Federman DD: Medical student education in dermatology. *Arch Dermatol* 1985;**121**:1503.
22. Elias PM, Epstein JH: American dermatology training programs and the foreign medical graduate from less advantaged geographical areas. *Arch Dermatol* 1986;**122**:405–406.
23. Sutnick AI: First symposium on the problems of foreign medical graduates. *JAMA* 1970;**213**: 2241–2246.
24. Sutnick AI, Reichard JF, Angelides AP: Orientation of foreign medical graduates. *Exchange* 1971;**6**:91–99.
25. Sutnick AI: The Philadelphia program for foreign medical graduates. *Bull Am Coll Phys* 1971;**12**: 410–411.
26. Sutnick AI, Kelley PR, Knapp D: The English Language and the FMG. *J Med Educ* 1972;**47**: 434–439.
27. Sutnick AI, Miranda M, Wilson MP: Tailor made training: The International Medical Scholars Program. *Int J Dermatol* 1990;**28**:416–417.
28. National Residency Matching Program. Results of the NRMP for 1991. *Acad Med* 1991;**66**: 372–373.

Part II

The Influence of Migration and Travel

8

Comments

Robin A. C. Graham-Brown

Our present world has, indeed become a global village. Modern technology has irrevocably altered our appreciation of the little planet we all share. The advent of jet travel has given us the means to move rapidly from one side of the world to the other, and the mass media have indicated many good reasons for doing so, to many people, in many parts of the globe. Famines in Africa are the accompaniment to our early morning cornflakes and have become an almost daily prick to our conscience as "citizens of the earth." We can watch the final of the Wimbledon tennis championships, or the Olympic 1500 meters final, or the World Series as they happen—virtually regardless of where we live. We are now so economically inter-dependent that interest rates in Bonn produce alterations in the shopping habits of the American, British, and Japanese homemaker. We are all increasingly capable of affecting, or being affected by, each other. This is also reflected in the practice of medicine.

One important influence in our modern societies is that exerted by the movement of peoples. Some movements are quick, short, and temporary (the foreign holiday or the business trip); some are permanent. Throughout the history there have been movements of peoples and shifts in the state and nature of populations: Nations have invaded other nations, driving people from their homelands, but also often leaving their mark in the genes of the oppressed; groups have been persecuted and driven out of societies by the people with whom they live, often enduring appalling hardships in order to

seek refuge elsewhere; powerful nations have sent emissaries to far-flung parts of the world to bring back treasures like spices and gold; trade has involved vast numbers of human beings; economic, political, and natural disasters have forced huge populations to pick up their bags and walk (the Irish after the potato blights, the Jews of Eastern Europe, Germany, and Russia, the Vietnamese "boat people," and who knows who will be next?).

Absorption

Thus, societies have absorbed outsiders into their midst. Some societies are, of course, virtually founded on migration: the United States, Canada, Australia, South Africa. Some have "older" civilizations into which new blood has been injected. This part deals with some illustrative accounts of the effects that such movements and contacts may have on the practice of dermatology. It is not comprehensive (it could never be), but the chapters, when taken together, make a number of key points that all dermatologists should try to remember when dealing with "auslanders," whether temporary or permanent.

One of the tenets of the American state has always been the need to accommodate the disadvantaged and oppressed of the world, and we have an excellent account by Drs. Kim and Schwartz of the problems encountered by immigrants to the United States of America. The experiences of ethnic minorities in Western Europe and the United Kingdom are addressed in two chapters: those of Drs. Finzi and Fioroni, whose experience is naturally conditioned by their contacts in Italy; and that of Drs. Graham-Brown and Neame from Leicester, England, where there is a huge Asian ethnic minority in the city. Dr. Scholz discusses the situation in the former Eastern bloc countries. The chapter about Africa by Dr. A. George is intended to stand alongside those from the "developed" world to illustrate the sort of medical environment from which migrating patients may come, the differences in emphasis that they were accustomed to, and some of the reasons for those differences. In addition, we are fortunate to have an excellent account of the problems encountered by the traveler from Drs. Sigg-Martin, Eichmann, and Steffen.

Recommendation

Taken together, we hope that this part will provide interesting and stimulating reading. Further, we hope that dermatologists will be provoked into addressing the differences of disease expression and understanding occasioned by cultural, ethnic, and socioeconomic factors when dealing with patients from "immigrant" communities. Perhaps, also, reading these accounts may stimulate someone, somewhere to look hard at the problems in their community, collect some data, and contribute to the next edition of *Global Dermatology*.

9

The United States of America

Y. Alyssa Kim and Robert A. Schwartz

Dermatology in the United States is a dynamic field, largely due to the constant influx of newly arriving immigrants. These immigrants bring their endemic diseases with them, which changes the spectrum of the dermatologic diseases seen in the United States. For this reason, dermatologists practicing in the United States, especially in the large metropolitan cities where new immigrants tend to settle, need to be alert and to adapt to the changing trends of the dermatologic diseases as the medical field is influenced by immigrant populations.

According to the Department of Immigration and Naturalization,[1] the predominant immigrant populations are from North and Central America and from Asia, with Mexico being the leading source of both legal and illegal immigrants (see Figure 9.1). Mexicans accounted for 70% of the legal immigrants admitted in 1990. The next highest countries of origin were El Salvador, Philippines, Vietnam, and Dominican Republic during the fiscal year 1990. The top six leading states of intended residence for immigrants in 1990 were California, New York, Texas, Illinois, Florida, and New Jersey. These states accounted for over 80% of all immigrants admitted during 1990. Thus, the physicians practicing in these geographic regions are most likely to encounter the exotic diseases imported by these immigrants.

In addition, clinicians need to be aware that there are approximately 8000 foreign-born adopted children, almost all from the Third World countries. The study by Jenista and Chapman[2] of 128 children arriving from either Asia or Latin America noted that many of these children presented a variety of medical problems with 16% of the children having some type of skin diseases.

The predominant dermatologic diseases due to immigrants are primarily various infectious diseases that are brought to the United States from their native countries. Because of the broad range of the subject, we shall limit the scope of the topic to four diseases that had a major

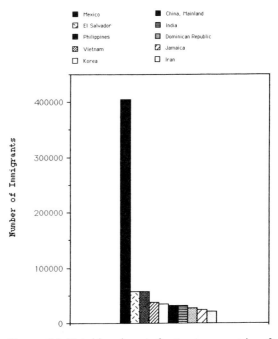

FIGURE 9.1. Total immigrants for top ten countries of birth of year 1990

45

impact on dermatologic trends in the United States rather than turning this chapter into a compilation of anecdotal case reports. These four diseases are: leprosy, chancroid, Chagas' disease, and cysticercosis cellulosae cutis.

Leprosy

Leprosy is one of the most ancient diseases known to afflict humanity. The leprosy bacillus, *Mycobacterium leprae*, the first known bacterial pathogen of man, was identified in 1873 by Hansen;[3] hence, the eponym for leprosy, Hansen's disease. It presents a large public health problem throughout much of the world, but the bulk of the victims are found within the tropics, including Africa, the subcontinent of India, and the entire Southeast Asia. Relatively few cases have been observed in the United States, and of these cases, most of the patients were from the southern states. However, this traditional demography of the disease has been altered recently by the influx of leprosy patients into other than southern parts of the United States.[4-6]

According to the Epidemiology Department of the Gillis W. Long Hansen's Disease Center, 8501 cases have been reported between 1921 and 1989.[5] The bulk of the cases are observed in California (33%), Texas (16%), Hawaii (11%), New York (9%), Louisiana (8%), Florida (5%), and Illinois (2%). These six states account for 81% of the leprosy cases reported in the United States. Furthermore, according to the data from the Centers for Disease Control, the leprosy cases reported in the United States have increased from 50 to 60 cases per year 30 years ago to nearly 200 cases per year during the 1980s.[7] Leprosy patients in New York City include a large number of immigrant populations from the Caribbean and South America, whereas immigrants from Mexico are largely responsible for the leprosy cases seen in California and the southwestern United States. The United States Public Health Service Hospital of Staten Island, New York, has reported that 99% of the patients were foreign-born, and the trend was almost exclusively a reflection of immigration pattern.[6]

The majority of the patients were asymptomatic at the time of entering the United States. The average latent period from the time of entering the United States until onset of symptoms was 4.8 years and there was a lag of 5.4 years before these patients sought medical attention and the diagnosis was established.

Because the majority of leprosy patients tend to have no clinical manifestations of the disease at the time of entry, simply preventing the immigration of those patients with clinical signs will not be an effective method of disease control. In addition, due to the long latency of infection, the immigrants from the endemic regions should be followed for at least 5 years. The majority of people exposed to *M. leprae* probably endure subclinical infection because a high prevalence of antibody titer is discovered in people living in endemic areas.[8] Furthermore, the family members of newly diagnosed patients should also be monitored for possible development of the disease because genetic factors determining resistance or susceptibility have been established by the concordance rate of 80% in monozygotic twins[9] and also by the occurrence in families.[10] It has been estimated that the disease will develop in as many as 10% of household contacts of lepromatous patients living in the endemic areas; although this figure should be lower for family members living in the United States, cautions still need to be employed. In our own institution, a few leprosy patients we have encountered had a family history of the disease: One was a young Puerto Rican man with lepromatous leprosy,[11] and the other was an Indian man with histoid lepromas of lepromatous leprosy.[12] Both patients had a parent who was also diagnosed with leprosy. Prophylactic dapsone twice weekly has been recommended for household contacts of lepromatous patients, but the efficacy of this regimen is poorly documented;[13] however, most patients can be treated safely in their own homes. According to the data from Shepard et al.,[14-17] bacilli from even severe lepromatous cases cannot be grown in the mouse footpad after as little as 3 days' treatment with rifampin. This implies probable nontransmissibility, thus eliminating the question of isolating lepromatous patients being treated with rifampin.

Chancroid

Chancroid, also known as soft chancre, is an ulcerative sexually transmitted disease that is caused by a small, pleomorphic gram-negative coccobacillus called *Haemophilus ducreyi*.[18] Chancroid has been traditionally considered a venereal disease of tropical and subtropical regions and rather an uncommon phenomenon in the United States. Recently, however, this trend has been altered by continuing immigration from the endemic countries, and, subsequently, there have been reports of urban outbreaks throughout the United States.

Approximately 800 cases of chancroid have been reported in the United States annually between 1971 and 1980,[19] with clusters of cases focused in seaports, especially among persons recently returning from the endemic areas in the tropics. In 1977, the smallest number of annual cases, 455, was recorded.[20] Then, beginning in 1980, immigrants from Southeast Asia, Mexico, and the Caribbean reintroduced the disease into the United States.[21] Outbreaks have been reported in California,[22] Boston,[23] Florida,[24] New York,[25] and Dallas.[26] The outbreaks in the United States have been associated with prostitute contact.[22,23,27] Most patients are heterosexual young black or Latino men.[22,26] Symptomatic women tended to be prostitutes;[22,26] in addition, some evidence suggests that female prostitutes constitute a major reservoir for the organism.[28]

In Orange County in southern California, there has been a report of an outbreak of chancroid due to the heavy influx of laborers from Mexico. Five years prior to 1981, the average number of cases of chancroid reported annually in California was 21, during which time the incidence in the United States was 646.[2]

The Orange County Special Diseases Clinic (OCSDC), which is the primary diagnostic and treatment facility for sexually transmitted diseases in the county, reported 923 cases of either confirmed chancroid or genital ulcers of unknown etiology during May 1981 through February 1983; no patients were diagnosed as having chancroid by the OCSDC in 1980. The OCSDC began to note an increase in the number of Spanish-speaking patients with darkfield-negative smears from penile lesions in the spring of 1981.

Through interviews, many of the patients were found to be undocumented aliens who commonly lived in groups of five or more in apartments in central Orange County. To avoid deportation by the Immigration and Naturalization Service, these people maintained a "low profile," socializing only within their hidden environments. Many of the married men left their wives and children behind in their homelands and came alone to the new country to find work. In this closed community, prostitutes who solicited door to door were readily available. These prostitutes most likely served as the reservoir for the organisms and were able to transmit the infection in rapid progression, leading to the outbreak of chancroid in Orange County, California.

Chancroid can be easily confused with other sexually transmitted diseases including syphilis, lymphogranuloma venereum, granuloma inguinale (Donovanosis), genital herpes simplex, and secondarily infected traumatic abrasions. Darkfield examination of the lesion and repeated serologies are needed to rule out a primary syphilis. A history of recurrency, Tzanck smear from the exudate to search for multinucleated giant cells, and a culture for herpes simplex should aid in eliminating genital herpes simplex infection. The lymphogranuloma venereum complement-fixation test and a tissue smear for Donovan bodies should help in ruling out lymphogranuloma venereum and granuloma inguinale, respectively. In spite of previously mentioned diagnostic tools, clinicians should keep in mind that a mixed infection is always a possibility.

Only a systemic antimicrobial regimen is effective in eradicating *H. ducreyi*. The susceptibility of the organism to antibiotics differs among geographic regions, and this should be taken into account when selecting therapy. Use of erythromycin and trimethoprim–sulfonamide preparations has been effective in the United States;[20,29,30] however, resistance to trimethoprim has been growing, and therapy may be ineffective in patients who contract their infection outside the United States.

Chagas' Disease

American trypanosomiasis, or Chagas' disease, is a parasitic disease caused by the protozoan hemoflagellate, *Trypanosoma cruzi*, which is transmitted from infected sylvatic and domestic mammals to humans by blood-sucking reduviid bugs of the family Triatomidae, order Hemiptera or kissing bugs.

Chagas' disease poses a major public health problem in Latin America, where an estimated 10 to 20 million people are infected in endemic areas from Mexico to southern Argentina.[25] In spite of the presence of insect vectors as well as *T. cruzi*-infected wild mammals in Texas and the southwestern United States, indigenous Chagas' disease is a rarity in the United States, with only three known acute cases.[31–33]

Infection with *T. cruzi* is apparently lifelong in untreated patients. Most inhabitants in the endemic regions enter the indeterminate phase of *T. cruzi* infection after spontaneous resolution of the acute illness or without even experiencing the acute phase.[37] The indeterminate phase is characterized by lifelong, low-grade parasitemias, the presence of antibodies to many parasite antigens, and an absence of symptoms. An estimated 10% to 30% of those who are in the indeterminate phase eventually develop symptoms, but, generally, years to decades after the infection is acquired.[35]

Many of the immigrants arriving in the United States come from Latin America, particularly from Central America, in which Chagas' disease is endemic. In a study of El Salvadoran and Nicaraguan immigrants living in the Washington, D.C., area, 5% of this population was found to be infected with *T. cruzi*.[36] This suggests that there may be upwards of 50,000 immigrants infected with the parasites residing in the United States. In addition, another study at a blood bank in Los Angeles demonstrated that one asymptomatic El Salvadoran donor, of the 988 voluntary donors, had clear seropositive evidence for *T. cruzi*.[37] The risk for transmission for transfusing each unit of contaminated blood is estimated to be 13% to 23%.[35] There have actually been three reported cases of transfusion-associated development of acute Chagas' disease in the United States[36,38]

and Canada.[40] Even though the trypanosomiasis-transmitting vector may have lost its role in linking the parasite-host chain with the migration of its hosts to nonendemic areas, the disease persists, through an iatrogenic route of transmission.

Typically, the lesions begin at the site of inoculation, within 5 days of the initial bite. Most commonly, the initial presenting features in Romaña's sign, which is unilateral inflammation of the lacrimal glands, edema and erythema of the eyelids, and conjunctivitis. This sign is a result of conjuctival entry of parasites. If Romaña's sign is combined with the presence of tender preauricular adenopathy, the two features characterize Parinaud's syndrome.

Less frequently, if the port of entry occurs through skin, tender erythematous tumorlike lesions called chagomas may appear. These can necrose and ulcerate. Other nonspecific skin findings are transient morbilliform, urticarial, and erythema multiformelike eruptions.

Children are prone to acquiring acute Chagas' disease and development of myocarditis and encephalitis. Thus, infected children have higher morbidity and mortality rates than infected adults, who often remain asymptomatic during acute infection and tissue invasion. The chronic stage is characterized by myocarditis leading to fibrosis and chronic congestive heart failure in the late stage,[41] as well as megacolon or megaesophagus.

To prevent further spread of Chagas' disease in the United States, several measures need to be adopted. First, immigrants from endemic regions should be screened for the presence of *T. cruzi* antibodies, and those with positive serologies should be monitored for late complications of the disease. Infants of infected women should be examined for a possible transplacental infection and development of acute Chagas' disease. Lastly, public health agencies should establish tighter screening methods for possible *T. cruzi*-infected blood donors to avoid transfusion-related transmission of the disease.

Cysticercosis

Cysticercosis is a parasitic infection that is acquired primarily by ingesting inadequately cooked pork that contains encysted larvae of tapeworm, *Taenia solium*. This infection is prevalent in Central and South America, eastern Europe, Africa, India, and China.[42] This disease is, however, rare in the United States, presumably because of the sanitary precautions against feeding human feces to hogs.[43] The incidence of cysticercosis has been rising in recent years due to the increased number of immigrants from endemic areas[42-45] and as Americans increase their scope of international travel.

Infected patients are likely to present with seizure disorders or with asymptomatic, firm subcutaneous nodules that may undergo caseation and calcification. Because calcification of the subcutaneous cysticerei occurs, on average, 5 years after the onset of the infection and the larvae can remain in the inert cyst forms for as long as 56 years,[46] a careful history by clinicians is crucial in determining the diagnosis.

The best method of establishing the diagnosis is by surgical biopsy and by confirming the presence of an encysted larvae histologically.

To prevent further development of the disease, clinicians must remain alert and informed to establish an early diagnosis and educate the patients of the importance of sanitary measures and avoidance of ingesting poorly cooked pork.

References

1. US Department of Justice, Immigration and Naturalization Service. Immigration statistics: fiscal year 1990. Washington, DC: US Government Printing Office, 1991. Available from: Statistics Division, Immigration and Naturalization Service, Washington, DC 20536.
2. Jenista JA, Chapman D: Medical problems of foreign-born adopted children. *Am J Dis Child* 1987;**141**:298–302.
3. Hansen GA: Undwersogelser angaende spedalskhedens arsager. *Norsk Mag Laegevid* 1874; **4**:1–88.
4. Barrett-Connor E: Latent and chronic infections imported from southeast Asia. *JAMA* 1978; **239**:1901–1906.
5. Fleischer AB Jr, Maxwell BA, Baird DB, Woosley JT: Hansen's disease (leprosy): The North Carolina experience. *Cutis* 1990;**45**:427–434.
6. Levis WR, Schuman JS, Friedman SM, Newfield

SA: An epidemiologic evaluation of leprosy in New York City. *JAMA* 1982;**247**:3221–3226.
7. Morbidity and Mortality Weekly Report, Annual Summary, 1979. Atlanta, Centers for Disease Control, 1980.
8. Abe M, Minagawa F, Yoshi Y, et al: Fluorescent leprosy antibody absorption (FLA-ABS) test for detecting subclinical infection with Mycobacterium leprae. *Int J Lepr* 1980;**48**:101–119.
9. Chakravatti MR, Vogel FA: A twin study on leprosy. In: Baker PE, ed: Topics in Human Genetics. Vol. 1. Stuttgart: Georg Thieme Verlag, 1978: 1–23.
10. Kluth FC: Leprosy in Texas: Risk of contacting the disease in the household. *Texas Med* 1956; **52**:785–789.
11. Bucci F, Jr, Mesa M, Schwartz RA, McNeil G, Lambert WC: Oral lesions in lepromatous leprosy. *J Med* 1987;**42**:4–6.
12. Janniger CK, Kapila R, Schwartz RA, et al: Histoid lepromas of lepromatous leprosy. *Int J Dermatol* 1990;**29**:494–496.
13. Filice GA, Fraser DW: Management of household contacts of leprosy patients. *Ann Intern Med* 1978;**88**:538–542.
14. Shepard CC, Levy L, Fasal P: Further experience with the rapid bactericidal effect of rifampin on Mycobacterium leprae. *Am J Trop Med Hyg* 1974;**23**:1120–1124.
15. Shepard CC, Levy L, Fasal P: Rapid bactericidal effect of rifampin on M. leprae. *Am J Trop Med Hyg* 1972;**21**:446–449.
16. Levy L, Shepard CC, Fasal P: The bactericidal effect of rifampicin on M. leprae in man: (a) Single doses of 600, 900 and 1,200 mg; and (b) daily doses of 300 mg. *Int J Lepr* 1976;**44**:183–187.
17. Shepard CC, Ellard GA, Levy L, et al: Experimental chemotherapy in leprosy. *Bull WHO* 1976;**53**:425–433.
18. Goens JL, Schwartz RA, De Wolf K: Mucocutaneous manifestations of selected sexually transmitted diseases: chancroid, lymphogranuloma venereum, and granuloma inguinale. *Am Fam Phys* 1994;**49**:415–18, 423–25.
19. Faro S: Lymphogranuloma venereum, chancroid and granuloma inguinale. *Obstet Gynecol Clin N Am* 1988;**10**:517–520.
20. Boyd AS: Clinical efficacy of antimicrobial therapy in Haemophilus ducreyi infections. *Arch Dermatol* 1989;**125**:1399–1405.
21. Fiumara NJ, Rothman K, Tang S: The diagnosis and treatment of chancroid. *J Am Acad Dermatol* 1986;**15**:939–943.
22. Blackmore CA, Limpakarnjanarat K, Rigua-Perez JG, et al: An outbreak of chancroid in

Orange County, California: descriptive epidemiology and disease-control measures. *J Infect Dis* 1985;**151**:840–844.

23. Chancroid—Massachusetts. *MMWR* 1985; **34**:711–718.

24. Becker TM, DeWitt W, Van Dusen G: Haemophilas ducreyi infection in south Florida: a rare disease on the rise? *South Med J* 1987; **80**:182–184.

25. Sexually transmitted disease statistics. Atlanta, GA: Centers for Disease Control, 1987:2,37. Publication 136.

26. McCarley ME PD, Jr, Sontheimer RD: Chancroid: clinical variants and other findings from an epidemic in Dallas County, 1986–1987. *J Am Acad Dermatol* 1988;**19**:330–337.

27. Schmid GP, Sanders LL, Jr, Blount JH, Alexander ER: Chancroid in the United States: reestablishment of an old disease. *JAMA* 1987;**258**:3265–3268.

28. Khoo R, Sng EN, Goh AJ: A study of sexually transmitted diseases in 200 prostitutes in Singapore. *Asia J Infect Dis* 1977;**1**:72–79.

29. Schmid GP: Treatment of chancroid, 1989. *Rev Infect Dis* 1990;**12** (suppl 6):5580–5589.

30. Richman TB, Kerdel FA: Amebiasis and trypanosomiasis. *Dermatol Clin* 1989; **7**;301–311.

31. Woody NC, Woody HB: American trypanosomiasis (Chagas' disease). First indigenous case in the U.S.A. *JAMA* 1955;**159**:676–677.

32. Greer DA: Found: Two cases of Chagas' disease. *Texas Health Bull* 1955;**9**:11–13.

33. Schiffler RJ, Mansur GP, Navin TR, Limpakarnjanaat K: Indigenous Chagas' disease (American trypanosomiasis) in California. *JAMA* 1984;**251**:2983–2984.

34. Kirchhoff LV, Neva FA: Chagas' disease in Latin American immigrants. *JAMA* 1985;**254**:3058–3060.

35. Kirchhoff LV: Is Trypanosoma cruzi a new threat to our blood supply? *Ann Intern Med* 1989;**111**: 773–774.

36. Kirchhoff LV, Giam AA, Gilliam FC: American Trypanosomiasis (Chagas' disease) in Central American immigrants. *Am J Med* 1987;**82**:915–920.

37. Kerndt P, Waskih M, Shulman T, et al: Trypanosomia cruzi antibody among blood donors in Los Angeles, California. *Transfusion* 1988;**28**(suppl):315.

38. Grant IH, Gold JW, Wittner M, et al: Transfusion-associated acute Chagas' disease acquired in the U.S.A. *Ann Intern Med* 1989;**111**: 849–851.

39. Geiseler PJ, Ito JI, Kerndt PR, et al: Program & Abstracts: Twenty-seventh Interscience Conference on Antimicrobial Agents and Chemotherapy. Washington D.C.: American Society for Microbiology, 1987:169.

40. Nickerson P, Orr P, Schroeder ML, et al: Transfusion-associated Trypanosoma cruzi infection in a non-endemic area. *Ann Intern Med* 1989;**111**:851–853.

41. Hagar JM, Rahimtoola M: Chagas' heart disease in the United States. *N Engl J Med* 1991;**325**:763–768.

42. Wortman PD: Subcutaneous cysticercosis. *J Am Acad Dermatol* 1991;**25**:409–414.

43. Schlossberg D, Mader JT: Cysticercus cellulosae cutis. *Arch Dermatol* 1978;**114**:459–460.

44. King DT, Gilbert DJ, Gurevitch AW, et al: Subcutaneous cysticercosis. *Arch Dermatol* 1979; **115**:236.

45. Raimer S, Wolf JE, Jr: Subcutaneous cysticercosis. *Arch Dermatol* 1978;**114**:107–108.

46. Tschen EH, Tschen EA, Smith GB: Cutaneous cysticercosis treated with metrifonate. *Arch Dermatol* 1981;**117**:507–509.

10

Western Europe

Aldo F. Finzi and Alberto Fioroni

In European countries, before immigrants are officially recognized by host governments and can benefit from the various national health services, they receive medical assistance from humanitarian (particularly religious) organizations. This makes it difficult to carry out accurate epidemiological surveys; however, it is known that more than half of the immigrants are younger than 30 years old and that they initially came from those parts of Africa, Asia, and Latin America that have had close (usually colonial) ties with the chosen European country. Consequently, at first there were a significant number of East Africans emigrating to Italy and North African Arabs emigrating to France. It was not long, however, before this kind of "directed" immigration was overwhelmed by an immigration based on the geographical proximity of Mediterranean Africa to Italy, France, and Spain, and on that of Eastern Europe and Turkey to Germany. Subsequently, immigrants from more distant, particularly Asian countries, such as the Philippines, have settled in various countries throughout Europe[1] (Table 10.1).

These migratory waves have caught western European governments and their national health organizations by surprise, and there are fears that they will be unable to continue to provide all of their resident citizens with the existing first-class level of care if the threatened invasion of immigrants from North Africa and the former Soviet Union (the latter estimated by the Soviet government itself as being in the order of 20 million people) should take place.

Current national government and European Economic Community (EEC) data on extra-European immigration are only partial and do not reflect the real dimensions of the problem[2] insofar as a large number of immigrants, perhaps the majority, are clandestine and, consequently, not included in the statistics.

At the moment, there are about 900,000 immigrants in refugee camps in Germany waiting to have their requests for asylum examined. This large and ever-increasing number of people is creating such logistical problems that, in addition to requisitioning school gymnasiums and prefabricated buildings, the federal police have even equipped container ships in Bremen and Hamburg.

At the end of August 1991, from the southern Italian ports of Bari and Brindisi, the Italian government completed the repatriation of 17,000 Albanians who, driven by the hope of being accepted in the same way as 20,000 of their

TABLE 10.1. Place of origin of foreigners officially resident in Italy (October 1990).

Maghreb	45.5%
Far East	18.6%
Africa (other countries)	18.2%
Eastern Europe	9.1%
South America	3.8%
Middle East	3.0%
North America	1.8%

Source: Observatory on Immigration. Italian Prime-Minister's Office.

fellow-countrymen during an earlier exodus in March 1991, had crossed the Adriatic in old and overcrowded ships. In order to prevent any subsequent mass exodus, the Italian authorities organized a massive air bridge consisting of more than 50 Alitalia and military aircraft, returning all of the refugees back to Albania in 3 days. In exchange for enormous food and financial supplies, the Italian army and navy are now in Albania to organize assistance and prevent new large-scale attempts at emigration.

But it should not be forgotten that, as the 500th anniversary of the Christian reconquest of Granada approaches, Europe is being faced by a new Muslim invasion driven by the powerful force of demographic growth which, in the Maghreb, is more than 2.5% a year—compared with only 0.2% in Europe. The populations of Great Britain and France now include, respectively, 8% and 11% of people born overseas (versus 6% in the United States of traditional immigration and wide open spaces). As the then British Home Secretary, Kenneth Baker, has said: "Europe is becoming an economic magnet; migration on this scale has never been experienced in recent European history."

In confronting the concrete aspects of the dermatological problems related to immigration, we can perhaps divide them into three groups:

1. common dermatoses found throughout the world whose presentation and treatment do not vary from one geographical area to another (e.g., common warts, contagious molluscum, scleroderma, dermatitis herpetiformis, mycosis fungoida);
2. diseases that are equally widespread but that have different aspects or require a different therapeutic approach according to geographic area (e.g., polymorphous acne, lupus vulgaris, psoriasis), or where the natural color of the skin makes diagnosis difficult;
3. diseases that are acquired as a result of living in or coming from tropical areas (Buruli ulcer, leishmaniasis, rhinoscleroma, pemphigus foliaceous-Brasiliensis).[3–5]

Regional Variations in Ubiquitous Dermatoses

Polymorphous Acne

It is known that the higher temperatures in tropical countries not only lead to greater perspiration, but also to increased greasiness of the skin.

Therefore, there is usually a spontaneous improvement in the acne of young immigrants from the tropics. Furthermore, there are many tropical races (particularly from Southeast Asia and the whole of the Amazon region) that are relatively less hirsute than Caucasians and, consequently, have fewer sebaceous glands; as a result, there is a natural tendency for them to develop less severe forms of acne.

Bacterial Infections of the Skin

Pyogenic infections, particularly from streptococci and staphylococci, are very common in the tropics and usually lead to impetigo and ecthyma.

Young immigrants, especially those coming from rural areas, have been exposed to a wide variety of skin lesions (insect stings or accidental wounds, scratches and burns), especially if they walked bare-legged or without shoes. All of this has often led to the overlapping of bacterial infections that, if not treated (unfortunately, often the case) can lead to hypopigmented scarring that remains indefinitely because it is frequently mistaken for depigmenting active dermatitis.

Cutaneous Tuberculosis

This disease, the incidence of which has been dramatically reduced in Western Europe over the last few years, to the extent that it has now become a rarity, is being represented by Third World immigrants (particularly those coming from areas without *M. tuberculosis* who, consequently, do not have any basic immunity).

All of the other forms of skin turberculosis are associated with visceral infections. Scrofuloderma covers a lymphoglandular colliquative necrosis, usually in the neck, which presents fluctuant nodes and gathered fistulae. Sometimes, tubercular ostitis spreads to the overlying skin and causes a tubercular ulcer, the granulation tissue on the floor of the ulcer being surrounded by a bluish-white border. Lupus vulgaris manifests itself when a microorganism enters the skin of a patient who is already positive to Mantoux's test. In this way, a tuberculoid dermal granuloma is produced, initially presenting as a small brick-red nodule (which under diascopy, takes on a characteristic yellow color), but subsequently extending outward in a centrifugal manner and leaving a central area of atrophic epidermis that may ulcerate and eventually cause malignant degeneration.

In subjects coming from the Third World, the most frequent form of tuberculosis is warty tuberculosis of the skin. This is similar to lupus vulgaris in that a tuberculoid granuloma appears on the dermis after a traumatic inoculation in an already immune patient but, in addition to the dermal granuloma, there is reactive hyperplasia of the epidermis that leads to a markedly verrucous lesion.

Nummular Dermatitis

This form of endogenous dermatitis, which frequently involves the upper and lower limbs, often affects young adults from tropical areas where it is both more common and severe enough to make tropical treatment inadequate. Transfer to temperate zones leads to spontaneous improvement and increases time to relapse.

The same applies to dyshidrosis.

Kaposi's Sarcoma

From the exceptionally severe cases involving Nigerian men, described in 1935, the incidence of Kaposi's sarcoma has increased (particularly in Africa) with the development of AIDS in the Third World. African cases of AIDS associated with Kaposi's sarcoma are less frequent than those in the United States or Europe but, nevertheless, still represent 15–20% of the total.[3]

In addition to the classical form which presents small achromatous nodules particularly in the legs and feet and is sometimes associated with a very slowly progressing articulatory edema, there is a more florid form that involves large, ulcerated skin tumors with a local invasiveness that may extend to the osteroarticular system and, often, the presence of visceral localizations and lymph node metastases. Mucous membranes of the mouth, eyes, and genitals may also be affected. Finally, particularly in children, a form without skin lesions but with generalized lymphadenopathy and visceral localization may develop and have a fatal outcome within a few months. Recently, in Africa, there has been the spread of an aggressive and rapidly fatal form of Kaposi's sarcoma, localized in the lymph nodes, lungs, and soft tissue, and associated with the presence of the acquired immunodeficiency virus. This opens the way to other concomitant, particularly cytomegaloviral, infections in these patients.

Keloids

Spontaneously appearing keloids, occurring especially in the thoracic region, should not be confused with hypertrophic scars due to wounds, traumas, and even vaccination, which are quite common in the Third World. A keloid can be distinguished from a hypertrophic scar, because it extends beyond the area of a possible triggering trauma and often has pseudopodal extrovert characteristics.

Psoriasis

Although it is often wrongly thought to be less frequent in the tropics, perhaps because of the beneficial climatic effect of greater exposure to the sun, there is a high incidence of psoriasis in the Third World (with the exception of Africa). Immigrants quite frequently develop guttate or large patchy lesions accompanied by severe itching, either because of reduced solar exposure or because of the known triggering effects of the stress associated with emigration and the need to adjust to a new environment.

Hypertrophic Lichen Planus

In immigrants from Southern India and Sri Lanka, lichen ruber planus skin eruptions (especially on the legs) takes on a hypertrophic appearance, with strongly hyperpigmented and pruritic nodules. Left untreated, these lesions can last for years. In treatment, intralesional steroid infiltration is to be avoided, because it easily gives rise to skin atrophy; systemic therapy is preferred.

Actinic Lichen Planus

These eruptions, also incorrectly called tropical lichen planus (which was the term used during World War II to describe lichenoid eruptions due to the administration of the antimalarial agent, mepacrine), affect the face with hyperpigmented pruritic papulae that progressively become larger and take on an annular appearance with a shallow central depression. It is frequent along the Mediterranean coasts of Africa, along the Egyptian Nile, and in the Near East.

A similar but milder condition is described in Kenya as lichenoid melanodermatitis.

Superficial Mycosis

A large number of immigrants, particularly those from North Africa, the Middle East, and southeast Europe, are reintroducing into western Europe some previously eradicated mycoses, such as tinea favosa due to *T. schoenleinii* or scalp kerion, mainly caused by *T. violaceum* and *T. tonsurans.*

After a brief incubation period of about 2 weeks, small erythematous zones form around the base of the hairs and soon begin to flake; the subsequent pustules are followed by scutuli in the carbuncles. These are small (just a few millimeters), round yellowish concretions, concave at the top, with the characteristic smell of mouse urine. They are firmly attached to the underlying tissue and, if removed, leave the skin erose, erythematous, and sometimes serogenetic. The final result is permanent alopecia, and so the need for early treatment cannot be overstressed.

In addition to endothrix tinea capitis, foot and nail infections due to *Hendersonula* are not infrequent.

Deep Mycosis

Both subcutaneous and systemic mycosis are still rare in Europe, with the exception of the ubiquitous sporotrichosis and all of the systemic mycoses accompanying AIDS. Only sporadic cases are currently reported, the most frequent being mycetoma (also known as Madura foot because of its classical location), which is reported primarily in patients from equatorial Africa.[7]

Infestation of Ectoparasites

Scabies and pediculosis are historically widespread in periods of social instability and intense and disordered migration. Among the 17,000 Albanian refugees who landed on the coast of Puglia in Italy, these were the most frequent diseases (approximately 10% of the refugees).

Tungiasis

This is the infection caused by the female *Tunga penetrans* in the skin of man. In the past, it was limited to broad areas of Central and South America but, in 1873, the insect was transported by a British ship from Brazil to Angola, from where it spread rapidly throughout equatorial Africa (thanks, it is said, to Stanley's expeditions) and to India.[8] In Europe today, it is commonly found not only in immigrants but also in tourists who become infected by walking or lying stretched out on the beaches. *Tunga* feed on the blood of any warm-blooded animal. After having been fertilized, the female attaches itself to the skin of humans or other animals (especially pigs) and, for a week, its abdomen grows to about the size of a pea; within a week's time up to 200 eggs are laid. The main problem with this infestation is the fact that complications such as tetanus or gangrene can set in.

Cutaneous Larva Migrans

This is due to the entry of *Ancylostoma brasiliense*, *A. caninum*, and *Strongyloidea* sp., which fail to complete their life cycle in man and, consequently, remain under the skin. They are common in all hot, damp, tropical, and subtropical climates.

Just a few hours after the larva penetrates the skin, an erythematous papule appears, accompanied by itching symptoms. A serpiginous trace corresponding to the tunnel excavated by the larva is then formed and may progress a number of centimeters a day. The surrounding skin appears erythematosus edematous. Itching can be severe and lead to additional infections. The larva is difficult to remove because it is often outside the area of the visible lesion. Unless treated with thiabendazole, infestation can continue for a number of months.

Leprosy

This disease, caused by the specific microorganism, *Mycobacterium leprae*, is characterized by an extremely variable incubation period that can be very long. This makes the infection particularly dangerous and insidious. It accounts for one of the major fears among European populations in the face of health risks from immigrants, particularly those coming from the Indian subcontinent, tropical Africa, Southeast Asia, and South America (where there are estimated to be 15–20 million lepers).[7]

Leprosy has been classified into two main types, lepromatous (LL) and tuberculoid (TT), with intermediate (BB), borderline lepromatous (BL), and borderline tuberculoid (BT) forms. In lepromatous leprosy, cell resistance against *M. leprae* is minimal, whereas in tuberculoid leprosy, cellular immunity is pronounced and manifested by the widespread reaction of epithelial cells and lymphocytes even in the presence of just a few bacilli.

Both clinically and histologically, borderline leprosy has the characteristics of both forms.

Lepromatous leprosy patients may present with a wide variety of slightly erythematous or hypopigmented lesions, ranging from maculae to papulae to nodules, and to patchiness and nodosity; frequently, nerve sensitivity transmission in these lesions is damaged right from the beginning. Tuberculoid leprosy lesions are often slightly erythematous or hypopigmented maculae with altered cutaneous sensitivity.

Leprosy is often difficult to diagnose, and a number of specific diagnostic criteria need to be taken into account: sensory alterations, nerve thickening, and the presence of acid-resistant bacilli or typical histopathological lesions. Differential diagnosis concerns a wide range of dermatological conditions: hypopigmented macular lesions can be confused with superficial mycoses, and pityriasis allia and infiltrated lesions with psoriasis, lupus vulgaris, syphilis, lupus erythematosus, annular granuloma, polymorphous erythema, neurofibromatosis, sarcoidosis, and cutaneous lymphoma.

Consequently, great care must be taken in all suspect forms found in individuals coming from risk zones.

References

1. Bastenier A, Dassetto F: Italia, Europa e nuove immigrazioni Edizioni della Fondazione Agnelli, Turin, 1990.
2. Moretti E: I movimenti migratori in Italia in un quadro di rifermimento internazionale. Cooperativa Libraria Universitaria Ancona, Ancona, 1990.
3. Manson–Bahr PEC, Bell DR: Manson's Tropical Diseases, 19th ed. London: Bailliére-Tindall, 1987.
4. Pettit JHS: Manual of Practical Dermatology. New York: Churchill Livingstone, 1985.
5. Pettit JHS, Parish LC: Manual of Tropical Dermatology. New York: Springer-Verlag, 1984.
6. Hay RJ: Personal communication, 1991.
7. Maegraith B: Clinical Tropical Disease, 9th ed. Oxford: Blackwell Scientific Publications, 1989.
8. Binford CH, Connor DH: Pathology of Tropical and Extraordinary Diseases. Armed Forces Institute of Pathology, Washington, D.C., 1976.

11

The United Kingdom

Robin A. C. Graham-Brown and Rebecca L. Neame

The United Kingdom of Great Britain and Northern Ireland is, as the country's official title suggests, a state composed of different parts. England, Scotland (including many far-flung Hebridean islands, Orkney, and the Norse Islands of Shetland), Wales, part of Ireland, the old Celtic Kingdom of Cornwall (Kernow), the Channel Islands, and the Isle of Man are all bound together by a form of parliamentary democracy within a constitutional monarchy. It may be a surprise to some that within this "federation" there are, in fact, substantial legal and constitutional differences: abortion and homosexuality remain illegal in Northern Ireland; Scottish law and educational systems are completely different from the rest of the United Kingdom; there are much lower income tax rates in the Channel Islands and the Isle of Man.

As a member of the "Old World," we have an extensive and well-documented history of internecine squabbles, invasions, wars, occupations, and colonial expansion. Much of it is well known far beyond our shores, disseminated through the (not always strictly factual) vehicles of the theatre, books, movies, and television. Our myths and legends (e.g., King Arthur and Robin Hood) are probably more real to many than the truly historical characters portrayed in Shakespeare, like Macbeth and King Richard III.

The islands that make up the United Kingdom (and the Republic of Ireland) have seen many changes. There have been many movements of their peoples and of others who have, at various points, expressed an interest in the United Kingdom. For example, the Romans found their way there under the leadership of Julius Caesar. The arrival of invaders from Scandinavia resulted in wholesale repopulation of the east and north of England and the movement of the Celts into the western reaches of the islands. The occupation by the Duke of Normandy in 1066 resulted in a substantial and lengthy mixing of British and French interests, which produced one of the longest running soap operas in history. This ended officially when the British finally withdrew from Calais during the reign of Queen Mary (although the continuation of scraps such as the Napoleonic Wars and the refusal of General de Gaulle to countenance British membership of the European Community may indicate that the British and French still enjoy the odd skirmish).

The British were, of course, great explorers and invaders themselves. Usually driven by financial motives (but occasionally by altruism), British sailors, merchants, and military men set out to as many parts of the globe as they could reach. The result of this was the establishment of a massive empire with components in every continent. We even had an interest for a while in a small piece of real estate that in 1776 became the United States of America.

One of the consequences of the United Kingdom's complicated history is that, particularly in the last 100 years, there have been substantial migrations both to and from these islands. Emigration to the United States, Canada, Australia, New Zealand, South Africa, and elsewhere has been going on for years and has often provided part of the core population of those "New World" states. This is not the concern of this chapter, however; here we examine the problems produced by migration into the United Kingdom.

Migration into the United Kingdom

In 1981, the largest "immigrant" group in the United Kingdom was from Ireland,[1] although there have been small migrations from many other parts of the world. Notable among these was the influx of Jewish settlers escaping persecution in Eastern Europe and Russia, which occurred at the end of the nineteenth century and the early part of the twentieth century. Further population movements occurred from Europe, particularly during the turmoil of the Nazi invasions of Czechoslovakia and Poland, and during and after the Second World War. Small numbers of people have also moved from Italy, Cyprus, and other European countries, largely for economic reasons.

More recently, however, there has been a large influx of migrants from the Commonwealth (as the British Empire came to be known). There were peaks and troughs in this process, but the first groups came from the West Indies and from India in the early 1950s. Migration from the Indian subcontinent accelerated in the 1960s, despite (or possibly partly because of) the introduction of legislation to control immigration.[1] Another huge surge occurred when the then-President Idi Amin threw the Asian population out of Uganda in the early 1970s.

Strict immigration laws now control the number of people from Africa, India, Pakistan, Bangladesh, and other former colonies who may take up residence in Britain. This has not been universally popular. There was a significant outcry, for example, when it was announced recently that only a very small proportion of the residents of Hong Kong would be entitled to full British citizenship when the colony returns to Chinese ownership in 1997. In direct contrast to this, however, is the fact that frontiers within the European community (of which the United Kingdom is now a member) will completely disappear as far as rights of residence and work are concerned. Thus, a citizen of Italy, Denmark, Portugal, or Greece may move at any time to the United Kingdom and seek work, and vice versa. As an aside, it is interesting to note the paradox that such freedom will produce. Portugal has granted citizenship to a large number of the residents of its Chinese colony Macao, which also faces a return to Chinese rule. This means that migrants from Macao will be able to move to Europe and then live in Britain, if they so wish, although most residents of Hong Kong cannot.

Medical Problems Among Ethnic Minorities in Britain

Thus, the United Kingdom has an ever-changing ethnic landscape that provides a wide variety of diagnostic, therapeutic, and cultural challenges for British doctors. It has increasingly been recognized that ethnic minorities pose a number of special problems; however, there are two important, and interrelated, points that need to be borne in mind in any discussion on this subject.

First, it has become apparent that settlement of immigrants within the United Kingdom has been far from uniform.[2] This should not have been a surprise in view of the propensity of peoples of like mind and cultural tradition to want to be near each other. "Birds of a feather flock together" says the old proverb! The well-established American concept of "neighborhoods" composed of different ethnic mixes has only been properly addressed in the United Kingdom in the relatively recent past. For many years it was almost taboo to discuss the idea that a multiethnic society could function on the basis of a measure of separation instead of a complete mixing and integration. Integration was the buzz-word of the sixties.

In Leicester, it has long been realized that this was not how things would develop. When Amin gave the Asian population orders to leave, they, not unnaturally, headed for places where they had some contacts. The United Kingdom agreed to resettle a substantial number of people and there were already areas of the country in which relatives and friends of the business community of East Africa lived and worked. One of these was Leicester. The net result is that Leicester now has a large ethnic group whose origins lie in an Indian/East African heritage. Furthermore, the majority of this community derives from immigrants to Africa from the area of India now known as Gujarat. The Asian population of Leicester currently stands at 18%, with three-quarters of that group being Gujarati.[3]

Second, the concept of "ethnicity" is a difficult one to define.[1] It is simply not enough to record an individual's country of birth when considering disease statistics. Many members of "ethnic" minorities have been born in the country to which their parents, grandparents, or even earlier generations moved, but still consider themselves as being ethnically separate from other groups in society. This is already highly developed in the United States where concepts of Irish-Americans, Polish-Americans, African-Americans, native Americans, and so on are now accepted descriptive terms. It is, however, taking time for similar ways of thinking to be adopted in the United Kingdom. Some of our politicians appear to find it surprising that Asians still cheer for India or Pakistan when England plays them at cricket.

That there are specific medical problems among immigrant communities and different ethnic groups is well illustrated by the list of contents of important books such as *Ethnic Factors in Health and Disease*, edited by Cruikshank and Beevers[4] and Polednak's *Racial and Ethnic Differences in Disease*.[5] Topics covered in these works include genetic disorders such as sickle cell disease and thalassemia, rheumatic and autoimmune disorders, cancer, viral infections, psychiatric disease, cardiovascular disease, and diabetes. Studies in our own city have revealed important differences in the white and Asian populations in regard to pulmonary tuberculosis, obstetric and contraceptive practices, diabetes mellitus, and rheumatic disease, and large studies are currently underway to examine differences in cardiovascular mortality.

Strikingly, as far as dermatologists are concerned, there is practically nothing in either Cruikshank and Beevers' or Polednak's books about skin disease, apart from brief brushes with dermatology in discussions on HIV infections, scleroderma, and sarcoidosis.[4,5] This glaring omission has to be set against the fact that cutaneous morbidity is substantial in all societies where records exist. Skin infections, both acute and chronic, are undoubtedly a major burden in the developing world. It has been estimated that as many as 30% of the U.S. population has a skin condition at any one time.[6] Figures from the United Kingdom, where health care is "filtered" by a network of general (family) practitioners, have indicated that at least 6–8% of patient consultations in general practice are for skin problems, and that many skin patients have to be referred to the hospital unnecessarily because of the lack of dermatological training available to family doctors.[7] It is presumably because there has been so little attention paid to the true incidence and prevalence of skin disease among the different groups in our communities that so little has found its way into the books. More recently, however, some information about skin disease in ethnic minority populations has begun to emerge.

Skin Problems Among Ethnic Minorities in the United Kingdom

London is one of the largest cities in the world and contains citizens of many colors, creeds, and cultures. A recent estimate suggested that schoolchildren within the Inner London area used as many as 147 different first languages.[3] Dermatologists serving the large Jewish communities of North London (and similar communities in provincial cities such as Manchester, Leeds, and Glasgow) have long been aware that they were more likely to see classical Kaposi's sarcoma than their colleagues elsewhere, and to have more trouble with pemphigus.

In areas such as South London, where there are sizeable Afro-Caribbean groups, dermatologists report several distinct differences in the way patients from the white and black communities present to the skin clinic.[3] There are virtually no skin cancers in the black patients, and they present much less frequently with nevi and other benign skin lumps. Infestations, especially pediculosis, are rarer and verrucae are reported to be less common in Afro-Caribbean children in South London.[3]

Much commoner, however, are presentations with abnormalities of pigmentation and hair. Pigmentary abnormalities are clearly exaggerated in pigmented skin and both blacks and Asians in Britain present difficult management problems. Vitiligo is extremely unsightly in black skin. Notably, it may also assume a "trichrome" pattern in Afro-Caribbeans.[8] Other pigmentary conditions are also seen commonly:[8] Futcher's lines (which are, of course, physiological); hyperpigmentation of the palms and soles; pigmented nail bands; and dermatosis papulosa nigra. Sadly, skin lightening creams are still available, popular, and used widely. The results of these, including full-blown ochronosis, are still seen in the United Kingdom skin clinics that have large colored populations in their drainage areas.

The tendency for curly hair to produce folliculitis of the beard and scalp is a particularly common presenting feature in black men, who often also develop folliculitis (acne) keloidalis as a result.[8] Afro-Caribbeans are still also seen with traction alopecia, to which their hair seems to be more prone. Other skin conditions that are seen more often in Afro-Caribbeans in Britain include cutaneous sarcoidosis, lichen striatus, keloid scars, eczematides, and lupus erythematosus.[3]

Another problem, which was stressed by Pembroke in an address to a meeting on immigrant communities in western environments in Oxford, is that many young British dermatologists are trained in areas with virtually exclusively white populations.[3] They are often ill-prepared for the differences in physical signs that are presented by black skin. For example, atopic dermatitis is common in Afro-Caribbean children, but the clinical picture may be dominated by a micropapular appearance strongly resembling lichen nitidus.

Finally, it is important that dermatologists be aware of the need for special care with certain management techniques in black skin. Acne should be treated more energetically to avoid scarring and postinflammatory hyperpigmentation and surgery needs to be carefully considered because of keloid formation. The terminology, explanations, and discussion used with the patient should reflect the fact that many British Afro-Caribbeans have suffered considerable racial discrimination over the years. Patients may be extremely sensitive to phraseology that suggests "difference" when used by individuals who are part of "the establishment." Paradoxically, however, West Indians are reported to have unrealistically high expectations of modern medicine and may be very disappointed when they are informed that, for example, folliculitis keloidalis is difficult to treat.[3]

The other major ethnic minority on whom there is useful information available is the British Asian population. It is important to stress for readers from other countries that the term "Asian," when used in Britain, generally means someone whose roots are in the India subcontinent, rather than Southeast Asia, China, Korea, or Japan. As we have already mentioned, there are cities in Britain with large Asian minorities. Some have communities that have largely migrated from Pakistan or Bangladesh and are, consequently, overwhelmingly Muslim. Some have communities that are predominantly Hindu, and others Sikh. Thus, a specifically religious dimension may be superimposed on other cultural differences. For example, many Hindus are vegetarian (and even vegan), and iron deficiency is common among the women. Asian women do not like to be examined by male doctors at the best of times, but some Muslim women are particularly resistant and may not present for help at all if they cannot see a woman physician.

Unlike the Afro-Caribbean community, where exotic or tropical diseases are now rare in Britain, there is still a fair chance of seeing chronic infections in Asian patients. Leprosy is still a significant problem, unusual forms of tuberculosis still occur in Asian patients,[9,10] and most centers of Asian population will have a few patients with Madura foot. Because many of these diseases take years to develop and the people affected grew up in endemic areas, this is to be expected for the lifetime of this generation at least.

Of more interest, however, are findings that suggest that there may be differences in disease prevalence, or the ways in which diseases are seen and dealt with in the Asian community. There has been some controversy about this, with some studies maintaining that eczemas of various kinds were more common in Indians and Pakistanis,[11] whereas others found that atopic disease in general was actually less prevalent among children born overseas.[12] In our own skin clinic, we have observed and reported a very marked difference in the pattern of skin disease referred to us in the Asian and white communities.[13] We looked at nearly 1000 new referrals to our department in two separate months. We found that pigmentary disorders were more common among Asian referrals, whereas skin cancers were, as expected, seen almost exclusively in whites. There were other more minor differences, but the most striking, by far, was that atopic dermatitis was much more common in the Asian group. We stratified part of the sample by age (in the children this had the effect of excluding the possible effect of skin cancers as a complicating factor) and discovered that atopic dermatitis was three times as common in Asian children aged 0–9 years as compared to white children of the same age. This was highly statistically significant ($p < .001$).

Such findings do not mean, of course, that the true prevalence of atopic dermatitis is different between the two groups. The disparity could be accounted for by a combination of factors, including differences in prevalence, severity of disease, an increased tendency for Asian parents to demand hospital treatment, and alterations in referral patterns by those doctors looking after Asian children. We had already shown that Asian parents were less likely than white parents to subject their children with atopic dermatitis to exclusion diets.[14] Although this tends to confirm the notion that there might be differences in the way in which the disease is perceived in the two communities, it could be interpreted as implying that Asian families are actually less anxious about the condition than whites. We had also observed (but did not publish) the fact that there was no statistically significant difference in the severity of atopic dermatitis between the Asian and white children in the same study (Webber et al, unpublished observations).

In an attempt to investigate further the possibility of differences in the prevalence and/or expression of atopic dermatitis in the Asian ethnic minority in Leicester, we have recently completed a field survey. The findings are yet to be published in full at the time of writing but are presented in thesis form.[15] This study has established an overall prevalence of atopic dermatitis at 14% in children aged 18 months, but interestingly showed no difference in prevalence of severity between white and Asian children. Thus, if these findings are correct, we have to look elsewhere for an explanation of the extraordinary disparity in referral pattern.

Finally, it is important to emphasize the need for all those dealing with ethnic minorities to understand and respect the cultural traditions. Indeed, an understanding of this area is essential to good clinical management. We can, perhaps, illustrate this and end the chapter with an instructive story:

A young Asian girl was brought to the skin clinic by two female relatives (or so they appeared), complaining of excessive hair. The girl was a few months past her sixteenth birthday and was perfectly normal, apart from prominent facial hair. This was carefully explained to her and the two attending ladies, but they were not satisfied, demanding that something should be done. The doctor (RACG-B) then asked more about the family history, hoping to lead them to see that the "problem" was basically genetic but soon discovered that one of the women was not a relative at all, but the matchmaker who had recently flown in from Pakistan to assess the girl's marriage prospects.

With social pressures like this, skin complaints that are there for all to see assume an importance far beyond that which would be the case of someone from a different ethnic and cultural group.

References

1. Webster J, Fox J: The changing nature of populations: the British example. In: Cruik-

shank JK, Beevers DG, eds. Ethnic Factors in Health and Disease. London: Wright, 1989.

2. Brown C: Black and White Britain: The Third PSI Survey. London: Heinemann, 1984.

3. Graham-Brown RAC, Berth-Jones J, Dure-Smith B, et al. Dermatologic problems for immigrant communities in a western environment. *Int J Dermatol* **29**:94–101.

4. Cruikshank JK, Beevers DG. Ethnic Factors in Health and Disease. London: Wright, 1989.

5. Polednak AP: Racial and Ethnic Differences in Disease. Oxford: Oxford University Press, 1989.

6. Johnson M-LT: Skin conditions and related need for medical care among persons 1–74 years. United States. 1971–74. Vital Health Statistics: Series 11, Data from National Health Survey; no. 212. Hyattsville, MD:US Dept of Health Education and Welfare, 1978. DHEW Publication No. (PHS) 79-1160.

7. Sladden MJ, Graham-Brown RAC: How many GP referrals to dermatology outpatients are really necessary. *J R Soc Med* 1989;**82**: 347–348.

8. Gawkrodger DJ. Racial influences on skin disease. In: Champion RH, Ebling FJG, Burton JL, eds. Rook, Wilkinson and Ebling's Textbook of Dermatology. Oxford: Blackwell Scientific 1992:2859–2875.

9. Graham-Brown RAC, Sarkany I: Lichen scorfulosorum and tuberculosis dactylitis. *Br J Dermatol* 1980;**103**:561–564.

10. Milligan A, Chen K, Graham-Brown RAC: Two tuberculides in one patient—a case report of papalonecrotic tuberculide and erythema induratum occurring together. *Clin Exp Dermatol* 1990;**15**:21–23.

11. Bowker NC, Cross KW, Fairburn EA, Walls M: Sociological implications of an epidemiological study of eczema in the City of Birmingham. *Br J Dermatol* 1976;**95**:137–140.

12. Morrison-Smith J, Cooper SM: Asthma and atopic diseases in immigrants from Asia and the West Indies. *Postgrad Med J* 1981;**57**:774–776.

13. Sladden MJ, Dure-Smith B, Berth-Jones J, Graham-Brown RAC: Ethnic differences in the pattern of skin disease seen in a dermatology department—atopic dermatitis is more common among Asian referrals in Leicestershire. *Clin Exp Dermatol* 1991;**16**:348–349.

14. Weber SA, Graham-Brown RAC, Hutchinson PE, Burns DA: Dietary manipulation in childhood atopic dermatitis. *Br J Dermatol* 1989;**121**:91–96.

15. Neame RL: A population-based prevalence study of atopic dermatitis. BSc Thesis, University of Leicester, 1992.

12

Immigrants in Eastern Europe

Albrecht Scholz

The political situation in Eastern Europe in relation to tourism has various specific characteristics. Although the government and the political leaders always spoke about friendship between countries, the borders were closed. The people had to apply for travel licenses, and private travel from one country to another was a problem. Normally, traveling was organized and supervised by the government and general supervision was perfect and omnipresent. Citizens of socialist countries rarely received official permission for visiting Western Europe; far more seldom was traveling to America, Africa, or Asia allowed. For that reason, international contacts between people were limited. According to agreements between several socialist and developing countries, inhabitants of Africa (especially Mozambique, Angola, and Ethiopia) and Asia (especially Vietnam and Cambodia) visited the former Soviet Union, Czechoslovakia, and East Germany. Generally, these foreigners had only rare contacts with the people. Social contact was only possible in factories, where they were trained. There were no official statistics on diseases of foreigners.

My inquiries on this subject to the ministries of Eastern European countries were not answered. My knowledge comes from publications on rare dermatological diseases in journals and by personal contacts with colleagues in Budapest, Prague, and Warsaw. Colleagues from Moscow, Leningrad, and Sofia did not respond.

Prague, Czech Republic

Patients of an area representing half a million people were sent to the dermatological university clinic of Prague if outpatient treatment was difficult or impossible. If compliance was not guaranteed, foreigners were immediately sent to the clinic. In 1987 through 1990 (until September), 10 to 15 foreign patients per year were treated. All of them were men except for one woman. The mean age was 20 to 25 years. Their native countries were Yemen, Syria, and Lebanon, and very often African countries (Angola, Mozambique, Zambia, and Sudan).

They were most frequently treated for venereal diseases:

1. lues latens (including tropical treponematoses),
2. gonorrhea,
3. chancroid (1 in 55 cases),
4. scabies with pyoderma (8 cases). Only a few patients suffered from dermatological diseases like urticaria, zoster and, in one case, leishmaniasis.[3]

Budapest, Hungary

In 1989 and 1990, about 5000 patients were examined in an outpatient department for foreigners at the University of Budapest. Most of them came from Romania, with a few from African countries. About 5% of the patients (100 persons) suffered from dermatosis. The order of frequency was

1. dermatitis (contact and atopic dermatitis),
2. verrucae vulgaris,
3. tinea versicolor,
4. psoriasis vulgaris.

Only eight cases of gonorrhea or syphilis were observed. All of the Romanians were HIV-seronegative. Five HIV-seropositive Africans without signs of illness were sent home. Until 1990, in Hungary 260 HIV-seropositive cases in the general population were known; 20 of them suffered from AIDS.[1]

Warsaw, Poland

From Poland, we have good information about deep mycoses among workers from Africa and about leishmaniasis among workers from Arabic countries. In 1990 93 HIV-seropositive foreigners lived in Poland.[4]

Dresden, Germany

Unfortunately, there were no official statistics about foreigners in the German Democratic Republic (GDR). The Ministry of Health did not answer my inquiries on this topic. For that reason, I can only report on the situation in the district of Dresden. In 1988, 12,220 foreigners from Vietnam, Mozambique, Cuba, Poland, and China worked in the district of Dresden (2 million inhabitants; GDR, 16 million). In 1989, 15,422 foreigners from these countries lived in the district of Dresden. Dermatological diseases were seldom: we saw some cases of leishmaniasis cutis, leprosy and deep mycosis.[2,6]

The diagnosis of dermatosis papulosa nigra was rather new for us.[5]

Problems were caused by venereal diseases: Syphilis was often imported from Vietnam to East Germany (coming to South Vietnam from American soldiers to prostitutes). Tropical treponematosis came from Africa. Each year, some patients with ulcus molle were treated.

Among the cases of gonorrhea, which decreased at the same rate as AIDS campaigns increased, only a few penicillinase-producing *Neisseria gonorrhoeae* (PPNG) were found. During the last 6 years in the GDR a total of 110 patients suffered from PPNG. In 1985 and 1989, 50,000 and 23,000 cases, respectively, of gonorrhea were registered per year. Because of the isolation of the GDR until now, the PPNG was no problem.

All foreigners who lived for more than 3 months in the GDR were tested for HIV infection, and if they tested positive, they were sent back to their native countries. In the whole of the GDR (now the eastern part of Germany), at present 100 German citizens and 120 foreigners were HIV-seropositive. Twenty Germans and 2 foreigners suffer from AIDS. The opening of the border changed the situation. It is said that the only positive effect of the wall is the small number of AIDS cases. Foreigners were not sent home because of dermatological diseases but because of tuberculosis, carcinoma, and hepatocirrhosis (about 30 patients each year).

Conclusions

Diseases of immigrants are no problem for Eastern Europe, but we must

- learn to diagnose dermatological diseases on black skin,
- pay attention to rare diseases such as leishmaniasis and deep mycosis and leprosy,
- know the different epidemiology of treponematosis in Africa and Asia (especially regarding the PPNG in gonorrhea).

References

1. Balo-Banga JM: Personal communication, 1992.
2. Barth J, Voigt R, Jacobi H: Leprosy—Facts and Trends. *Med Aktuell* 1987;**13**:64–65.
3. Frey T: Personal communication, 1992.
4. Jablonska S: Personal communication, 1992.
5. Jacobi H, Härtel S: Dermatosis papulosa nigra. *Dermatol Monatsschr* 1987;**173**:264–267.
6. Meinhof W, Wolff HH: Dermatomykosen aus dem Mittelmeerraum in Deutschland. *Dtsche Med Wochenschr*: 1991;**96**:234–237.

13

Africa

Adekunle O. George

Diseases, ignorance, and poverty abound in the developing countries of Africa, and they have much influence on dermatology in this sector of the world. It can be said without exaggeration that tropical diseases have had a determinant role in history as explained by Darlington in 1969, in relation to Africa.

Diseases has [sic] obstructed every racial and cultural development in Africa. It has damaged Africans. It had deferred or destroyed immigrants and invaders of Africa who did not protect themselves from diseases by hybridization.[1]

Skin diseases are drawn into the vicious web by the triad above, encouraged by the low literacy level, fueled by governmental policies that place priorities on other areas at the expense of health, and compounded by the adherence of the people to superstitious beliefs.[2] It is important to appreciate some basic data about Africa to assess the nature and magnitude of the problem if practical and meaningful solutions are to be offered. Ryan[3] has clearly summarized some of these relevant data:

- 25 of 50 countries in Africa have no dermatologists;
- 60–80% of skin diseases encountered in rural populations are preventable, curable, and controllable;
- skin problems (for example, onchocerciasis) are among the five most common causes of morbidity and loss of man power in rural areas;

- 90% of skin diseases are first attended by auxilliary health workers with virtually no dermatologic training;
- more than 80% of children in some desperate communities are afflicted with infection of the skin;
- fewer than 150 recognized dermatologists are looking after the skin health of all sub-Saharan countries in Africa.

Understanding Cultural Practices

Tribal marks are common in many areas in Africa. Scarification of the body may be accompanied by rubbing in materials obtained from burnt leaves or wood over which incantations have been made. These marks were useful for identifying people from the same areas or families during wars, and for beauty. The traditional doctor also scarifies the skin over lumps and areas of tenderness to drive off evil. In recent times, names and dates of birth have been scarified on the abdominal wall of children in the rural and semiurban areas as a permanent record. The Yorubas were aware of diseases associated with swellings of scarification marks as evidenced from Ifa Corpus, the most important genre of Yoruba oral literature.[4] Some of the diseases—sarcoidosis,[5] lichen planus, and psoriasis—have frequently become localized to these areas of trauma many years after, making diagnosis easier as investigative facilities are generally lacking in the tropics. Tribal marks have declined in popularity for cosmetic reasons. A mark of beauty in the past is being avoided. Instead, many educated Africans, especially women, now seek plastic surgery for the removal of facial marks.

Breast-feeding in the rural areas (where the majority of Africans still live) may continue with or without mixed feeding until another conception, when the child is then abruptly weaned. This is the usual period for the occurrence of the protein–calorie deficiency disease kwashiokor (with its skin manifestations).

Traditionally, a girl may go about unclothed until the age of 8–9 years and a boy until the age of 10 years, after which it becomes mandatory that the girl should cover herself with a "Tobi" and the boy with a "Bante."[6] This practice is now dying out, and even in the very poor families, infants and children are clothed. One can thus appreciate the change in the distribution of papular urticaria, which was more generalized compared to the involvement of mainly the exposed areas of limbs and faces in recent time. Certain traditional practices are carried out in some places before marriage. Some girls are kept in "fattening houses" and forcefully overfed, and annointed with various types of oils to achieve soft, smooth glistening skin. Female circumcision may be carried out at this period as well. Intertrigo in the natural body folds—under the breasts, genito-femoral areas, and gluteal cleft as well as in between layers of skin folds from excessive fat (a semblance to the Michelin tire mascot)—can result in the hot humid African clime. Secondary infection by bacteria and *Candida* is a common occurrence. Atrophic scars with hypopigmentation after circumcision of the girl could be confused with lichen sclerosus et atrophicus by medical personnel alien to the local tradition.

There is a 15-fold increase in the prevalence of albinism in the more settled close community of the southeastern part of Nigeria (the Igbos), compared with the Fulanis and the Hausas to the north (Fig. 13.1) who are more nomadic.[7] Marriages within the towns and villages are highly encouraged by the Igbos who could disown offsprings who marry outside this social barrier. The trend has maintained the high prevalence of albinism. Nowhere in the traditional views of the Igbos on albinism is

inbreeding implicated. They have, instead, weird etiological theories ranging from punishment from the gods to conception during pregnancy or the observation of frightening sights during pregnancy. Albino children are less treasured because the inherent problems of albinos are fairly well known. Albinos are taunted at home and at school and have poor marital and occupational prospects. Some of the local names for albinos are rather derogatory. The Efik name means literally "a white man from the bush." Other names include "D.O"—District Officer, a reference to the days when District Officers were Europeans.

Microfilarial skin density in patients suffering from onchocerciasis in a study in the Kwara State area of Nigeria was found to be highest in male adults and least in children.[8] The reason for this has been linked to the role played by the various genders and age groups in the community. The male adult has much exposure as he goes about with cattle-rearing, fishing, farming, or hunting. The women help on the farm mainly in the harvesting season and could be seen at other times picking mushrooms and wild berries or washing clothes in the river. The child gets bitten as he or she sits under the tree waiting for the mother. This member of the family who could be as young as one and one half years cannot be disregarded as a source of infection in control measures in epidemiological studies in the management of onchocerciasis.

The clapping of hands is a new trend in religious worship in Africa. Following independence in many African states and the return of white colonialists to their home countries, many Africans gave up traditional religion entirely or still supplemented traditional worship with some form of Christian worship. Emotional excitement is usually high and manifested by the clapping of hands and stamping of feet as they sing. Purpura on the palmo-plantar areas has been documented in such religious zealots.[9]

Social and Economic Factors

A study was carried out to find the prevalence of sand fleas (*Tunga penetrans*) among primary and postprimary school pupils in the Choba

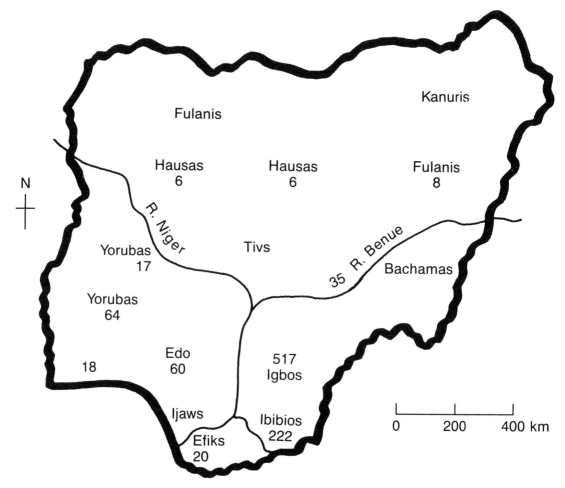

FIGURE 13.1. Distribution of albinos in major tribal groups in Nigeria, (Modified from Ref. 7).

area of the Niger River delta.[10] The high prevalence of *Tunga penetrans* infestation is believed to be associated with the large number of goats and other domestic animals that are allowed to roam the area. Animal husbandry practice in the area is still fairly primitive. Most of the domestic animals in the area fend for themselves.

Onchocerciasis—"river blindness"—is not a sudden killer. It insidiously erodes health and by its effect on the eyes removes the contribution of a sizable number of the adult population to the working force. This has qualified it as one of the six diseases engaging the attention of the World Health Organization.

There is a relationship between sociology and sexually transmitted diseases (STDs). In 1961, an average syphilis infection rate of 13–51% was found in the various provinces of Ethiopia.[11] One reason adduced for the spread was uncontrolled prostitution and this was related to the existing marriage laws. The commonest marriage law allowed easy dissolution by the man with no provision for settlement for the woman or for their children's maintenance. Sexually transmitted diseases remain high in other African countries. The cost of treatment of STDs continues to remain high because of the emergence of resistant strains, especially to cheap and well-established drugs like the penicillins. It is not unusual to see some petty traders sitting by the roadsides in some African towns selling capsules of tetracycline and ampicillin, as well other antibiotics and analgesics such as acetylsalisylic acid tablets, openly displayed on trays alongside sweets and packets of biscuits. Clients come along to buy as little as two capsules for headache, fever, and other complaints. It is a frequent practice for some men to buy and gulp a capsule or two of antibiotics before visiting nearby brothels.

Traumas (thorns and the like) have been documented in up to 70% of patients who developed malignant melanoma in a study from Africa.[12] Malignant melanoma occurs mainly in the legs and especially on the feet in up to 90% of cases. Walking barefooted cannot solely account for the etiology as most low-income people now wear some form of footwear, especially cheap rubber slippers. Chromium in cement is one of the commonest contactants in occupational medicine in Nigeria.[13] Often these lowly workers acknowledge the relationship of the cement to the flare up of their dermatitis. Many, nevertheless, wrap empty cement packag-

ing paper around the legs and feet, hoping to minimize exposure to the cement dust, not realizing the detrimental effect of such occlusive cement contaminated paper.

Many countries in Africa, have not established dermatology as a specialty in their health services, and the general physician has to cope as much as he can. In Nigeria, the most populous country in Africa with a population of approximately 100 million people, there are only about 20 dermatologists with the majority working within 5 large towns (Fig. 13.2). This has resulted in some patients traveling over 900 km for consultation. The plight of such patients are highlighted by Vollum in Uganda[14] and Russel in Nigeria.[15] The cost and availability of drugs are other thorny issues.

Leprosy is officially treated free of charge; nevertheless, many government-owned hospital

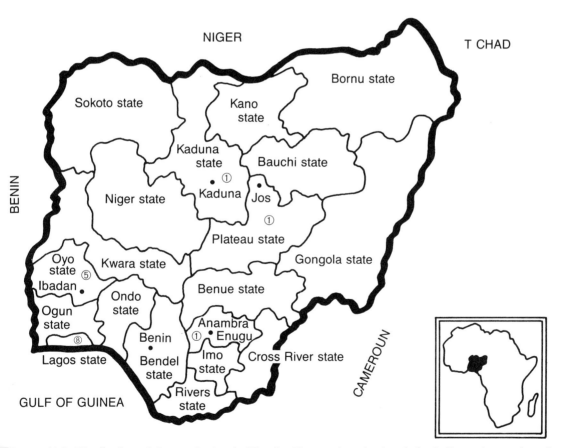

FIGURE 13.2. Distribution of dermatologists in Nigeria. The numbers in the circles indicate the number of dermatologists in the states.

pharmacy departments only stock drugs that will allow them to generate funds for replenishing their supply. The purchase of drugs given free is not given a high priority. One can appreciate the reasoning behind this practice because the government has not provided adequate money for health care. Leprosy patients ultimately have to look around for money and this adversely affects the management of leprosy with an increased predisposition to the development of drug resistance.

The cost of intralesional triamcinolone acetonide has increased on the average from ₦5.00 to about ₦80.00 for 2 ml (1600% increase) in 5 years! Wages have only increased by 50% in the same period. To avoid the high cost of drugs, some patients visit traditional doctors and pharmacies for consultation and treatment. This has resulted in the alteration of the appearance of some diseases. Vitiligo, for example, may have textural changes due to the employment of irritants or abrasives. Diseases may be seen at a very late stage when there may be little to offer in terms of cure.

Political events, wars (e.g., in Ethiopia, Niger, and Chad), and natural disasters (famine, earthquakes) have had much influence on dermatology in Africa. The influx of refugees from famine-striken or war-torn areas causes severe congestion and poor living conditions in refugee camps, and with overcrowding, periodic increases in the incidence of scabies, pediculosis, and pyodermas occur. The tough economic situation in tropical countries has caused emigration of many of the few dermatologists to the oil-rich, tax-free Gulf states and other overseas countries.

The construction of dams for hydroelectricity across the Volta River in Ghana and the Niger River in Nigeria has influenced the epidemiology of onchocerciasis and schistosomiasis. Deportations of thousands of Nigerians some years ago from endemic areas in the Volta River basin and from other West African countries had a significant impact on the transmission of onchocerciasis. The incidence of noninfective skin conditions like the dermatitis group is on the increase. This may be due to increase in the importation of cosmetics (soap, bleaching creams) and the establishment of new industries.

Preventive Dermatology

Preventive measures for preventable diseases are the mainstay for reducing the problem in dermatology in tropical Africa. The mucosal and skin changes of protein-calorie malnutrition, such as kwashiokor, can be eradicated with increased food production, family planning methods, and nutritional advice. The need to impart health education rather than health information can be appreciated from the account of Shrank, an expatriate dermatologist who worked in Nigeria about 3 decades ago.[16] He wrote:

From the survey it seemed that the most useful improvement in Ikereku would be an adequate supply of clean water: the villages would be able to keep their homes and themselves cleaner, and also avoid typhoid, dysentery and guineaworm infestation. The elders of the village agreed to the idea, and after some publicity a fund for the building of a deep well costing £300 was launched. This sum was well within the means of the community. After 3 months only £4:10s has been collected in addition to my original contribution of £5. They had not understood its importance. Education is the key. If the simple mechanisms of diseases are understood then much can be avoided; clean wounds would reduce pyoderma, dramatically. Clean water prevents guinea worm. Clean barber's instrument might abolish tinea capitis, footwear would limit damage to the feet . . . .

The emphasis given to preventive medicine has remained small and has not changed much since Shrank wrote the above account 3 decades ago. There is the need to identify which traditional practices should be encouraged. Some practices evolved to meet a purpose and must have sufficed at some point to have survived in the community. Protective clothes and headgear (cap or wide-brimmed hat) can minimize actinic damage to the skin of the albino. Family planning and genetic advice can reduce the number of affected siblings in a family. Choice of vocation, such as avoidance of farming (as practiced in the rural areas), can prevent further lesions in mechanobullous diseases like epidermolysis bullosa. Adaptation to change in social customs is important for containing all infectious processes including sexually transmitted diseases. Reducing the pool of infectious agents either by the use of drugs or by personal or public hygiene can contain the infection processes.

There is need for case notification and contact tracing for some infectious diseases like leprosy. The Department of Health, Information, and Education needs to work together to bring health education to the people. In schools, for example, examination of the scalp for tinea capitis and the glabrous skin for hypochromic patches of leprosy can help detect early cases. In a survey of school children aged 10–19 years in Bombay, India,[17] 2012 had leprosy out of 415,419 students examined. Seventy-eight percent were in the clinical stage and 97% had no deformities yet. Only 2.1% were positive for acid fast bacilli. If not for this survey, most of these patients would have been missed until adult life with disastrous consequences to them and their contacts over the years. The need for surveillance is made obvious by a recent report[18] of an alarming resurgence of yaws observed in several countries in the tropics.

The contribution to medical knowledge from dermatologists in Africa in recent times will depend on original simple, inquisitive, and relevant research based on sound clinical investigation with the simplest possible equipments because well-organized and well-equipped laboratories and adequate financial support are lacking.[19] The etiological factors and treatment of acne keloidalis nuchae, which affects mainly blacks, will have to be addressed. The regimen of treatment for tinea versicolor, common in the hot humid tropic, will need to be looked at to reduce the time of recurrence of the dermatitis. It is hoped that further basic research, especially in the tropics, will lead to the development of a specific test for the diagnosis of yaws in the individual and for epidemiological purposes. This approach to research will allow a breakthrough in the common medical problems of the developing world.

Financial and material aids will still be required from colleagues working in the economically advanced countries. For example, the American Academy of Dermatology has established a task force to provide educational materials to developing countries throughout the world—asking for contributions from colleagues in the developed nations for teaching materials such as books, journals, slides, instruments, and other materials in great demand in all developing countries.[20]

The impediment to the advancement of health comes from economic pitfalls tied to political intrigues locally and abroad. The reviewer of Graham Hancock's book *Lord of Poverty* commented thus:[21]

Poverty is getting worse in many underdeveloped countries in Africa, Asia and Latin America in spite of the $45–60 billion given annually by Western financed institutions. First, although the aid money is allegedly spent to help underdeveloped countries, much of it is actually spent in the West either to finance the purchase of Western goods or to finance the bureaucracy of the aid administration. Two-thirds of FAO employees work at its Rome headquarters. Secondly there are too many instances of vast sums of money being spent on projects doomed to be "white elephants," because of lack of common sense or homework before the scheme was started. The World Bank's own internal assessment is that, on average, 60% of development projects are failures, rising to 75% in the poorest countries. The USAID fish-farming programme in Mali produced fish at a cost of $2,000 per pound in a country where the average annual income is $400; the massive sugar complex in the Sudan, built at a cost of $613 million by the World Bank and which was sited 1000 miles over difficult desert from the nearest seaport.

Conclusions

Less arrogance on the part of the aid agencies and a willingness to conduct on-the-spot assessments and consultation with local people as well as locally based aid workers could avert such appalling mistakes and allow the vast sums of money so wasted to be put to appropriate use.

References

1. Kerdel-Vegas F: The Proser White Oration at the Royal College of Physicians on October 5, 1972. *Trans St. John's Hosp Dermatol Soc* 1973;**59**:1–9.

2. Ezenwa AO: The role of traditional medicine in the developing countries. *Postgrad Doctor* (African edition) 1985;**7**:363–366.

3. Ryan TJ: A fresh look at the management of skin disease in the tropics. *Int J Dermatol* 1990;**29**: 413–415.

4. Omo-Dare P: Yoruban contributions to the literature on keloids. *J Nat Med Assoc* 1973;**65**: 367–406.

5. Alabi GO, George AO: Cutaneous sarcoidosis in West Africa and tribal scarifications. *Int J Dermatol* 1989;**28**:29–31.

6. WHO/EMRO Technical publication No. 2 Vol. 2, Baasher T, Bannerman RHO, Rushman H, Sharaf I, eds: Traditional Practices Affecting the Health of Women and Children. 1982:7–20.

7. Okoro AN: Albinism in Nigeria; Clinical and social study. *Br J Dermatol* 1975;**92**:485–492.

8. Edungbola LD: Prevalence of onchocerciasis in Ile-Ire District, (Ifelodum) Kwara State, Nigeria. *Trop Geogr Med* 1982;**34**:231–239.

9. Williams CKO, Olofin AA, Durosimi MA: Haemoglobinuric episodes following vigorous ritual dancing. *E Afr J Med* 1986; **63**:182–186.

10. Arene FOI: The prevalence of sand flea (tunga penetrans) among primary and post-primary school pupils in Choba area of the Niger Delta. *Publ Hlth* 1984;**98**:282–283.

11. Marchionini A: Relationship of sociology to dermatology and venereology (The Proser White Oration, October 1963). *Trans St John's Hosp Dermatol Soc* 1964;**50**:1–8.

12. Otu AA: Injury and melanoma. *Lancet* 1985;i: 220–221.

13. Olumide YM: Dermatitis in Nigeria. Hand dermititis in men. *Contact Dermatitis* 1987;**17**: 136–138.

14. Vollum DI: An impression of dermatology in Uganda. *Trans St John's Hosp Dermatol Soc* 1973;**59**:120–128.

15. Russel BF: A visit to University College Hospital, Ibadan. *Trans St John's Hosp Dermatol Soc* 1961;**47**:166–170.

16. Shrank AB: A field survey in Nigeria. *Trans St John's Hosp Dermatol Soc* 1965;**51**:85–94.

17. Koticha KK: School surveys in Bombay. *Int J Leprosy* 1979;**47**:333–338.

18. Programme for the Control of the Endemic Treponematoses. Geneva: World Health Organization, 1987 (VDT/EXBUD/87:1).

19. George AO: Skin diseases in tropical Africa: Medical, social and economic implications. *Int J Dermatol* 1988;**27**(3):187–189.

20. Shaw JM: Donate your old books and journals. *Int J Dermatol* 1991;**30**:68.

21. The results of aid. *Int Hlth Dev* 1991;**1**:27–29.

14

Travel Medicine

Rita Sigg-Martin, Alfred Eichmann, and Robert Steffen

Travel medicine, occasionally called emporiatrics (from *emporos*, Greek for traveler), is an interdisciplinary field, based mainly on epidemiology, preventive medicine, infectious diseases, tropical medicine, and dermatology. The primary goal of travel medicine is the reduction of morbidity and mortality in travelers; the secondary goal is the reduction of the impact of illness and accidents that travelers have suffered and were later aggravated by self-medication. The importance of travel medicine is reflected by the fact that each year 30–35 million persons are at particular risk as they travel from industrialized countries to developing countries where hygienic conditions may be unsatisfactory.

Epidemiology

Only a few studies have addressed the question of health impairments in international travelers, including dermatological problems. Among 2445 travelers interviewed prior to departure, 31 (1.3%) reported a chronic dermatological condition, necessitating treatment or ongoing evaluation.[1] In a follow-up study on 7886 travelers to developing countries, 1.2% reported dermatological problems; about one-third each was ill abroad only, during and after the journey, or had symptoms only on returning home.[2] Many anecdotal reports but no extensive epidemiological data differentiating between dermatological diagnoses in travelers are available to date.

Due to "sex tourism," sexually transmitted diseases (STDs) continue to be imported even with a risk of HIV transmission; for example among all Swiss tourists to tropical Africa, 4% had casual sexual contacts with the locals, half of the encounters without condoms as late as 1988.[3] This rate is likely to be higher among visitors to Southeast Asia and South America. According to the above-mentioned follow-up study, 0.6% of tourists to the tropics report vaginal or urethral discharge during or after their exotic journey.[2] Various reports document how HIV infections[4] or other STDs, particularly gonorrhea with resistant *Neisseria gonorrhea*, continue to be imported[5] following international travel.

Influence of Travel on Preexisting Dermatoses

Sunlight, heat, and moisture, as well as a cold, and similarly, positive or negative emotions may aggravate or alleviate some skin diseases. A few people have a genetically determined higher susceptibility to sunlight.

Dermatosis Usually Improved by Travel

Psoriasis is usually improved by ultraviolet light, but a sunburn of the untanned skin may cause a Köbner phenomenon and lead to exacerbation.[6,7] Ultraviolet light induces peeling of the skin and thus, improves acne vulgaris; however, a minority of patients report an aggravation. Patients with atopic dermatitis usually observe a reduction of their skin lesions in summer,[8] but again, perspiration may aggravate the disease. As ultraviolet light improves T-cell lymphomas of the skin, this is used therapeutically.[9] Curiously, urticaria may improve during a vacation.

Aggravated Dermatosis by Travel

Sunlight may provoke symptomatic herpes simplex infection.[10] This occurs often in people skiing in the sun (herpes solaris). Sunlight, or more specifically ultraviolet light, may also aggravate seborrheic dermatitis, rosacea,[11] Mallorca acne, and transient acantholytic dermatosis (Grover). Mallorca acne (acne aestivialis) consists of itching papules on the sun-exposed areas of the face and the lateral aspects of the arms. There are no comedones or pustules as in acne vulgaris. Photosensitivity is 1 of the 11 inclusion criteria for systemic lupus erythematosus.[12] Sunlight can also provoke discoid lupus erythematosus, subacute discoid lupus erythematosus,[13] and recurrent erythema multiforme.[14,15] Bullous pemphigoid, pemphigus vulgaris,[16] and pemphigus erythematosus and foliaceus are generally aggravated by sunlight. Pityriasis alba, characterized by hypopigmented macules mostly in the face or arms, has no known cause, but dry skin and sun seem to be risk factors.[17] Rarely atopic dermatitis and Darier-White disease (keratosis follicularis) may be unfavorably influenced by the sun.[18] Porphyria cutanea tarda is a photosensitive disease with bullae formation on the light-exposed areas.[19] Erythropoietic protoporphyria is characterized by variable degrees of sun susceptibility.[20] Patients with white skin and a lack of pigmentation tend to burn their skin easily, such as in vitiligo,[21] Vogt-Koyanagi-Harada syndrome, Chediak-Higashi syndrome, Cuna moon disease of children, albinism, oculocutaneous albinoidism, Tietz' syndrome, and piebaldism. Patients with dermatomyositis may be sensitive to light. Photophobia and acute sunburn are the earliest symptoms of xeroderma pigmentosum; later freckles, teleangiectasia, and tumors appear on the sun-exposed skin, due to damage in the DNA repair mechanism.[22] Freckles are brownish macules on the sun-exposed skin of fair or red-haired people. The freckles are more prominent in summer, when they are exposed to sunlight.[23] Reticular erythematous mucinosis or plaquelike mucinosis can be induced by ultraviolet phototesting.[24] Psoriasis is only rarely aggravated. The same applies to chronic venous insufficiency, tinea pedis, tinea versicolor, and actinic porokeratosis. Patients taking oral retinoids should be aware that they may easily sunburn in the mountains due to the higher amount of UV radiation at a higher altitude.

Dermatoses with light intolerance include Bloom's syndrome, Cockayne's syndrome, and Rothmund-Thomson's syndrome. Hartnup's disease is a defect of tryptophan excretion with pellagralike dermatitis after sun exposure. People with phenylketonuria have fair skin and are very sensitive to light. Pellagra, a niacin deficiency characterized by diarrhea, dermatitis, and dementia, may also be aggravated by sunlight. The same applies for carcinoid syndrome which can have pellagralike skin lesions.

Heat plays a prominent role in intertrigo and hyperhidrosis. Persons with anhidrotic ectodermal dysplasia have no eccrine sweat gland and show heat congestion when exposed to sun and heat. Travel to tropical countries may be life threatening in such cases.

Dry climate may unfavorably influence ichthyosis vulgaris and atopic dermatitis.

Cold will aggravate Raynaud's disease and syndrome, peripherial vascular malperfusion, vasculitis due to cryoglobulins and cryofibrinogens, erythrocyanosis crurum, acrocyanosis, and cold panniculitis.[25]

Dermatoses Induced by Travel

Light may induce photoallergic and phototoxic reactions, polymorphous light eruption, persistent light reaction, hydroa vacciniform, solar urticaria, actinic reticuloid, and phytophoto-dermatitis.

Phototoxic Dermatitis

Phototoxic dermatitis occurs after the use of drugs and sun exposure. The drug molecules absorb energy; this energy is transmitted to the tissue and causes an alteration of the skin. Phototoxic dermatitis occurs on the sun-exposed areas. In contrast to photoallergic dermatitis, prior sensitization is not required. Phototoxic dermatitis can occur in any individual, depending on the dose of light and the dose of medication. The signs are a sunburn type of reaction, with erythema only in the sun-exposed areas. The onset of the erythema is 5–20 h, and worsens within 48–96 h. Thereafter, the sunburn may persist with racemose, bluish, erythematous, and pigmented. Nails may also be involved (photoonycholysis). Drugs that may frequently cause phototoxic reactions are tetracycline,[26] phenothiazines, nalixidine acid, nonsteroidal anti-inflammatory drugs, and psoralens. Sulfonamides, griseofulvin, calcium cyclama, amiodarone,[27,28] captopril, chlorpromazine,[29] clofazimo, dacarbazine, 5-fluoroura-cil, furosemide, levomepromazine, naproxen,[30] piroxicam,[31] promazine, thioridazine, as well, and vinblastine have been implicated also. Treatment consists of elimination of the drug and the sunlight, followed by therapy similar to that for a sunburn.

Phototoxic contact reactions are primarily due to topical agents, such as furocoumarins, which are found in plants and fragrances. Berloque dermatitis is a phototoxic contact reaction due to 5-methoxypsoralen in the oil of bergamot. Its signs are a subclinical inflammatory reaction and postinflammatory hyperpigmentation on the site of application. Bergamot oil containing perfume as well as plants like lime, orange, celery, parsnip, fig, rue, mokihhana berry, and anise can cause phototoxic reactions. The same applies to topical application of dyes such as eosin or methylene blue, which all contain 5-methoxypsoralen. Furocoumarins in plants can cause erythema, blistering, or bullae on exposed areas (phytophotodermatitis or dermatitis bullosa striata pratensis). Coal tar can cause phototoxic dermatitis with residual hyperpigmentation.

Photoallergic Dermatitis

Photoallergic dermatitis is an eczematous reaction on the skin caused by a photosensitizing substance and sunlight exposure, after sensitization by a drug has occurred. Drugs that can induce photoallergy include chlorthiazides,[32] carbamazepine, chlorpropamide, tolbutamide, chlorpromazine,[29] promazine, chloroquine,[33] amitriptyline, chlorthalidone, piroxicam, diphenhydramine, glibenclamide, sulfanilamide, sulfonylureas, griseofulvin, indomethacin, and nalixidic acid. Topical inducers of photoallergy (photocontactallergy) are bithionol, sulfathiazole, salicylanilides, carbanilides, and hexachlorophene.

Clinical signs are similar to contact dermatitis. The papulovesicular eczematous or exudative dermatitis occurs after 24–48 h, mostly on the sun-exposed areas, but also on other parts of the body. The causative drug is altered by light and acts as hapten. The low-molecular hapten reacts with a high-molecular protein and becomes an allergen that induces the antigenic response.

The diagnosis of photoallergy is performed by phototesting. Photoallergy can be produced by topical exposure to chemicals and is then called photoallergic contact dermatitis. This is often induced by chemical substances in sunscreens such as PABA (paraaminobenzoic acid) and PABA esters and benzophenones, and by fragrances (musk ambrette, methylcoumarin).[34] Because some drugs can provoke both phototoxic and photoallergic reactions, there exists a confusion in the use of the terms "phototoxic" and "photoallergic"; more appropriate would be the term photosensitive.

Polymorphous Light Eruption (PLE, "Sun Allergy") and Sunburn

This occurs mainly when unadapted skin is exposed to strong sunlight. The term PLE describes a group of heterogenous, idiopathic, acquired photodermatoses. They are acute, recurrent, and characterized by delayed abnormal reaction to ultraviolet radiation. The lesions on the skin are various: erythematous macules, papules, plaques, and vesicles; however, in each patient the eruption is consistently monomorphous. In some countries, canthaxanthine has been recommended against PLE, however, this agent may cause retinal deposits.[35]

Sunburn is an acute, delayed inflammation of the skin following exposure to ultraviolet radiation obtained from sunlight or artificial sources. Sunburn usually presents as erythema and if severe, with vesicles and bullae, edema, tenderness, and pain.

Tumors

Various tumors show an increased incidence after chronic UVB exposure. These include actinic keratosis, basal cell cancer, melanoma,[36] and Bowen's disease.

Infections

Frequent bacterial infections include impetigo, furunculosis, erysipelas, ecthyma, cellulitis, tropical ulcer, erythrasma, intertrigo, pitted keratolysis, cat-scratch disease, borreliosis, and venereal diseases such as gonorrhea, syphilis, and chancroid. Atypical mycobacterioses, such as aquarium granuloma or mycobacterial ulcus (Buruli), are possible. Among the viral infections, herpes, condylomata acuminata, common warts, and HIV transmission are of greatest importance. Fungi and yeasts include tinea corporis, faciei, barbae, cruris, pedis, manum and unguium, perlèche, candida intertrigo, candida paronychia, tinea nigra, and pityriasis versicolor. A variety of parasitic diseases are frequently transmitted, including trichomoniasis, cutaneous leishmaniasis, and creeping eruption. Epizoonotic infestation is possible by pediculosis; stings by bee, wasps, ants, and scorpions; bites by flea, tick, and snakes; or also by contact with a jellyfish.

Dermatological Side Effects of Prophylactic Measures and of Drugs Frequently Used Abroad

Vaccination, Chemoprophylactic Agents, Medication for Self-Treatment

A variety of vaccinations are recommended for travelers with destinations in developing countries.[37] They are usually well tolerated; few dermatological adverse events are to be expected as smallpox vaccination now is obsolete and BCG vaccine is rarely indicated.[38]

In contrast, all agents used for malaria prophylaxis (chloroquine, amodiaquine, mefloquine, proguanil, doxycycline, and sulfadoxine/pyrimethamine) are associated with cutaneous adverse drug reactions (pruritus, exacerbation of psoriasis, and discoloration of skin and hair) in 4.7–10.9% of users according to a recent survey.[39] More important are erythema multiforme, Stevens-Johnson's syndrome, or toxic epidermal necrolysis reported after the use of sulfadoxine/pyrimethamine. The incidence rate varies between 1 in 5,000[40] to 1 in 80,000.[39] Other agents have also been associated with severe cutaneous adverse reactions, such as chloroquine[33] and mefloquine.[41]

Some researchers recommend antimicrobiols for prophylaxis of traveler's diarrhea, including sulfamethoxazole/trimethoprim, doxycycline, or quinolones. These may also be associated with dermatological adverse reactions.[42]

Side effects of frequently prescribed medication, including drugs that are often prescribed by dermatologists, are listed in Table 14.1.

Interactions of Prophylactic and Therapeutic Drugs

Allopurinol, chloramphenicol, phenylbutazone, indomethacin, salicylates, and sulfonamides interact with the protein binding of coumarin in the plasma. The effect of coumarin is enhanced and leads to purpura due to increased coumarin action. Mefloquine should not be given simultaneously with quinine to avoid potentiation of neuropsychiatric side effects.

TABLE 14.1. Side effects of drugs frequently used during travel.

Medication	Side effects
Acetylsalicylic acid	Urticaria, angiodema, purpura, morbilliform erythema nodosum, erythema multiforme, bullae (palms), agranulocytosis, drug-induced pemphigus, prurituers, fixed drug eruption, TEN, vasculitis, eosinophilia, hyperhidrosis.
Ampicillin	Morbilliform or maculopapular eruption, eosinophilia, urticaria, angioedema, bullae, TEN, erythema exudativum multiforme, pustular exanthemas, pruritus.
Beta-blockers	Induction of psoriasis and pustular psoriasis.
Chloroquine, amodiaquine	Hyperpigmentation, aggravation of psoriasis and porphyria, exfoliative dermatitis, fixed drug eruption, erythema annulare centrifugum. After use of 3–4 months, 25% of users have gray-brown, brown, or black-brown pigmentation on the face, the neck, the gum, subungually or pretibially. Medication for less than 3 months should induce no hyperpigmentation. These side effects are more frequent with mepacrine and amodiaquine than with chloroquine. A yellow pigmentation occurs after 2–6 months of mepacrine or amodiaquine medication. Chloroquine may cause a depigmentation of the hair after 2–3 months. Albinis, edema, exfoliative dermatitis, lichen planuslike dermatitis, pruritus ani may occur.
Clindamycin	Diarrhea, clostridium difficile colitis vasculitis, jaundice, morbilliform eruption, pruritus.
Coumarin	Alopecia, ecchymosis, gangrene, bullae, necrosis, petechiae, purpura fulminans, urticaria, vesicles, burning of the tongue, hypogeusia, angioedema, pruritus.
Cyclamate	Cold urticaria, photosensitization.
Dapsone	Fixed drug eruption, TEN, methemoglobin with cyanosis, motor neuropathy, maculopapular exanthemas, erythema multiforme, erythema nodosum, erythroderma, lichenoid drug eruption bullae.
Estrogens and progesterone in anticonception pills	Symmetric brown hyperpigmentation on cheeks, front, and around the mouth. Sun increases the pigmentation (melasma or chloasma).
Furosemide	Urticaria, pruritus, exfoliative dermatitis, pustular exanthema, lichenoid exanthemas, bullae, photosensitivity, pseudoporphyria, purpura.
Nonsteroidal anti-inflammatory drugs	Urticaria, fixed drug eruption, morbilliform eruption, TEN, erythema multiforme, vasculitis, photosensitivity.
Penicillin	Anaphylaxis, angioedema, urticaria, black hairy tongue, glossitis, edema, ecchymosis, erythema multiforme, morbilliform erythema, fixed drug eruption, TEN, pruritus, scarlatiniform erythema, papules, erythema nodosum, pruritus, bullae.
Sulfonamides including pyrimethamine/sulfadoxine (Fansidar)	TEN, fixed drug eruption, morbilliform eruption photosensitivity, erythema multiforme, lichenoid eruptions. Trimethoprim-sulfamethoxazole: SLE-like syndrome, fever, pancytopenia, hepatitis, Stevens-Johnson's syndrome, vasculitis, urticaria, lichenoid drug eruption, erythema multiforme.
Tetracyclines	Fixed drug eruption, phototoxicity reactions, pseudoporphyria, staining of teeth in children, pigmentation of oral mucosa, nails, conjunctivae, gums, scars, sun-exposed areas. Minocycline can cause a pigmentation of conjunctivae, mouth, nails, and teeth. The pigmentation occurs after a cumulative dose of 50 g, rarely after 4–5 g. Rare: urticaria, morbilliform eruption.

Prevention and Self-Therapy of Dermatological and Venereological Problems Occurring During Travel

Phototoxic and Photoallergic Reactions, Polymorphous Light Eruption, Sunburn

In general, travelers to the tropics should try to avoid excessive sun exposure. Persons prone to phototoxic or photoallergic reactions should try to avoid ultraviolet light irradiation. Agents that have previously caused phototoxic or photo-allergic reactions should be avoided.

Several reports indicate that chloroquine may be partially effective in the prevention of PLE at a dosage of 200 mg chloroquine base daily.[43] Beta-carotene, however, may be of value for patients with abnormal reaction to UV-A and visible light (erythropoietic protoporphyria); however, this may lead to retinal deposits.[44,45] Antimalarials and beta-carotenes do not protect against sunburn, because their spectrum of absorption is not within the UV-B zone.

Adverse Reactions

One of the advantages of initiating malaria chemoprophylaxis 1 week prior to departure is the ability to change the agent should adverse events occur. Travelers need to be instructed that they should contact a doctor abroad if moderate to severe skin reactions occur.

Frostbite

Warm and dry clothing along with avoidance of smoking and alcohol are the most effective measures.

Skin Infection

Skin infection in tropical climates is avoided by frequent washing and the wearing of cotton clothing. Persons with hyperhidrosis should use baby powder. Travelers must know that wounds tend to get severely infected following injury in a warm and humid climate. Utmost care should be given to disinfection and regular wound dressing.

Herpes infection is best prevented by applying sunscreeens with a sun protection factor (SPF) of at least 20. Kissing of persons with herpes labialis should be avoided.

Fungal infections of the feet and groin may be avoided by wearing sandals and cotton underwear, which allow perspiration.

Insect bites are avoided by wearing clothes that cover arms and legs; this is recommended particularly for the night. Because the anopheles mosquito may bite through fabrics that are less than 1 mm thick or not closely woven, it is recommended to impregnate clothing or to spray the fabrics with an insecticide containing permethrine or a repellent containing DEET. Uncovered parts of the skin, particularly the ankles, hands, and the face, should be covered with a repellent during night hours in areas with malaria transmission. In rooms without air conditioning, a mosquito net should be used. If a person is allergic to stings of bees or wasps, they should carry an appropriate emergency kit.

Sexually Transmitted Diseases

Avoidance of casual sexual contacts is necessary; if the traveler is unwilling to do so, the rules of safe sex should be applied (condoms). It is recommended that this be discussed with all travelers, especially those going abroad without their spouse.

Preexisting Dermatological Ailments

Persons with dry skin should use a body lotion after showering, taking brief showers and using soap only in the intertriginous areas.

Dermatological Travel Kit

- Sunscreen lotion/or cream (SPF 30 or higher)
- Repellent
- Hydrocortisone cream
- Antifungal powder or cream
- Antihistamine tablets
- Disinfectant

References

1. Hill DR. Pre-travel health, immunization status, and demographics of travel to the developing world for individuals visiting a travel medicine service. *Am J Trop Med Hyg* 1991;**45**:263–270.
2. Steffen R, Rickenbach M, Willhelm U, et al: Health problems after travel to developing countries. *J Infect Dis* 1987;**156**:84–91.
3. Stricker M, Steffen R, Hornung R, et al: Flüchtige sexuelle Kontakte von Schweizer Touristen in den Tropen. *Münch Med Wochenschr* 1990;**132**:175–177.
4. Mitchell S, Band B, Bradbeer C, Barlow D: Imported heterosexual HIV infection in London. *Lancet* 1991;**337**:1614–1615.
5. De Schryver A, Meheus A: International travel and sexually transmitted diseases. *World Health Stat Qt* 1989;**42**:90–99.
6. Farber EM: Recent advances in the treatment of psoriasis. *J Am Acad Dermatol* 1983;**8**(3):311–321.
7. Halprin KM, Comerford M, Taylor JR: Constant low-dose ultraviolet light therapy for psoriasis. *J Am Acad Dermatol* 1982;**7**:614–619.

8. Midelfart K, Stenvold SE, Volden G: UVB and UVA phototherapy of atopic dermatitis. *Acta Derm Venereol (Stockh)* 1985;**171**:95–98.
9. Rosenbaum MM, Roenigk HH Jr, Caro WA, Esker A: Phototherapy in cutaneous lymphoma and psoriasis in plaques. *J Am Acad Dermatol* 1985;**13**:613–622.
10. Perna JJ, Mannix ML, Rooney JF, et al: Reactivation of latent herpes simplex-virus infection by ultraviolet light. *J Am Acad Dermatol* 1987;**17**:473–478.
11. Wilkin JK: Rosacea. *Int J Dermatol* 1983;**22**:393–400.
12. Tuffanelli DL: Lupus erythematosus. *J Am Acad Dermatol* 1981;**4**:127–142.
13. Callen JP: Chronic cutaneous lupus erythematosus. *Arch Dermatol* 1982;**118**:412–416.
14. Fitzpatrick JE, Thompson PB, Aeling JL, Huff C: Photosensitive recurrent erythema multiforme: a critical review of characteristics, diagnostic criteria and causes. *J Am Acad Dermatol* 1983;**9**:419–423.
15. Huff JC: Erythema multiforme: a critical review of characteristics, diagnostic criteria and causes. *J Am Acad Dermatol* 1983;**8**:763–765.
16. Korman N: Bullous pemphigoid. *J Am Acad Dermatol* 1987;**16**:907–924.
17. Zaynoun ST, Aftimos BG, Tenekjian KK, et al: Extensive pityriasis alba. *Br J Dermatol* 1983;**108**:83–90.
18. Baba T, Yaoita H: UV radiation and keratosis follicularis. *Arch Dermatol* 1984;**120**:1484–1487.
19. Eubanks SW, Patterson JW, May DL, Aeling JL: The porphyrias. *Int J Dermatol* 1983;**22**:337–347.
20. Murphy GM, Hawkk JL, Magnus IA: Late-onset erythropoietic protoporphyria with unusual cutaneous features. *Arch Dermatol* 1985;**121**:1309–1312.
21. Nordlung JJ, Lerner AB: Vitiligo: it is important. *Arch Dermatol* 1982;**118**:5–8.
22. Robins JH: Xeroderma pigmentosum. Defective DNA repair causes skin cancer and neurodegeneration. *JAMA* 1988;**260**:384–388.
23. Azizzi E, Lusky A, Kushelevsky AP, Schwach-Millet M: Skin type, hair color, and freckles are predictors of decreased minimal erythema ultraviolet radiation dose. *J Am Acad Dermatol* 1988;**19**:32–38.
24. Bleehen SS, Slater DN, Mahood J, Church RE: Reticular erythematous mucinosis; light and electron microscopy, immunofluorescence and histochemical findings. *Br J Dermatol* 1982;**106**:9–18.
25. Becham BE: Equeatrian cold panniculitis in women. *Arch Dermatol* 1980;**116**:1025–1026.
26. Sanders CV, Saenz RE, Lopez M: Splinter hemorrhages and onycholysis: unusual reactions associated with tetracycline hydrochloride therapy. *South Med J* 1976;**69**:1090–1092.
27. Zachary CB, Slater DN, Holt DW, et al: The pathogenesis of amiodarone-induced pigmentation and photosensitivity. *B J Dermatol* 1984;**110**:451–456.
28. Walter JF, Bradner H, Curtis GP: Amiodarone sensitivity. *Arch Dermatol* 1984;**120**:1591–1594.
29. Menz J, Muller SA, Conolly SM: Photopatch testing. A six-year experience. *J Am Acad Dermatol* 1988;**18**:1044–1047.
30. Shelley WB, Elpern DJ, Shelley ED: Naproxen photosensitivity demonstrated by challenge. *Cutis* 1986;**38**:169–170.
31. Serrano G, Bonillo J, Aliaga A, et al: Piroxicam-induced photosensitivity. In vivo, in vitro studies of its photosensitizing potential. *J Am Acad Dermatol* 1984;**11**:113–120.
32. Addo HA, Ferguson J, Frain Bell W: Thiazide-induced photosensitivity: Study of 33 subjects. *Br J Dermatol* 1987;**116**:749–760.
33. Kligman AM: The identification of contact allergens by human assay. 3. The maximation test: a procedure for screening and rating contact sensitizers. *J Invest Dermatol* 1966;**47**:393–409.
34. Giovinazzo VJ, et al: Photoallergic contact dermatitis to musk ambrette. Clinical report of two patients with persistent light reactor patterns. *J Am Acad Dermatol* 1980;**3**:384–393.
35. Rousseau A: Canthaxanthine deposits in the eye. *J Am Acad Dermatol* 1983;**8**:123–124.
36. Longstreth J: Cutaneous malignant melanoma and ultraviolet radiation: a review. *Cancer Metast Rev* 1988;**7**:321–333.
37. Travel and Health. Geneva: World Health Organization. 1992.
38. Centers for Disease Control. Update on adult immunization: recommendations of the Immunization Practices Advisory Committee (ACIP). *MMWR* 1991;**40**:45–46.
39. Steffen R, Heusser R, Mächler R, et al: Malaria chemoprophylaxis among European tourists in tropical Africa: use, adverse reactions, and efficacy. *Bull WHO* 1990;**68**:313–322.
40. Miller KD, Lobel HO, Satriale RF, et al. Severe cutaneous reactions among American travelers using pyrimethamine-sulfadoxine (Fansidar) for malaria prophylaxis. *Am J Trop Med Hyg* 1986;**35**:451–458.
41. Van den Enden E, Van Gompel A, Colebunders R, Van den Enden J. Mefloquine-induced Stevens-Johnson syndrome. *Lancet* 1991;**337**:683.

42. Bigby M, Jick S, Jick H, Arndt K. Drug-induced cutaneous reactions. A report from the Boston Collaborative Drug Surveillance Program on 15,438 consecutive inpatients, 1975 to 1982. *JAMA* 1986;**256**:3358–3363.

43. Jansen CT: Oral carotenoid treatment in polymorphous light eruption: a cross-over comparison with oxychloriquine and placebo. *Photodermatol* 1985;**2**:166–169.

44. Weber U, Kern W, Novotny GE, et al: Experimental carotenoid retinopathy. I. Functional and morphological alterations of the rabbit retina after 11 months dietary carotenoid application. *Graefes Arch Clin Exp Ophthalmol* 1987;**225**:198–205.

45. Holzle E, Plewig G, von Kries R, Lehmann P: Polymorphous light eruption. *J Invest Dermatol* 1987;**88**:32s–38s.

Part III
Variables in Dermatology

15

Comments

Joseph L. Pace

Rarely can a section editor have been asked to comment on contributions so diverse as those found here. Indeed, the only common thread is this diversity and their relationship to dermatology is with respect to natural variables such as heat and cold, compounded by man-made folly such as the Korean conflict. Finally, the apparently obscure subject of veterinary dermatology masterfully gives fascinating insight into just how far veterinary medicine has progressed both in general terms and specifically in skin problems.

Diversity

Diverse and apparently unrelated as they seem, all the contributions in this part succeed in imparting new light on the topic. The respective authors had a fairly "wide" brief, resulting in different emphasis being given by the different writers.

Heat

In "Diseases Affected by Heat" for example, Bose and Ortonne have given a scholarly and exhaustive account of heat-related diseases. A discussion of the mechanisms of heat regulation and possible disturbances thereof is followed by details of all the dermatoses that may be affected or precipitated by heat. Finally, some modalities of heat as a treatment of skin disease are discussed. The chapter is well referenced and will be appreciated as a reference by all dermatologists.

Cold

Diseases Affected by Cold: Arctic and Subarctic Areas by the late Gunnar Lomholt gives a fascinating insight into life and cultural practices in Greenland. Waiting for a patient to arrive by dog sled is not an everyday occurrence for most dermatologists! Treatment of dermatoses related to occupations such as seal hunting and fishing makes interesting reading, although we read that psoriasis is apparently very common indeed in the Arctic Circle.

Injuries caused by cold are, of course, expected, particularly the "red cheeks with telangiectasia" even seen in young children. Visitors will find it salutary to know that most severe cold injuries are found in newcomers rather than well-protected Eskimos.

The data given for sexually transmitted diseases (STDs) are quite extraordinary. Cultural and/or environmental reasons may contribute to the astonishing statement that "26% of male teenagers and 42% of female teenagers had intercourse more than 15 times each month; over 50% had their first sexual encounter before the age of 15, and 28% of boys admitted to over 10 different partners annually." With high gonorrhea infection rates and an increasing number of HIV positives being reported, perhaps due to sex with visiting foreign workers, sexual education is being given a huge push for fear of an HIV epidemic based on heterosexual transmission.

War

Lee and Ku Ahn remind us of the serious conflict dangers to health posed by war situations, using the Korean conflict experience as an example. Normally accepted standards of living and hygiene break down, and the way is paved for an outbreak of epidemics of known (lack of immunization program for smallpox, hunger-pellagra, tuberculosis, injury, etc.) or previously unknown diseases, for example, Korean hemorrhagic fever.

War may actually contribute to the advancement of science because of the intensive study of any conditions affecting the military with resulting impairment of efficiency. This was the case with Korean hemorrhagic fever when the causative agent, the Hantaan virus, was discovered after many cases appeared in U.S. personnel. Tsutsugamushi fever appeared during this conflict and continues today in certain areas. It has been traced to a rickettsia, *R. tsutsugamushi.*

Not unexpectedly, STDs increased with the amount of free time available to the military personnel, whereas scabies, pediculosis, and typhus made their perennial appearance in

situations of misery, as they do in similar situations, even today.

Comparative Dermatology

For dermatologists, who, like this author, were fairly ignorant of the advances in veterinary medicine in the last few years, Ihrke's paper "Global Veterinary Dermatology" is a veritable eye-opener. We find that veterinary dermatology is an independent specialty with "residency programs" being organized in several countries. An international journal, Veterinary Dermatology, is valuable and two world congresses have been held, the more recent in May 1992.

The subject is being given very serious consideration indeed, although great variation exists in different parts of the world. These veterinary problems are of importance to the practicing dermatologist, because they may affect humans directly or indirectly, for example, cutaneous leishmaniasis and cat scratch fever. Alternatively, research on these diseases may shed light on similar, if not exactly identical processes, occurring in human beings. One must conclude that even a limited reference to animal dermatology is necessary even in undergraduate teaching and should certainly play a greater role in dermatology residencies than it currently does.

16

Diseases Affected by Heat

S. Bose and J. P. Ortonne

Heat affects man in different ways. By disturbing thermoregulation, it causes heat syncope, heat cramps, heat edema, heat stroke, and heat hyperpyrexia. It may induce anhidrotic heat exhaustion secondary to severe miliaria. It affects human beings psychologically, causing acute and chronic fatigue. Reaction to acute extreme heat causes burns, whereas abnormal reactions to chronic heat exposure causes erythema ab igne, heat-induced cancers, and erythermalgia. Certain diseases improve with heat therapy, whereas others become worse. Some occupations show premature cutaneous aging due to chronic heat exposure. Heat augments the ultraviolet damage induced by sun, thus accelerating cutaneous photoaging.[1]

Disturbances of Thermoregulation

The Skin in Thermoregulation

The skin is a barrier and a homeostatic organ between man and his environment. Thermoregulation of skin is maintained by cutaneous blood flow, basal metabolic rate, and sweating in the advent of environmental change. Core temperature of skin varies from 20°C to 40°C. It is maintained by variations in cutaneous blood flow, which is about 200 ml/min. The cutaneous circulatory system, with its arteriovenous anastomoses in acral areas and the parallel arrangement of arteries and veins in the limbs, permits countercurrent exchange of heat,

thus allowing maintenance of cutaneous temperature.[2] The intricate mechanism of temperature regulation includes detection of perfusion blood temperature by neurons in the preoptic area of the hypothalamus followed by the signals integrated in the posterior hypothalamus where appropriate heat-generating or heat-dissipating mechanisms are put into effect. With a rise in core temperature in a hot environment, inhibition of sympathetic output occurs, resulting in cutaneous vasodilatation. The rise in cutaneous temperature and sweating results in heat loss. The core temperature of the body is maintained at approximately 37°C from a range of external temperature between 15°C and 54°C by several mechanisms, which include a variation in cutaneous blood flow.[2,3]

Reactions to Extremes of Heat

Extremes of heat result in burns. Cutaneous injury by heat is influenced by duration of exposure, type of heat, and skin thickness. Burns may occur at 44°C. Transepidermal necrosis occurs in 1 s at 70°C but takes almost 45 min at 47°C. Pathogenesis involves denaturation and coagulation of cellular proteins and enzyme inactivation. Increased capillary permeability in burned tissue results in edema and an increase in interstitial osmotic pressure. In addition, vasoactive mediators, including prostaglandins, kinins, serotonin, histamine, oxygen radicals, and various lipid peroxides are released from burn tissue. Extensive burns predispose to infections by an alteration of immunologic, hemodynamic, and metabolic states. There is impaired phagocyte and neutrophil function with an increase in T-cells. The basal metabolic rate increases with a 1–2°C increase in core temperature. Burn patients are kept at an ambient temperature of 30°C to prevent heat loss and stress response. Experimentally, heat stress proteins are produced, known as heat shock proteins, but their role in thermotolerance is unknown.

Acclimatization to Heat

Repeated exposure to a hot environment produces physiological changes that lead to a greater degree of thermoregulatory fitness.

People exposed to hot, wet conditions become flushed rapidly. Their respiratory rate increases with hyperventilation. They may suffer from postural hypotension, resulting in hypotensive collapse. Both skin and body temperatures rise due to peripheral vasodilatation in the unacclimatized person. Onset of sweating is delayed and cardiovascular collapse may occur before sweating. During acclimatization, plasma volume increases, with salt retention both by urine and sweat as a consequence of increased aldosterone secretion. In response, sweating increases and commences at lower · rectal temperatures. Vasomotor responses also improve and vasoconstriction increases. There is a progressive decline in peripheral blood flow. The skin temperature is 2–3°C lower when an individual is fully acclimatized.[1]

Heat Syncope

Heat syncope is the sudden faintness and other signs of circulatory instability brought about in an unacclimatized individual subjected to heat stress. (See Table 16.1.)

Heat Cramps and Heat Exhaustion

Cramping pains in the muscles, low blood pressure, pallor, vertigo and nausea, vomiting, and fainting can occur in an individual engaged in prolonged, very active heat-producing work.

TABLE 16.1.

1. Disorders secondary to disturbances of thermoregulation
   Heat syncope. Fainting due to loss of vasomotor tone in the absence of gross water or salt depletion; common and mild.
   Heat edema. Water depletion heat exhaustion, that is, dehydration, salt depletion heat exhaustion.
   Heat cramps. Similar to and usually part of salt depletion heat exhaustion, but clinically a distinct syndrome that may occur by itself.

   Miliaria. Anhidrotic heat exhaustion—the anhidrosis is usually considered secondary to severe miliaria.

2. Failure of thermoregulation
   Heat stroke and heat hyperpyrexia.
   Sudden failure of sweating due to either failure of the thermoregulatory center, sweat gland fatigue, or, in some cases, water depletion.

3. Psychological effects
   Acute heat fatigue.
   Chronic heat fatigue.

Source: Reference 1, p. 1893. (With permission of Blackwell Scientific Publications, Ltd.)

Symptoms are caused by sodium chloride depletion that accompanies profuse sweating. These abnormalities are relieved by taking salt. These symptoms can occur even after acclimatization. In cystic fibrosis of the pancreas, the ability of the sweat glands to conserve and reabsorb sodium is defective. Consequently, patients with this disorder produce abnormally salty perspiration and, under severe heat stress, can suffer massive salt depletion and extreme symptoms.

Heat Stroke or Hyperpyrexia

After exposure to extreme body temperatures, people may collapse. They become unconscious and die within a short time with temperatures over 41°C. Symptoms are related to rapid decline and cessation of sweating. This is related to sweat gland fatigue, but the actual pathology is not understood. Hot dry skin, an increased internal temperature, delirium, and unconsciousness are signs of this dangerous syndrome. Individuals with hereditary anhidrotic extodermal dysplasia are naturally vulnerable due to the absence of sweat glands.[1]

Heat-Related Skin Diseases

Miliarias

This is a group of diseases characterized by vesicular dermatitis due to the blockage of sweat excretion at some point in the skin. Usually thermoregulation is well maintained as few sweat glands are involved except in miliaria profunda associated with tropical anhidrotic asthenia.[5] (See Table 16.2.)

Miliaria Crystallina or Sudamina

This disease is produced by the obstruction of the sweat duct within stratum corneum due to alteration in the surface keratin layer.[5] It is

TABLE 16.2. Heat-related skin diseases.

Miliaria
  Miliaria crystallina (1,5)
  Miliaria rubra (1)
  Miliaria pustulosa (1)
  Miliaria profunda (1)
  Occlusion miliaria (6)
  Tropical anhidrotic asthenia (5)
Urticaria induced by heat
  Cholinergic urticaria (2, 12–14)
  Cholinergic pruritus (1)
  Localized heat urticaria (2, 15–19)
Cumulative insult dermatitis (1)
Erythema ab igne (1, 2, 7, 20)
Heat-induced cancers (1, 2, 7–9, 21)
Erythermalgia (2, 22, 23)
Actinic granuloma and giant cell temporal arteritis (9)
Transient acantholytic dermatosis (10)
Occupational heat diseases
  Glass blowers, furnace workers, engineers (7, 9)
    Cutaneous aging
  Bakers and kitchen workers (1, 2, 7)
    Cutaneous aging
    Telangiectasia
    Elastosis
    Erythema ab igne
  Silversmiths and jewelers (1)
    Erythema ab igne
  Foundrymen (1)
    Erythema ab igne
  Farmers and athletes (6, 24)
    Elastosis
    Cutaneous aging
  Users of hair dryers (7)
    Elastosis cheeks

Note: Reference numbers in parentheses.

commonly seen the the neonatal period and is precipitated by sun or mild thermal damage.[5] Clinically, it presents as crops of clear thin-walled superficial vesicles 1–2 mm in diameter occurring predominantly on the head, neck, and upper trunk. Rupture of these vesicles is followed by branny desquamation. Pathologically, it is characterized by intracorneal or subcorneal vesicles in communication with sweat ducts. It is clearly differentiated from viral exanthem by the lack of erythema, the absence of giant epidermal and inflammatory cells.[1,5] Generalized involvement may interfere with thermoregulation. This is a self-limiting disease that improves with climatotherapy.[1]

Miliaria Rubra (Prickly Heat)

This is an erythematous papulovesicular eruption accompanied by pricking or stinging sensations, encountered only in situations provoking sweating.

Prickly heat is a common disorder of hot and humid environments. The blockage of sweat delivery is found at the granular layer.[1] The real cause of sweat obstruction is not clear. It could be due to excessive hydration, hypertonic solutions of sodium chloride resulting from partial drying of sweat, staphylococcal infection, or the action of sweat itself or other unknown factors. The clinical condition itself may have a damaging effect on the sweat gland. Lesions tend to appear in a few days to months after exposure to a hot humid environment. The palms and soles are spared. Patients complain of a prickling, mildly stinging sensation in the skin with the initiation of sweating. Symptoms extend beyond the area of involvement and is worst with profuse sweating but subsides when in cooler quarters. Individual lesions consist of small papulovesicular lesions with surrounding erythema on the skin surface. Lesions may be pustular and may be complicated by secondary infection. Microscopically, the vesicle is situated just under the stratum granulosum. Serial sectioning will, however, reveal its continuity with the sweat duct. Diagnosis depends on its typical symtoms. Patients improve with climatotherapy and cooling drying lotions.[1]

Miliaria Pustolosa

This disease is usually preceded by some other dermatitis that has produced injury, destruction, or blockage of the sweat duct. Pustules are distinct, superficial, and independent of hair follicle. The pruritic pustules occur most frequently on the intertriginous areas, on the flexure surfaces of the extremities, and on the scrotum.[1] Some of the associated diseases are contact dermatitis, lichen simplex chronicus, and intertrigo. Pustular miliaria may occur several weeks after the associated disease has subsided.[1] Usually, the pustules are sterile, but they may contain nonpathogenic cocci. Post-miliarial hypohidrosis occurs, due to occlusion of sweat ducts and pores all over the body, severe enough to impair man's ability to perform sustained work in heat. Affected persons may show decreasing efficiency, irritability, anorexia, drowsiness, vertigo, and headache. They may wander about in a haze.[1]

Occlusion Miliaria

Occlusion miliaria occurs due to long-standing poral occlusion with the application of extensive polyethylene film occlusion for 48 h or more hours. Thus, there is a local increase of heat. Miliaria may be produced with accompanying anhidrosis and increased heat stress susceptibility.[6] Giant centrifugal miliaria profunda[11] has been reported from occlusion from tape applied on the site of venous or arterial punctures.

Miliaria Profunda

This condition nearly always follows repeated attacks of miliaria rubra and is uncommon except in the tropics. The lesions are easily missed. The affected skin is covered with pale firm papules 1–3 mm across, especially on the covered areas, but sometimes also on the limbs. There is no itching or discomfort from the lesions.[1]

Tropical Anhidrotic Asthenia

Tropical anhidrotic asthenia is a state of exhaustion and heat intolerance affecting man exposed several months to a hot climate. It is characterized by the appearance of discrete vesicular lesions in the skin (miliaria profunda) and diminished or absent sweating in these areas. During the Second World War, generalized vesicular lesions of skin with hydohidrosis or anhidrosis were noticed when soldiers were exposed to heat.[5] They also had symptoms of acute fatigue, nausea, dizziness, palpitations, tachycardia, and malaise.

Urticaria Induced by Heat

Cholinergic Urticaria

This disease is common in young adults and is triggered by exercise, heat, and emotion. A sensation of warmth is followed by the development of pruritic 1–3 mm wheals with a surrounding erythematous flare.[2] This most often involves the chest and back and, in several cases, can be generalized. Uncommonly, wheezing and other systemic symptoms, such as nausea, abdominal pain, and headaches, may occur.[2] Angiodema may also be present and cholinergic urticaria may co-exist with other physical urticarias. Cholinergic urticaria may be produced by taking a hot bath or exercise until sweating. An intradermal test with mecholyl[2] is positive only in patients with severe cholinergic urticaria and is not a reliable means of diagnosis. Treatment includes avoiding triggering factors; i.e., heat, aspirin,[12] exercise, etc., and use of hydroxyzine or danazol.[13]

Cholinergic Pruritus

Cholinergic pruritus[1] or itching without whealing may be due to a slightly different mechanism. After a severe attack of cholinergic urticaria, further exertion may fail to cause urticaria, lasting 24 h or more. This condition may be induced by heat and tends to last for months to years and may improve spontaneously.

Localized Heat Urticaria

It is a rare entity having urticaria on the skin in direct contact with heat.[2] Women are commonly affected, and systemic symptoms may occur if large areas of skin are exposed to heat. A rare delayed type of localized heat urticaria was described in one family[18], in whom wheals developed 1.5 to 2 h after heat exposure. Pathogenesis is not understood. Histamine and nonhistaminic substances with the ability to cause smooth muscle contraction have been recovered from heat urticaria skin,[17] and histamine release into venous blood of the heat-challenged arm has been documented. Recently, increased plasma levels of prostaglandin D_2[16,17] have been identified in affected individuals. Biopsies after local heat challenge have revealed mononuclear perivascular inflammation within 6 h, with degranulated mast cells detected by electron microscopy. Treatment includes avoidance of precipitating factors, administration of antihistaminics, and induced tolerance[19] either by emersion of the hand in hot water for 1 min every hour until it stops reacting, or taking a hot water bath every 12 h until the reaction ceases.

Hydroxyzine plus cimetidine completely abolishes symptoms.[15] Adding indomethacin shows additional benefits.[2]

Cumulative Insult Dermatitis: Chronic Irritant Dermatitis

This type of dermatitis develops after series of repeated and damaging insults to the skin. These include chemical irritants and physical factors such as friction, microtrauma, low humidity, heat, cold, solvents, soap, detergents, powder, soil, or water.[1] Susceptibility depends on level of exposure, age, site of onset, and individuals with impaired skin resistance such as atopics.[1] Other factors such as skin temperature and repair capacity are probably important. Treatment includes removing all adverse factors, cleaning with isotonic saline, and use of emollient hand creams.[1]

Erythema ab Igne

This condition, once common in Europe, is now rare since the introduction of central heating, though it is sometimes seen in rural areas among elderly who sit close to the fire or who are habituated to using heating pads or hot water bottles for ailments such as chronic backache.[1] Similar changes can be seen on the faces of bakers and silversmiths and on the palms of older people and others working over a heat source.[1] It may also be seen in mentally disturbed patients with thermophilia, having bizarre areas of erythema ab igne.[1] Clinically, it presents as reticulate erythema, hyperpigmentation, epidermal atrophy, scaling, and telangiectasia, which eventually resemble features of poikiloderma.[1,10] Histologically, epidermal atrophy, dermal pigmentation, vasodilatation, vacuolar change in the basal cell layer, and degeneration of connective tissue with fragmentation of collagen bundles are seen.[1,7,20] Focal hyperkeratosis and epidermal dysplasia occurs later. There is accumulation of elastic tissue, but unlike the changes seen in solar elastosis, there is no basophilia.[1,7,20]

Heat-Induced Cancers

Acute heat exposure, severe enough to cause ulceration, can also produce squamous cell cancers.[7] Evidence is convincing that infrared radiation along with heat can cause a variety of skin cancers.[1] In northern China, the Kang cancer is produced by sleeping on hot bricks. In India, the Kangri cancer of Kashmiris arises from the habit of wearing pots containing hot coals next to the skin.[1,2] Even in modern Japan, pocket-sized metallic benzene-burning flasks are available to maintain skin warmth in freezing weather. The tumor induced by this practice is called Kairo cancer.[21] Turf or peat fire cancer is seen in rural Irish women who spend hours at chores in front of an open hearth containing burning peat.[1,2] It is also reported on the legs of older women in Japan produced by thermal irradiation from a sunken hearth (Irori).[21] Invariably, the tumors arose in skin that showed the hallmarks of erythema ab igne. Basal cell cancer developing in sites of focused infrared radiation in patients wearing rimless glasses has been described.[7] Long-term movement of a pipe stem on the lower lip[8] along with the high thermal temperature generated within the stem may cause irritation sufficient to induce carcinomatous degeneration.

Erythermalgia

Erythermalgia or erythromelalgia is characterized by erythema and burning distress in the feet or hands with an increase in local temperature precipitated by heat. It was first described in 1878[2] as "erythromelalgia" which was subsequently changed to erythermalgia in 1938.[2] The disorder was further divided into primary (idiopathic) and secondary forms.[2] Recently, however, idiopathic erythermalgia is considered to be a congenital disorder.[23] Symptoms usually involve lower extremities with patients seeking relief by walking in snow or using a fan or ice packs. Men are affected twice as often as women. Secondary erythermalgia is seen in older people, equally between the sexes, associated with mild symptoms and asymmetry. It is commonly associated with polycythemia rubra vera but may also be associated with myeloid metaplasia, hypertension, venous insufficiency, diabetes mellitus, rheumatoid arthritis, systemic lupus erythematosus, and thrombocytopenia with or without polycythemia rubra vera. Erythermalgia often precedes the diagnosis of myeloproliferative diseases by several years. Temperature studies show an increase in induced burning distress at 32–36°C and disappearance at cooler temperature. Relief of symptoms is noticed upon taking aspirin or moving to a cooler area. Pathogenesis is not known, but a primary or secondary vascular abnormality with endothelial swelling and platelet aggregation is proposed. Prostaglandins from activated platelets result in pain and erythema. Pathologically, arterioles show endothelial cell swelling and proliferation of smooth muscle cells in the vessel walls, resulting in narrowing of the lumen. There is a reduction of nerve terminals in the periarterial and sweat gland plexus.[22] Aspirin gives maximum benefit, followed by methysergide maleate in some. Other treatments used include epinephrine, nitroglycerin ointment, sublingual isopranolol, and in severe cases, lumbar ganglionectomy and peripheral nerve division. Underlying polycythemia has to be treated.

Actinic Granuloma and Giant Cell Temporal Arteritis

Actinic granuloma is an annular superficial dermal thickening with slight atrophy and hypopigmentation developing in areas of actinic elastosis.[19] The initial lesions are papules that gradually enlarge and clear in the center to form rings. The lesions are persistent and asymptomatic. Pathologically, the dermis shows histiocytes and giant cell inflammatory reaction around elastic fibers and the center of the lesion. Elastic fibers are removed from the center by elastosis. Infrared radiations might cause elastosis, and radiant heat other than sun produces elastotic degeneration.[9] The condition has to be differentiated from granuloma annulare, sarcoidosis, and necrobiosis lipoidica. Typical histology and site can easily distinguish these conditions from actinic granuloma. Patients improve with intralesional triamcinolone and photoprotection.

Similarly, in giant cell temporal arteritis, infrared (IR) may be a culprit because solar elastosis is commonly associated with this condition. However, damaged elastic tissue being a form of reaction is disputed.

Transient Acantholytic Dermatoses (Grover's Disease)

Grover's disease is characterized by transient elematous and excoriated papules and vesicles predominantly on the trunk and is related to heat or IR, for example, sun exposure, hot tub bath, hot water bottle, or steam bath.[10]

Occupational Heat Diseases

These diseases occur in people working in hot environments. Glassblowers, furnace workers, and boiler engineers[7,9] show severe cutaneous aging from early adulthood. It is related to elastic fiber damage and delayed DNA repair caused by infrared radiation. Similarly, bakers and kitchen workers,[1,2,7] due to prolonged exposure to heat, show thickened, leathery, elastic skin on the arms. There is enhanced cutaneous aging, telangiectasia, elastosis, and erythema ab igne. Silversmiths, jewelers, and foundrymen show features of erythema ab igne on exposed areas.

Infrared radiation may contribute to premature aging, especially in women using hood-type hair dryers for 1.5 h a day for 7 years.

Pouches of inelastic skin on both cheeks has been reported.[7] Farmers[6] and athletes[24] working all day in the sun for years are prone to cutaneous aging due to both IR and UVR. Infrared radiation may significantly enhance the aging and carcinogenic effects of ultraviolet radiation.

Heat-Exaggerated Skin Diseases

Many skin diseases are exaggerated by heat or IR. (See Table 16.3.)

A. Melanoderma, which has various etiologies, is also caused by long continued exposure to heat.[6] Postinflammatory hyperpigmentation, commonly seen in Asians and Africans, may get exaggerated by exposure to heat and sun.[6]
B. Hypohidrotic ectodermal dysplasia is a congenital skin disease consisting of a triad of hypotrichosis, anodontia, and anhidrosis. Clinically, there is reduced sweating, hypotrichosis, and partial or total anodontia. The skin is smooth, soft, and dry and finely wrinkled and prematurely aged. Alopecia is often noted with sparce, dry, fine, short hairs. It is due to lack of reduced sweat glands. These patients tolerate heat badly and are prone to heat stroke and fatigue in hot weather.[1]
C. Toxic erythema of the newborn is a benign self-limiting condition characterized by pustular erythematous macules, papules, and pustules that may be discrete or confluent. Histological examination of erythematous macular lesions shows a perivascular accumulation of eosinophils in the upper dermis. It is easily distinguished from bacterial, herpetic, or candidal lesions by its histology. Allergy may have a role due to frequent eosinophils. The intrafollicular location of mature pustules has led to the

suggestion that the inflammatory response is elicited by some component of sebum. It has been proposed that toxic erythema may be a response to mechanical or thermal skin trauma. Hence, heat has a role both as a precipitating and exaggerating factor.[1]
D. Livedo reticularis has a reddish blue, mottled, blotchy, and reticular appearance that does not disappear with either heating or cooling. Livedo may be an early manifestation of periarteritis nodosa or other vascular diseases. Specific forms of livedo reticularis includes the winter form and the form with summer ulceration affected by heat,[5] which may improve with low-molecular-weight dextran therapy.[25]
E. Hyperhidrosis or excessive sweating may be due to defective thermoregulation or may be emotional or mentally related. Heat increases thermoregulatory hyperhidrosis due to increased temperature of blood bathing the hypothalamus.
F. Ehlers-Danlos syndrome (EDS) type IV[26] is a severe variant of EDS that is characterized by excessive fragility of blood vessel and internal organs. Extremities show hyperelastic thin fragile skin with acrogerialike appearance. It is temperature dependent and is exaggerated by IR.

Heat Therapy for Skin Diseases

A. Infections: Heat therapy (Table 16.4) was used in the past for the treatment of syphilis.[27,28]

TABLE 16.3. Heat-exaggerated skin diseases.

Melanderma (6)
Postinflammatory hyperpigmentation (6)
Hypohidrotic ectodermal dysplasia (1)
Toxic erythema of newborn (1)
Hyperhidrosis (1)
Livedo reticularis (5, 25)

Note: Reference numbers in parentheses.

TABLE 16.4. Heat therapy for skin diseases.

Infections
  Syphilis (27, 28)
  Cutaneous leishmaniasis (29)
  Atypical mycobacteria (9, 34)
  Verrucae (9)
  Chromomycosis (9)
  Sporotrichosis (9)
Psoriasis (30, 31)
Atopic dermatitis (9)
Malignancy: melanoma, Kaposi's sarcoma (9)
Miscellaneous
  Cutis marmorata (5)
  Vascular anomalies and decorative tattoos (9)
  Laser CO_2 and YAG, low-energy laser therapy for wound healing (9)

Note: Reference numbers in parentheses.

It was called fever therapy. High body temperature, 40°C, was created with malaria to kill the treponemes; however, such therapies are obsolete now. Cutaneous lesions of leishmaniasis improved substantially with heat treatment by locally increasing the temperature to 55°C for 5 min.[29]

Chromomycosis,[9] verrucae,[9] sporotrichosis,[9] and atypical mycobacteria[9,34] improved with local heat, 40–42°C, several times a day, probably because of increased sensitivity of these organisms to heat and host response by heat shock protein production.

B. Psoriatic plaques treated with ultrasound[31] by raising the local temperature to 42–45°C for 30 min three times weekly for 4–10 treatments cleared the majority of the plaques. Palmoplantar psoriasis resistant to available treatment improved when adjunct hyperthermia therapy was given with ultrasound.[30] Similar results were obtained with exothermic pads at temperatures of 42–45°C on plaques. In psoriasis, heat therapy leads to increased vascular delivery of drugs to local areas by increasing the cell membrane permeability. Hyperthermia by stalling the cells in S-phage improves the efficacy of methotrexate, which is effective on cells in the S-phage.[30]

C. Atopic dermatitis[9] improved within 3 weeks with an IR lamp that raised temperatures to 42°C.

D. Hyperthermia in conjunction with radiation (total doses 3000–3200) has been used in the treatment of malignant melanoma and Kaposi's sarcoma.[9,28]

E. Miscellaneous

1. Acquired cutis marmorata is the term applied to transient reticular cyanosis of mixed bluish and pink pattern which appears on cold exposure but disappears with warming. The cyanotic component is supposedly caused by incomplete oxygen associated with cooling seen in overweight women with cooler skin over thicker adipose tissue.[5]

2. Use of IR coagulators showed substantial improvement with acceptable scarring in capillary haemangioma, spider vein, benign telangiectasia, and portwine stains.[9]

3. Lasers, a source of coherent monochromatic

radiation, used as a high-energy device to generate temperature from 50°C to several thousand degrees celsius resulting in tissue coagulation, vaporization, and cutting is used in various dermatological conditions from pigmented nevus to large tumors.[9] Low-energy red and IR lasers have been helpful in stasis and decubitus ulcers.[9]

Experimental Studies

IR radiation ranges from wavelengths of 700 to 1000 μm. Heat in the range of 41–43°C significantly inhibits DNA repair mechanisms.[7] Many biochemical reactions are amplified by heat and are heat dependent. Heat could contribute significantly to UV-induced aging changes, including precancers and cancers. Harmful effects of heat was noted as far back as 1978.[7] There was shortening of UV-induced tumors in mice at a temperature of 38°C.[7] It was also found that heat enhanced both the immediate and delayed effects of UV radiation in haired mice living at 34°C.[7] These animals developed intense erythema crusting and ulceration, whereas animals living at a lower temperature had only mild erythema with slight crusting. The latency period for UV-induced tumorigenesis was even shorter at the higher temperature. Heat is found to act synergistically to denature DNA in squamous cells of the buccal mucosa.[7] There was intensification of UV-induced dermal damage in guinea pigs by IR.[33] One of the markers of chronic actinic or thermal damage is elastic fiber hyperplasia. The fibers not only proliferate, they become thicker, branched, and twisted, resulting in the disordered overgrowth termed elastosis. Mice developed these changes along with tumors during the course of irradiation. Guinea pigs irradiated with UVB alone for 45 weeks showed quantity and thickness of elastic fibers. Infrared radiation alone produced dense skeins of fine feathery fibers, whereas UVB followed by IR resulted in substantial increased thickened fibers and formation of fine parallel skeins of elastic fibers. It was noted that guinea pig collagen was more resistant than mouse collagen. Increase in ground substance proteoglycans was noted when both UV and IR were used. Phototoxic reactions to topical methoxsalen were reduced by prior heating in a hot water chamber and 250-W red IR bulb.[9] Low-energy laser studies show a stimulatory effect on DNA, RNA, and protein synthesis in bacteria and transformed animal cells, fibroblast proliferation in humans, and hair growth in mice.[9]

Epidemiologically and with clinical evidence, IR radiation strongly contributes to chronic sun damage. These changes do not occur in protected skin. Sunbathing in midday, even using good UVA + UVB cream, will not protect against damaging IR. Future creams would include IR protective cream along with photoprotective cream.

References

1. Rook A, Wilkinson DS, Ebling RH, et al: Textbook of Dermatology 4th ed. Oxford: Blackwell Scientific, 1986.
2. Page EH, Shear NH: Temperature dependent skin disorders. Am Acad Dermatol 1988;**18**:1003–1019.
3. Scheuplein RJ: Mechanism of temperature regulation in the skin. In: Fitzpatrick TB, Eisen AZ, et al., eds. Dermatology in General Medicine, 3rd ed. New York: McGraw-Hill, 1987:347–357.
4. Demling RH, Burns. N Engl J Med 1985;**313**:1389–1398.
5. Cage GW, et al: Eccrine glands. In: Fitzpatrick TB, Eisen AZ, Wolff K, et al., eds. Dermatology in General Medicine, 3rd ed. New York: McGraw-Hill, 1987:701–703.
6. Domonkos AN, Arnold HL: Andrews' Diseases of the Skin, 7th ed. Philadelphia: W. B. Saunders, 1982:1049.
7. Kligman LH, Kligman AM: Reflections on heat. Br J Dermatol 1984;**110**:369–375.
8. Selden ST. Infrared radiation, Freud and lip cancer. J Am Acad Dermatol 1990;**22**:536–537.
9. Dover JS, Philips TJ, Arndt KA: Cutaneous effects and therapeutic uses of heat with emphasis on infrared radiation. J Am Acad Dermatol 1989;**20**:278–286.
10. Hu CH, Michel B, Farber EM: Transient acantholytic dermatosis (Grover's disease), a skin disorder related to heat and sweating. Arch Dermatol 1985;**121**:1439–1441.
11. Rogers M, Kan A, Stapleton K, Kemp A: Giant centrifugal miliaria profunda. Pediatr Dermatol 1990;**7**:140–146.
12. Doeglas HMG: Reactions to aspirin and food additives in patients with chronic urticaria including the physical urticarias. Br J Dermatol 1975;**93**:135–144.
13. Wong E, Eftekhari N, Greaves MW, Ward AM: Beneficial effects of danazol on symptoms and laboratory changes in cholinergic urticaria. Br J Dermatol 1987;**116**:553–556.
14. Lawrence CM, Jorizzo JL, Kobza Black A, et al: Cholinergic urticaria with associated angioedema. Br J Dermatol 1981;**105**:543–550.
15. Irwin RB, Lieberman P, Friedman MM: Mediator release in local heat urticaria: protection with combined H_1 and H_2 antagonists. J Allerg Clin Immunol 1985;**76**:35–39.
16. Levis RA, Soter NA, Diamond PT, et al: Prostaglandin D_2 generation after activation of rat and human mast cells with anti IgE. J Immunol 1982;**129**:1627.
17. Karo O, Dover JS, Francis DM, et al: Release of prostaglandin D_2 and histamine in a case of localized heat urticaria and effects of treatment. Br J Dermatol 1986;**115**:721–728.
18. Michaelsson G, Ros A: Familial localized heat urticaria of delayed type. Acta Dermatol Venereol (Stockh) 1971;**51**:279–283.
19. Leigh IM, Ramsay CA: Localized heat urticaria treated by inducing tolerance to heat. Br J Dermatol 1975;**92**:191–194.
20. Sharad P, Marks R: The wages of warmth: changes in erythema ab igne. Br J Dermatol 1977;**97**:179–186.
21. Akasaka T, Kon S: Two cases of squamous cell carcinoma arising from erythema ab igne. Nippon Hifuka Gakkai Zasshi 1989;**99**:735–742.
22. Uno H, Parker F: Autonomic innervation of the skin in primary erythermalgia. Arch Dermatol 1983;**119**:65–71.
23. Michels JJ, Van Joost T, Vuzevski VD: Idiopathic erythermalgia: a congenital disorder. J Am Acad Dermatol 1989;**21**:1128–1130.
24. Conklin RJ: Common cutaneous disorders in athletes. Sports Med 1990;**9**:100–119.
25. Issroff SW, Whiting DA: Low molecular weight dextran in the treatment of livedo reticularis with ulceration. Br J Dermatol 1971;**85**:26–31.
26. Furga AS, Steinmann B: Ehlers-Danlos syndrome type IV: Another temperature dependent skin disorder? J Am Acad Dermatol 1989;**21**:323.
27. Polla BS: Heat (shock) and the skin. Dermatologica 1990;**180**:113–117.

28. Malkinson FD: The heat's on. *Arch Dermatol* 1980;**116**:885–887.
29. Junaid AJN: Treatment of cutaneous leishmaniasis with infrared heat. *Int J Dermatol* 1986;**25**:470–472.
30. Colman WR, Lowe NJ: Ultrasound induced hyperthermia as adjuvant therapy for palmoplantar psoriasis. *J Dermatol Treat* 1991**2**:7–10.
31. Orenberg EK, Deneau DG, Farber EM: Response of chronic psoriatic plaques to localized heating induced by ultrasound. *Arch Dermatol* 1980;**116**:893–897.
32. Kaidbey KH, Witkowski TA, Kligman AM: The influence of infrared radiation on short-term ultraviolet-radiation-induced injuries. *Arch Dermatol* 1982;**118**:315–318.
33. Kligman LH: Intensification of ultraviolet induced dermal damage by infrared radiation. *Arch Dermatol Res* 1982;**271**:229.
34. Meyers WM, Shelly WM, Conner DH: Heat treatment of *Mycobacterium ulcerans* infections without surgical excision. *Am J Trop Med Hyg* 1974;**23**:924–929.

17

Diseases Affected by Cold: Arctic and Subarctic Areas

Gunnar Lomholt

The Arctic and Subarctic areas are sparsely populated, most people living at or near the coast. Even with a reasonable number of physicians, this makes coverage of medical care extremely difficult. It might even take days with small boats or on dog sleds to reach the clinic or the local hospital. In many areas, physicians periodically visit small villages to observe the medical conditions. Such visits are very time-consuming and a special challenge for the physicians working in these areas.[1-4] Consequently, the patients attending the clinics are often delayed and suffering from severe and extensive diseases. The development of radio and telecommunication and the use of helicopters have greatly alleviated the problems.

Dermatology

Most dermatological patients suffer from much more extensive conditions than usually seen in the industrialized parts of the world. In general, the diseases are more or less the same, but because of the great distances, several small hospitals are established in connection with health centers and more beds than usual are required, so a reasonable result of the treatment introduced can be expected.

The main occupation is fishery and seal hunting, often from very small boats and kayaks. Many women are occupied with preparing fish in small factories. This constant contact with cold water, fish products, and salt results in chronic dermatitis of the hands, often with development of perniotic changes. More commonly, women in the shrimp industry present with a chronic paronychia caused by damages of the shield.

Lapps and Eskimos live as nomads, following their herds of reindeer on their wanderings. In the northern part of Norway, however, many are farmers.

Only a few of the conditions seen are worth mentioning. Varicose veins and leg ulcers are astonishingly rare even though the pregnancy rate is high and the conditions in connection with delivery often unacceptable. Allergic contact dermatitis seems less frequent, but atopic dermatitis is presumably as common as elsewhere. A survey from Tromsoe University—the most northern in the world, approximately 400 km north of the Arctic Circle—seems to show a higher prevalence of psoriasis than demonstrated anywhere.[5]

A dermatologist visited the whole west coast of Greenland for the first time in the summer of 1958 to determine the cutaneous conditions.[7] Favus was known to exist and was especially traced. It was only found in the northern part where dogs are permitted and used for sledding. Seventeen cases of active favus and 25 with spontaneous healed favus were found. The patients with active favus were later sent to Copenhagen for treatment. For the first time, griseofulvin was found effective. Previously, the treatment was with X-ray epilation of the scalp. The patients with sequelae of favus presented a uniform picture of a nearly total, cicatricial alopecia with a narrow fringe of thin ruffled hair.[8]

Injuries caused by cold, wind, and sun are very common. The permanent red cheeks often with small teleangiectasies seen in young girls is most impressive. In older men, more or less pronounced rosacea is commonly seen. Severe cases of perniosis and frostbite are, however, unusual. Adiponecrosis e frigore in children is not common but occasionally seen during strong winters in the northern part of Europe. People living in this part of the world are dressed in warm clothing to protect themselves against cold. The Eskimo men, as well as women use trousers and anoraks of sealskin to protect the head and face, as did their ancestors.

Severe cold injuries are mainly seen among people who have lost their orientation because of dense fog, especially notable on the sea due to storms. Most of such cases are seen among visitors who are skiing and lose their way. This is not infrequent in tourist resorts outside the arctics. Frostbite and gangrene are well known among polar explorers and mountain climbers at high altitudes.

Lack of proper clothing, wind, moisture, circulatory diseases, anoxia, immobility, and poor general health in connection with prostation all potentiate the effect of cold, not necessarily very low temperatures. Lewis mentions that there is good evidence to support the view that some races, such as the Eskimos and Nepalese Sherpas, are more "immune" to cold injury than other races, and there is some evidence to suggest that personality factors such as poor motivation may increase the propensity to frostbite.[6] Exposure to very cold water by falling into the sea will only allow a few minutes for survival.

A meticulous description of cold in relation to skin diseases is given by Haxthausen.[4] This involves frostbites, perniosis, and chilblain with additional keratosis pilaris as well as acrocyanosis, levido reticularis, Raynaud's phenomenon, and cold urticaria.

Treatment of patients with acute frostbite and perniosis is with warm water ($\sim 42°C$) for approximately 20 min to the hands and feet, and in the case of hypothermia, a universal bath is recommended. The traditional rubbing of the affected areas with snow should be avoided because it only worsens the condition. Intake of alcoholic drinks should also be avoided until the person is indoors in a warm environment. No internal medication is really effective. Sympathectomy should not be given in the acute stage, and in the case of gangrene, amputation should be postponed as long as possible and not before demarcation of the affected area is evident.

Sexually Transmitted Diseases

In general, problems with sexually transmitted diseases (STDs) and their control are very similar thoughout the Arctic. The incidence is, however, much higher than in the industrialized parts of the world. The number of patients with gonorrhea in Alaska is three times as high as in the continental United States.[10]

The age of first sexual activity among arctic people is young, and the numbers of sexual encounters and partners is high. A school survey from Greenland has shown that more than half of the students indicated their sexual debut before the age of 15. In addition, the number of sexual partners is high: In 1989, 28% of the boys mentioned more than 10 contacts. Twenty-six percent of the boys and 42% of the girls had sexual intercourse more than 15 times each month.[11]

The incidence of gonorrhea is very high but has shown a great decrease since 1982 with 13,046 reported cases in Greenland compared with 2,474 in 1990 in a population of only 50,000. Among teenagers, not less than 57% are infected two or three times during a single year.[2]

Small epidemics of syphilis have occurred in Greenland since 1872, but were restricted by quarantine to the district involved. Epidemiological efforts disclosed 6 cases of syphilis in South Greenland in 1947 and 22 in 1965.[13] Since 1970, syphilis has, however, spread to the entire country. The highest number was registered in 1976 (707 cases), and in a new epidemic in 1987, 658 cases were registered. Since that time the number of cases dropped dramatically with only 34 cases during the first 9 months of 1991.[3]

Only a very few cases of late syphilis are registered, but during the years 1970–1987, 10 cases of congenital syphilis were recorded. Alaska registered only 25 cases of syphilis in 1988, and the last case of congenital syphilis was diagnosed in 1978.[10]

Chancroid was first reported in Greenland in 1976 and peaked in 1977 with 970 cases. An intensive campaign was introduced, and since 1980 it has disappeared. The reason for this is not well understood, but perhaps most of the infected patients came spontaneously for treatment because of the severe pain.[1]

Most of the people in Greenland with STDs are young teenagers, but Danish workers ($\sim$ 10,000) also play an important role. The distribution is nearly the same among men and women regarding syphilis, but for gonorrhea there is a predominance of men. Regarding patients with chancroid, the distribution was 1.7:1 for men and women. This is quite different from the usual. The reason is presumably the epidemiological treatment of all known contacts. Women usually have no or only slight symptoms in the early stage of the disease.[1]

Chlamydia trachomatis has presumably existed in arctic areas for years. Since 1977 when the first patient was diagnosed, it has been possible to investigate this disease.[12] A survey by From seems to show a very high prevalence.[1]

Statistics from Alaska and the Northwest Territories of Canada show very high prevalence of STDs, but the figures are lower. Sexually transmitted diseases is also a great problem in Russia and Siberia, but statistics are not available.[10] In contrast, the figures from the northern part of Norway and the Faroe Islands are impressively low; STDs are less frequent than in other parts of Europe.

HIV Infections

The first case of HIV infection was diagnosed in Greenland in 1985. With the high sexual activity and occurrence of STDs, especially genital ulcers, it might have great possibilities for spreading in the population. The health authorities have provided extensive information and education to the population and especially to the schools about this infection and the danger it might present for the country. At the end of 1991, approximately 30,000 tests for HIV have been performed on 17,721 persons. Up to that time, 32 cases of HIV were found—11 in women and 21 in men. Four patients have AIDS and two of them died. In Greenland, HIV is today, like STDs, mainly transmitted heterosexually.[11]

References

1. From E: Some aspects of venereal diseases in Greenland. *Br J Vener Dis* 1980;**56**:65–68.
2. From E: Venerea Groenlandica. Godthaab private printing 1990.
3. From E: Personal communication, 1991.
4. Haxthausen H: Cold in Relation to Skin Diseases. Copenhagen: Munksgaard, 1930.
5. Kavli G, Førde OH, Arnesen E, Stenvold SE: Psoriasis: Familial predisposition and environmental factors. *Br Med J* 1985;**29**:999–1000.
6. Lewis RB: Local cold injury: Frostbite. *Milit Surg* 1951;**110**:2.
7. Lomholt G: Report on dermatological conditions in Greenland to the Danish Government, 1958.
8. Lomholt G: Favus in Greenland. *Acta Derm Venereol (Stockh)* 1959;**39**:292–299.
9. Lomholt G, Berg O: Gonorrhoea situation in South Greenland in the summer 1964. *Br J Vener Dis* 1966;**42**:1–7.
10. Middaugh J, Gilchrist I, Misfeldt J, et al: Other sexual transmitted diseases. *Arctic Med Res* 1990;**49**(suppl 3):17–25.
11. Misfeldt J, Olsen J, Melbye M: AIDS/HIV-situation in Greenland 1991. *Ugesk Laeger* 1991;**153**:3630–3632.
12. Mårdh PH, Lind I, From E, Andersen AL. The prevalence of chlamydia trachomatis and neisseria gonorrhoea infection in Greenland. *WHO/VDT* 1980;**422**:1–9.
13. Olsen GA. Syfilisepidemien i Sydgrønland 1965. *Ugesk Laeger* 1966;**128**:1071–1076.

18

Diseases Affected by War: The Korean Experience

Sungnack Lee and Sung Ku Ahn

War and Medicine

War has existed from the beginning of history, and medicine has almost as long a history. During war, death, injury, and disease are inevitable, necessitating medical treatment. Thus, war and medicine have a close relationship. Experience obtained from wars has played a large role in the development of medical treatment. War also has influenced preventive medicine, the discovery of new disease entities, and the social status of doctors.

Especially during the Korean War (1951–1953), people were troubled by a great loss of manpower, an increase in urban population because of migrations, a decrease in employment, cultural conflict, lowered standards of living (economic loss), destruction of main industries, military and political conflict due to cold war tensions, and widespread infectious diseases.[1]

War and Skin Diseases

Between war and skin diseases, there is the same close relationship as between war and other infectious diseases. The similar factors include topographical and annual variation of temperature, amount of rainfall, humidity, worsening of living environment, individual nutritional state, hygiene, vaccination, and absence of concern for disease.

To understand a common skin disease in the Korean War, it is, of course, necessary to know the topographical characteristics of the Korean peninsula. The Korean peninsula is located in the northern hemisphere (north temperate zone), and there are four seasons: warm springs and fall, a very sultry summer (June–August), and a cold winter (November–February). Being a peninsula, it is surrounded by water on all sides but one and is composed of mouths of mountain area rather than plains. The temperature range is about 55°C (coldest in winter: −20°C; hottest in summer: 35°C) and there is a long and tiresome rainy season, starting in June and lasting for a month, when intensive rain includes half of the annual rainfall. During the war, many people suffered from frostbite in the frigid winter and from various infectious diseases in summer. Because of the war, new diseases, for example, tsutsugamushi disease and Korean hemorrhagic fever, became known.[2]

Viral Diseases

Korean Hemorrhagic Fever

In the spring of 1951, the United Nations was faced with an acute and severe infectious disease that had never been seen before. The allies opened a research center in the suburbs of Seoul and spent much money there to study the disease. At that time, the American medical team regarded it as a type of leptospirosis, relapsing fever, typhus fever, or hemorrhagic nephritis.[3] The etiologic agent (Hantaan virus) was not discovered until after the end of the war. This example shows how war contributes to the discovery of a new disease entity, the understanding of pathogenesis, and the development of treatment.

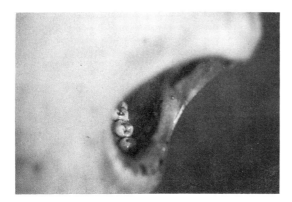

FIGURE 18.1. Multiple petechiae and purpuras

The disease was found everywhere within a 50-mile radius from the truce line and more often in the west rather than in the eastern mountainous region.[4] From 1950 to 1954, more than 2000 U.N. troops suffered from this disease of unknown cause. The mortality rate was about 6%. Beginning in 1956, it spread among civilians as well as military personnel and, at present, the distribution is nationwide except in the islands. Today, it peaks in frequency from May to June and from October to December.[2]

The hallmarks of clinical mainfestations are fever, thrombocytopenia, and acute renal insufficiency. The patients who survive progress through febrile, hypotensive, oliguric, and polyuric clinical stages and may require weeks or months to recover from general asthenia.

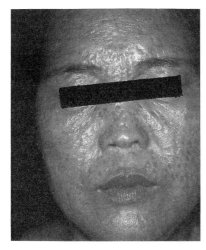

FIGURE 18.2. Scar of smallpox

In the toxic or febrile phase, patients complain of headaches, abdominal pain, dizziness, and blurred vision. Conjunctival infection and petechiae occur over the upper trunk and soft palate (Fig. 18.1).

An erythematous flush that blanches on pressure is characteristically seen on the torso and face. The Hantaan virus, the cause of severe hemorrhagic fever with renal syndrome in Korea and China, is found principally in the striped field mouse *Apodemus agrarius*.[5–7]

Smallpox

Smallpox (variola) no longer exists in an indigenous state in nature since the implementation of the successful worldwide eradication program. The last reported case was in Somalia in October 1977.[8]

In Korea, smallpox began an epidemic rise during the winter of 1945–1946. It occurred despite a prewar program of vaccination because apparently poor techniques had left many people unprotected. The military government ordered a nationwide program aimed at properly vaccinating every person south of the 38th parallel. As a result, only 113 cases were reported in 1947.

During the Korean War, about 47,000 people contracted smallpox and 12,000 died. Inadequate sanitation, hunger, and stress lowered resistance to the disease. Another factor contributed to the catastrophe: two large groups lacking immunization joined the population— refugees from the north and babies born after the outbreak of war.[3] Civilians, as well as the Korean and U.N. military forces, experienced outbreaks of smallpox. Even today, one can occasionally see the scarred faces of some people now over 50 years old (Fig. 18.2).

Diseases Caused by Environmental and Physical Factors

Frostbite (Cold Injury)

The winter in Korea lasts from November to February and the average temperature is −20°C with heavy snow and icy wind. Not surprisingly, frostbite was the most serious form of tissue injury during the war.[9,10]

It attacked many civilians as well as servicemen and occurred more in blacks than in whites. Occurrences were concentrated in December 1950 during a fierce battle in the region of the Yalu river, the most northern border of the peninsula, and in January 1951 during a retreat close to the intervention of the Chinese army.[3]

The war in Korea during the winter of 1950–1951 resulted in a high incidence of frostbite. More than 8000 cases of cold injury occurred during the Korean War (34 per 1000 troops per annum). Eighty percent of a group of patients with frostbite were exposed for 12 h or less, with a range of 2–72 h. The time duration necessary to incur frostbite is diminished by inactivity, inadequate clothing, or concomitant injury. The soldier having third degree frostbite, gangrene, and necrosis of the digit and fore part of the foot was treated with skin grafts and amputation and suffered a number of functional disturbances; for example, hyperhidrosis, pain, numbness, arthralgia, and residual abnormalities of the toe and fingernails.[11]

Immersion Foot

Immersion foot is a common disease in most wars. Even though the incidences of immersion or trench foot occurring at temperatures above freezing were not estimated accurately in the Korean War, many soldiers suffered because they had to stay in bunkers or trenches. The combination of prolonged exposure to nonfreezing cold and damp climate leads to the most serious situation. Other aggravating factors, such as exhaustion, trauma, dehydration, or constricting garments, also tend to decrease blood flow to the affected area. Vasoconstriction, as well as local anoxia, may produce a typical manifestation of cutaneous necrosis, ulceration, gangrene, and painful paresthesia. Non-caucasians are thought to have been more susceptible than whites during the Korean War. Thousands of cases occurred among U.S. military forces in Europe in the 1939–1945 war. Many of the affected men had loss of tissue and

permanent disability as a result of this kind of infection.[3,12]

Others

By the skin-breaking opportunities provided by the explosion of all sorts of bullets, shells, or cannon balls, various infectious diseases and trauma occurred on the battlefield.

Casualties were mainly victims of burns and frostbite, although accidental injuries were also common. For example, fatal tetanus, gas gangrene, and cellulitis were common afflictions.

Recorded at Osaka and Tokyo army hospitals during 1950 was an ever-increasing load of cases of gas gangrene, which gained its name from the bubbles of gas formed in the wound by anaerobic bacterial infection. Most unusual was Tetanus, a wound infection from which immunized U.N. soldiers are ordinarily free.[3]

Besides orthopedic injuries and shell fragment wounds, foreign body reaction and secondary skin diseases commonly occurred. To make things worse, malnutrition, poor hygiene, and improper treatment aggravated the above.[13,14]

Rickettsial Disease

Tsutsugamushi Disease

Tsutsugamushi disease is a febrile disease, characterized typically by a skin eruption and eschar, and accompanied by headaches and myalgias. This disorder is an acute, febrile illness of humans that is caused by *Rickettsia tsutsugamushi*. It is transmitted to humans by the bite of larval-stage trombiculid mites (chiggers). After about 5 days of illness, an eruption occurs on the trunk and spreads to the extremities. Most patients have a typical lesion; that is, eschar (Fig. 18.3).

Before the Korean War, there had been no reports of this disease; however, two English soldiers stationed at the western battle line (around the Imjin River) were found ill in 1951, and the first patient whose serum reacted with proteus OXK was reported. In the same year, four infected American soldiers were also reported.[2,15]

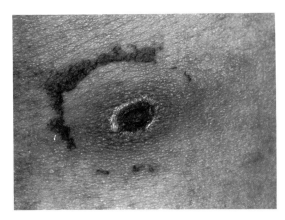

FIGURE 18.3. A typical eschar

In 1956, Jackson et al. separated the agent from the larva of *Trombicular pallida* being collected from wild mice living around the demilitarized zone.[16] Lee et al. first found the same agent in a Korean patient in 1986.[17] Presently, it occurs nationwide in the fall and early winter season, from October to November.

Sexually Transmitted Diseases in the Military

A sign of changing conditions in the Korean War was an evolution in the STD situation. During July and August in 1950, most cases among Americans in Korea resulted from the troop's flings in Japan. In September, rates were quite low, reflecting the rapid movement of forces through areas almost devoid of civilians. Beginning in October, STDs seemed to be acquired largely in Korea. In Pusan, for example, an area with a large concentration of troops and some 8000 prostitutes, numerous dance halls were opened to accommodate the troops.

Establishments, social breakdown associated with war, the poverty of the refugees, and the influx of professional prostitutes all contributed to the spread of syphilis, gonorrhea, pediculosis, and chancroid.[3]

Accuracy of reporting is somewhat of a problem. The reported rate was inversely proportional to the amount of field activity and combat. The Eighth Army reported that STD rates declined from 183 cases per 1000 troops per annum in 1949 to 143 in 1950; however, in the mid and late stage of the Korean War (1952–1953), the rate of STD moved gradually upward.[3,18]

Diseases Due to Animal Parasites

Scabies

Epidemics have long been associated with war, so conditions of poverty, poor hygiene, over-crowding, malnutrition, personal immunity, and sexual promiscuity are probably main contributing factors.

The disorder is worldwide in distribution. Even though the actual prevalence is unknown, Epstein reported that scabies occupied the third or fifth rank in 1955.[19] Today, it is markedly decreased due to improved environmental hygiene, development of DDT (which is not in use now) and new therapeutics. Still, the prevalence was as high as 1.1% in World Wars I and II, and the disease often struck in tandem with pediculosis during the Korean War.[20]

Pediculosis

Pediculidae are parasitic in humans. The species of importance are *Pediculus humanus* var. *corporis*, *Pediculus humanus* var. *capitis*, and *Pthirus pubis*.

Lice infestations have been observed in virtually every inhabited area of the world, and in times of war, with overcrowding or wide-spread inattention to personal hygiene, major epidemics have occurred.

In the Korean War, pediculosis corporis was seen in civilians, soldiers, and orphans.[3] Besides causing significant cutaneous disease, the human body louse is a vector for epidemic typhus, trench fever, and louse-borne relapsing fever.

Insect Bites

The summer season, lasting for 3–4 months in Korea, is very hot and humid. The hottest temperature can be over 35°C with 95%

humidity, especially after the end of the rainy season, which lasts about half a month. Therefore, the environment is very suitable for various species of insects.

One of the most troublesome insects of the war was the mosquito. It propagated encephalitis and malaria, and there was an outbreak of filariasis in Jeju Island.

Parasitic Diseases

People ate frogs or snakes because of the food shortage. They ate those as folk remedies, but it resulted in infection of sparganosis and occurrence of cysticercosis by *Taenia solium* during the Korean War. There were neither cutaneous leishmaniasis nor cutaneous creeping eruption from the infestation of *Strongyloides ancylostoma* in Korea, although it had spread to prisoners of war in Burma and Thailand in World War II.[21]

Nutritional Deficiency and Skin Disease

There is a close relationship between war, malnutrition, and disease; that is, war brings food shortages due to decreased production of food, distribution failure, and the destruction of factories.

The lack of food and especially of animal protein, when combined with a crowded, dusty environment and extreme cold, produce a new wave of deaths. At first, most occurred among the wounded. Then many who were uninjured died either from pneumonia, dysentery, or a combination of the two. Some who survived the first 5 or 6 months of captivity died later of deficiency diseases, mostly pellagra and beriberi.[3,21]

Pellagra

Vitamins are necessary organic molecules for human life and growth. As vitamins come from the diet, vitamin deficiency is secondary to nutritional deficiency. Nutritional deficiency states result in a diverse group of diseases with many distinctive cutaneous manifestations.

In recent times, isolated vitamin deficiency is uncommon. Multiple vitamins are usually involved.

Pellagra, which is the oldest known cutaneous manifestation among vitamin deficiency, was prevalent during the Korean War.[3,22]

Skin Diseases Caused by Biological and Chemical Warfare

There is no evidence of the use of chemical weapons, such as mustard gas, during the Korean War.

In the early period of 1952, the mutual slander about germ warfare between the U.N. allies and the North Korean government began.[3] Because numerous infections had simultaneously occurred on the Korean peninsula, the Chinese and North Koreans launched a massive effort to convince their own people that the U.N. command was engaged in the widespread use of biological weapons. The Americans counter-charged that real epidemics were occurring, was plausible because of the events of 1951 and the medieval disease environment that prevailed in most of China and North Korea.

Fungal and Mycobacterial Diseases

Although South Korea is a land of temperate climate with pleasant springs and falls, oppressive summers, and severe winters, its disease

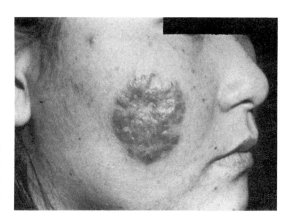

FIGURE 18.4. Lupus vulgaris

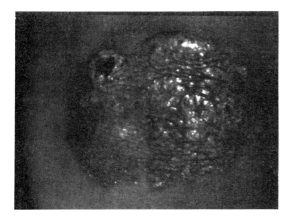

FIGURE 18.5. Tuberculosis verrucosa cutis

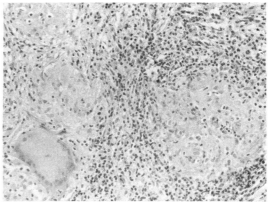

FIGURE 18.6. Lupus vulgaris showing typical tubercle formation with giant cells.

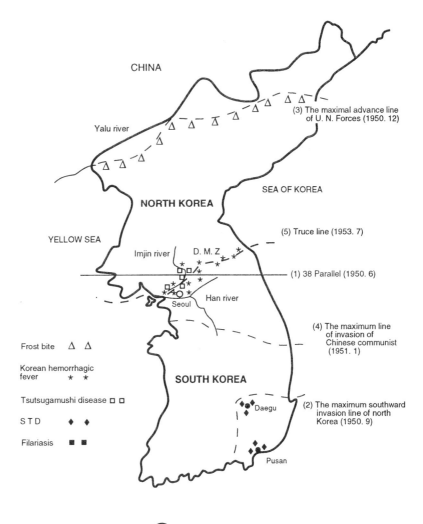

FIGURE 18.7. Sequential events of battle field and skin diseases (June 1950–July 1953).

environment emphasizes fungal and myco-bacterial infections. Especially high humidity, tiresome rainy days, and long-lasting hot temperature during the summer season leads to various kinds of dermatophytic infection.[14] It was nearly impossible to give statistical figures at wartime.

Far more tenacious was the slow and unspectacular killer "tuberculosis." It was a typical type of disease presentation especially in underdeveloped countries. It gained strength from malnutrition, crowding, exposure, and shortages of fuel and clothing brought about by the war. By late 1950, the death rate had reached 146 per 100,000.[3] Despite all efforts, tuberculosis remained the leading cause of death until 1960 in Korea.

Tuberculosis of the skin, which has been rare in developed countries, was declining the world over due to antituberculous medication and the elevation of living standards. Unfortunately, there is a resurgence of cutaneous tuberculosis. Today, lupus vulgaris and erythema induratum are the most common types of cutaneous tuberculosis found in Korea.[23] The former is characterized by reddish brown nodules that, when blanched by diascopic pressure, have an apple-jelly color (Fig. 18.4). Other lesions including tuberculosis verrucosa cutis (Fig. 18.5), lupus miliaris disseminatus faciei, and papulonecrotic tuberculids are commonly encountered. Histopathologically, the lesions show tubercules composed of epithelioid cells with or without caseous necrosis in the dermis (Fig. 18.6). The rate of prevalence and incidence cannot be precisely estimated due to the lack of statistics.

References

1. Kim HJ: Korean War, 1st ed. Seoul: Park Young, 1989.
2. Chun JH: Concept of Infectious Disease in Korea, 1st ed. Seoul: New Med, 1975.
3. Cowdrey AE: The Medic's War, 1st ed. Washington, DC: Center of Military History U.S. Army, 1987.
4. Paul JR, McClure WW: Epidemic hemorrhagic fever. Am J Hyg 1958;68:126–139.
5. Kim MY, Shin HK: An etioligic survey of the mites as a possible vector of epidemic hemorrhagic fever. Korean Army Med J 1963;9:64–69.
6. Lee HW, Lee PW: Korean hemorrhagic fever—demonstration of causative antigen and antibodies. Korean J Int Med 1976;19:371–383.
7. Andrew R: Epidemic hemorrhagic fever. Br Med J 1953;1:1063–1068.
8. Deria A, Jezek Z, Markvart M: The world's last endemic cases of small pox. Bull WHO 1980;58:279–283.
9. Ward M: Frostbite. Br Med J 1974;1:67–70.
10. Jarrett F: Frostbite. Current concepts of pathogenesis and treatment. Rev Surg 1974;31:71–77.
11. Edwards EA, Leep MRW: Frostbite. An analysis of seventy-one cases. JAMA 1952;149:1199–1205.
12. Allen AM: Tropical immersion foot. Lancet 1973;ii:1185–1189.
13. Rautio J. Paavolainen P: Afghan war wounded; experience with 200 cases. J Trauma 1988;28:523–525.
14. Ermakou MA: Experience with the treatment of skin disease of partisans during World War II. Vestn Dermatol Venerol 1976;7:81–85.
15. Munro FAD: Scrub typhus in Korea. J Roy Army Med 1951;97:227–229.
16. Jackson EB, Danaus Kas JX, Smaded JE: Occurrence of rickettsia tustsugamushi in Korean rodents and chiggars. Am J Hyg 1957;66:309–312.
17. Lee JS, Ahn C, Kim YK: Thirteen cases of rickettsial infection including nine cases of tsutsugamushi disease first confirmed in Korea. J Korean Med 1986;29:430–438.
18. Greenberg JH: Veneral disease in the armed forces. Med Aspects Human Sexual 1972;6:165–170.
19. Epstein E: Trends in scabies. Arch Dermatol 1955;71:192–196.
20. Epstein E: Scabies, ten years later. Arch Dermatol 1966;93:60–62.
21. Pelletier LL: Chronic strongyloidiasis in World War II Far East ex-prisoners of war. Am J Trop Med Hyg 1984;33:55–61.
22. Barthelemy H, Chouvet B, Cambazard F: Skin and mucosal manifestations in vitamin deficiency. J Am Acad Dermatol 1986;15:1263–1274.
23. Lee YB, Cho BK, Houh W: Clinical and histopathological study on skin tuberculosis during 5 years. Korean J Dermatol 1975;13:103–108.

19

Global Veterinary Dermatology

Peter J. Ihrke

The past two decades have been a time of extraordinary progress in the discipline of veterinary dermatology. Practitioner interest groups have grown in size and influence worldwide. During this time, veterinary dermatology has become recognized as an independent specialty, separate from internal medicine. Residency training programs have proliferated in North America, Europe, and the United Kingdom. Specialty colleges certifying diplomates through the process of examination have been active in the United States since 1974, and more recently in Australia; similar colleges are in the process of being organized in Europe.

Multiple major textbooks devoted to small animal dermatology, large animal dermatology, and dermatopathology have been published.[1-5] The first international journal devoted to veterinary dermatology, *Veterinary Dermatology*, was launched in 1989 by the European Society of Veterinary Dermatology (ESVD) and is now cosponsored by the ESVD and the American College of Veterinary Dermatology (ACVD). The First World Congress of Veterinary Dermatology, held in Dijon, France, in 1989, was attended by over 600 delegates from 35 countries and represented the work of 135 researchers. The Second World Congress of Veterinary Dermatology, held in Montreal, Canada, in May 1992 was sponsored by the ESVD, ACVD, American Academy of Veterinary Dermatology (AAVD), and the Canadian Academy of Veterinary Dermatology (CAVD).

Epidemiology of Skin Disease

Little hard data are available concerning the incidence or frequency of skin diseases in small or large domestic animals. It has been estimated that skin disease accounts for between 20% and 50% of the caseload in small animal hospitals in North America.[6-10] This range probably reflects differences in climatic conditions in the United States. These surprisingly high percentages of skin disease may be partially explained by the prominence of ectoparasitic skin diseases in veterinary medicine. Globally, the frequency of skin disease in large animals probably is higher than for small animals because of the impact of ectoparasitic disease in tropical and subtropical climates.

A recent study evaluated data from 17 veterinary medical teaching hospitals in North America to determine the most commonly documented causes of canine skin disease and the regional distribution of these diseases.[6] The 10 most common dermatologic diagnoses coded in order of occurrence were flea allergy dermatitis, skin neoplasia, pyoderma, seborrhea, allergy, demodicosis, scabies, immune-mediated skin disease, endocrine-related skin disease, and acral lick dermatitis. Some of the more surprising disease listings may be partially explained by inherent problems in this type of study. Coding and clinical interpretations may vary between institutions. In addition, regional differences in attitudes of the pet-owning population concerning veterinary care and attitudes of the general practitioner regarding referral would affect the study population. Perhaps most importantly, there probably is a bias toward more unusual cases in referral institutions. For example, even though auto-immune skin disease as a group was included among the 10 most common canine skin diseases, these are not common skin diseases. Because these diseases often are of great interest to referral specialists, bias may be introduced into the frequency of referral.

As would be expected, marked differences in the frequency of skin diseases were seen in different geographic locations in North America.[6] Flea allergy dermatitis was diagnosed more commonly in the southeast, southwest, west, and northeast. Seborrhea or scaling disorders were noted most frequently in the midwest and northeast, where the winters are long and dry heat indoors exacerbates or induces skin problems. Canine scabies was noted more frequently in the southeast and southwest. Pyoderma was diagnosed more commonly in the southeast, where higher humidity and warmer temperatures may create an environment more favorable for bacterial skin disease. The frequency of skin neoplasia correlated with probable increased sun exposure in warm, southern, and western climates and at higher altitudes such as in Colorado. Anecdotal information from veterinary dermatologists worldwide is in agreement with much of these data. Veterinary clinicians practicing in tropical and subtropical regions of the world attest to the increased frequency of skin disease in general and the enhanced importance of ectoparasitic and infectious skin diseases in these regions.

Marked breed predilections, indicating genetic susceptibility, have been reported for many skin diseases.[1,2,5] In addition, one study showed that breed was a marked risk factor for the development of skin disease in general.[11] Hospital data on the numbers of dogs of all breeds seen by the dermatology service and the entire teaching hospital at the University of California were compared for a 12-year time period. Thirty-one breeds of dogs were found to be statistically at elevated risk for the development of skin disease. Common breeds such as the Doberman Pinscher, Irish Setter, Dalma-

tion, Dachshund, Golden Retriever, and various small terrier breeds were at increased risk, and uncommon breeds such as the Chinese Shar Pei, Chow Chow, and Akita also were at increased risk. Decreased risk for skin disease was noted for crossbreed dogs and 12 purebred breeds including the common breeds, Saint Bernard, Standard Poodle, German Shorthaired Pointer, Beagle, Basset Hound, Afghan Hound, and Australian Shepherd Dog. The German Shepherd Dog, the most commonly seen purebred in both the dermatology and the general hospital population, was at average risk for the development of skin disease.[6]

Because animal breed popularity varies geographically for both the pet and livestock population, the frequency and type of skin disease observed will parallel these regional preferences. As an example, the dog breeds Akita and Sheba are popular in Japan; both of these breeds are at increased risk for the development of Vogt-Koyanaki-Harada-like syndrome (Ogata M, Kanagawa, Japan, personal communication, 1991). It is, therefore, not surprising that Vogt-Koyanagi-Harada-like syndrome in the dog is seen much more commonly in Japan than it is in North America or Europe.

An Overview of Veterinary Skin Diseases

To date, hundreds of different skin diseases have been identified in veterinary medicine. The commonality of skin diseases shared by human beings and all species of domestic animals that have been studied is striking. Veterinary counterparts to many of the bacterial fungal, ectoparasitic, immunologic, endocrine, hereditary, nutritional, environmental, metabolic, and neoplastic skin diseases seen in human beings have been documented. In addition, diseases without apparent counterparts in human medicine have been identified.

Certain categories of skin diseases are more important than others in both large and small animal dermatology based on their frequency of occurrence and severity. Globally, ectoparasitic skin diseases are of paramount importance.

In addition, substantial morbidity or mortality is associated with bacterial and fungal skin diseases.

Ectoparasitic Skin Diseases

Ectoparasites as a group are responsible for a wide variety of diverse skin diseases seen in all common species of domestic animals.[1,2,12] Viewed as a whole on a global basis, ectoparasitic skin diseases are the *most* important cause of morbidity in domestic animals. In small animal dermatology, canine flea allergy dermatitis is not only the most common canine skin disease on a worldwide basis but also the most common small animal disease affecting any organ system in much of the world (Fig. 19.1).

The magnitude of skin disease varies considerably from parasite to parasite and host to host. Animal irritability and annoyance associated with pruritus or pain also is highly variable. The effect of a solitary insect or arthropod may be mild and localized or a

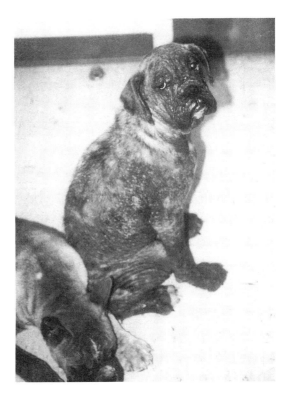

FIGURE 19.2. Severe generalized demodicosis with secondary deep pyoderma in two Boxer siblings. Note the generalized alopecia and nodular inflammation.

generalized hypersensitivity may occur. Other ectoparasitic skin diseases can cause severe generalized reactions and even death (Fig. 19.2). Secondary bacterial infection is a common sequelae to deeper penetration by ectoparasites. Local or systemic reactions can occur secondary to toxin injection as in the case with ticks and some spiders. Parasitic fly larvae can hatch from eggs laid in a wound and invade living tissue, causing extensive tissue necrosis.

The economic burden of ectoparasitic skin diseases is more readily quantifiable for food animals. Weight loss due to decreased food intake, diminished milk production, hide damage, wool loss, transmission of other diseases, and even death may be the direct results of ectoparasites. The cost of disease prevention programs, diagnostic testing, and therapy is substantial. Ectoparasites also can act as vectors or intermediate hosts for a variety of organisms including helminths, viruses, bacteria, fungi, protozoans, and rickettsia.

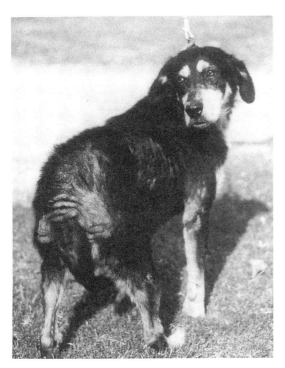

FIGURE 19.1. Chronic flea allergy dermatitis in a dog. Note the symmetric alopecia with lichenification and hyperpigmentation in the dorsal lumbosacral region.

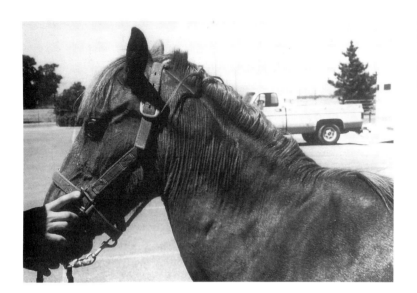

FIGURE 19.3. Culicoides hypersensitivity in an adult pony. The folding and thickening on the neck is due to chronic inflammation.

Important ectoparasites include mites (sarcoptes, notoedres, demodex, cheyletiella, psoroptes, chorioptes, psorergates, and otodectes), chiggers, ticks (soft and hard ticks, spinose ear ticks), spiders (black widow, brown widow, brown recluse), lice (biting and sucking), keds, fleas, biting flies [mosquitoes, culicoides (Fig. 19.3), black flies, horse flies, stable fly, horn flies, face fly], nonbiting flies (bots, hypoderma, blow fly, screw worm, cuterebra), bees, wasps, hornets, and helminths, such as pinworms, pelodera, habronema, onchocerca, stephanofilaria, parafilaria, dirofilaria, paralaphostrongylus, and hookworms.[1,2,12]

Bacterial Skin Diseases

Bacteria cause a wide variety of skin diseases in many species of domestic animals.[1,2,4,5,13–16] Relative importance varies considerably between different domestic species and with the degree of animal husbandry practiced. The economic loss due to bacterial skin diseases in large animals can be substantial. Abscesses and dermatophilosis (Fig. 19.4) in many large animal species and exudative epidermitis in pigs are common bacterial diseases of the skin and subcutaneous tissue. Exudative epidermitis of

pigs is of major economic importance in many parts of the world. Encouraging preventative research in bacterial interference (exudative epidermitis) and vaccination (dermatophilosis, fleece rot, and footrot) holds great promise in the future.[17–22] Bacterial infection of the skin (pyoderma) in dogs is the second most common canine skin disease worldwide (Figs. 19.5 and 19.6). Feline bite wound abscesses are among the most common feline diseases.

There is considerable variation in severity; bacterial skin diseases can be annoying, pruritic, painful, or life threatening. Bacterial skin disease can by primary or secondary to skin damage associated with trauma or other diseases such as ectoparasitism.[1,2,4,5]

Important bacterial skin diseases in domestic animals may be most efficiently grouped with respect to the causative organism, or group of organisms. *Staphylococcus* sp. is the causative agent in canine pyoderma, exudative epidermitis in pigs, and bacterial folliculitis in horses.[1,2,5] Feline abscesses are caused by a variety of organisms including *Pasteurella multocida*, beta hemolytic streptococci, fusiform bacilli, and *Bacteriodes* sp.[1] *Mycobacterium* sp. are the causative agents of feline opportunistic mycobacteriosis, feline leprosy, and opportunistic

FIGURE 19.4. Dermatophilosis in a horse. Alopecia and crusting are localized to the dorsal back. Courtesy of A. A. Stannard, Davis, CA.

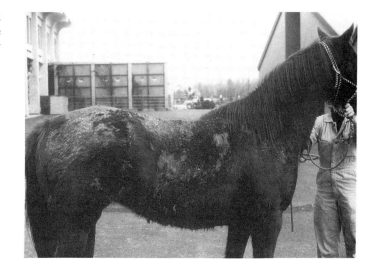

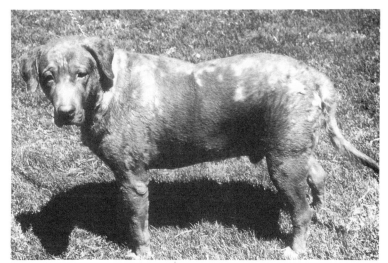

FIGURE 19.5. Superficial folliculitis in a Chesapeake Bay Retriever secondary to hypothyroidism. Moth-eaten alopecia is the most obvious clinical sign of the folliculitis.

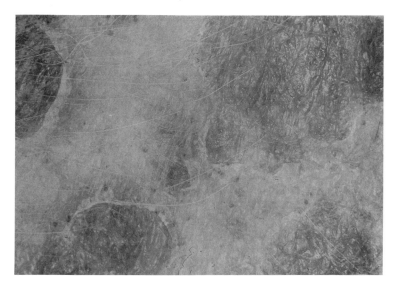

FIGURE 19.6. Superficial spreading pyoderma in a Springer Spaniel. Peripheral collarettes surround areas of severe erythema.

mycobacteriosis in cattle.[1,2,5] Subcutaneous abscesses in horses, ulcerative lymphangitis in horses and cattle, and caseous lymphadenitis in sheep and goats are caused by *Corynebacterium pseudotuberculosis*.[2,13,16] Various actinomycetes cause dermatophilosis in horses, cattle, sheep, and goats; actinomycosis (lumpy jaw) in cattle, actinobacillosis (big head) in cattle, nocardiosis in horses and cattle, and actinomycosis and nocardiosis in dogs.[1,2,6] Important clostridial infections include malignant edema (gas gangrene) and blackleg in cattle, sheep, horses, and pigs, and "bighead" in sheep and goats.[2,13]

Fungal Skin Diseases

Fungal skin diseases although common are frequently overdiagnosed in veterinary medicine.[1,2,5] Infections may be superficial (dermatophytosis), subcutaneous, or systemic with cutaneous involvement.[1,2,4,5,23–26]

Dermatophytosis is common in domestic animals worldwide (Figs. 19.7 and 19.8).[1,2,5] Wide variations in incidence exist globally as warm temperatures and high humidity encourage infection. The most commonly isolated species include *Microsporum canis* (cat, dog), *Trichophyton mentagrophytes* (dog, cow, goat, sheep, horse), *Microsporum gypseum* (dog, horse), *Trichophyton equinum* (horse), *Trichophyton verrucosum* (cow), and *Microsporum nanum*

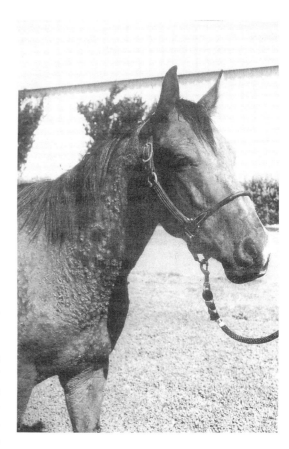

FIGURE 19.8. Generalized dermatophytosis due to *Trichophyton equinum* in a horse. Focal, alopecic nodular lesions are present.

(pig).[1,2,5] Feline dermatophytosis is the most common zoonotic skin disease.

Histoplasmosis, blastomycosis, and coccidioidomycosis are systemic mycoses that occasionally disseminate secondarily to the skin in a variety of species of domestic animals. The organisms (*Histoplasma capsulatum*, *Blastomyces dermatitidis*, and *Coccidioides immitis*) invade the normal immunocompetent host, usually via inhalation.[27–30] The dog is a natural host for systemic mycoses. The systemic mycoses are regional dermatoses with geographic restrictions to endemic areas. Cryptococcosis is uncommon to rare systemic mycoses caused by the encapsulated yeastlike fungus, *Cryptococcus neoformans* (a ubiquitous saprophyte found in nitrogen-rich debris such as pigeon droppings). The organism is an opportunist seen in association with coexistent debilitating or

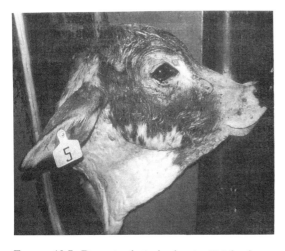

FIGURE 19.7. Dermatophytosis due to *Trichophyton verrucosum* in a dairy cow. Thickening and crusting is marked in bovine dermatophytosis.

immunosuppressive diseases.[1,31] Skin infection caused by other opportunistic fungi and algae are rare in most species of domestic animals.[4,32]

Sporotrichosis is an uncommon fungal disease of domestic animals caused by the dimorphic fungus, *Sporothrix schenkii.*[1,2] The organism is worldwide in distribution. Feline sporotrichosis exhibits large numbers of organisms in draining fluids and tissue. Consequently, extreme caution must be exercised as cats with sporotrichosis may more readily infect humans.[33,34]

Selected Skin Diseases

Dermatophilosis is the most common bacterial skin disease of large animals in much of the world. Horses, cattle, sheep, and goats are most commonly affected.[2,16,20] Because previous skin damage and moisture are marked predisposing factors, dermatophilosis is of greatest importance in tropical and subtropical regions of the world with heavy rainfall where ectoparasite control is problematic.

Flea allergy dermatitis is the most common canine skin disease on a worldwide basis.[1,4,5,9,10,35,36] In North Africa, it has been estimated to represent in excess of one-third of the total caseload in small animal practice.[8] Flea allergy dermatitis was the most commonly diagnosed skin disease at 16 of 17 North American veterinary schools surveyed and represented 34% of all diagnosed canine skin disease.[6] Hypersensitivity to flea bites is uncommon only in environments where temperature, humidity, and altitude preclude maintenance of the life cycle of the flea.

Solar induction of preneoplastic changes and skin tumors is seen in domestic animals.[1,2,5] Actinic keratoses, actinic comedones, and solar-induced squamous cell carcinomas, hemangiomas, and hemangiosarcomas should be seen with greater frequency in regions of the world receiving greater solar irradiation.

Nutritional skin diseases are uncommon in regions of the world where animals are fed either good-quality food formulated for a specific species or a balanced diet prepared for human consumption. A variety of nutritional skin diseases are reported when animals receive suboptimal nutrition.[1,2] Exfoliative skin diseases have been documented in various species of domestic animals receiving rations deficient in zinc or other micronutrients.[1–5] The author has been told by local veterinarians in developing and under-developed countries that nutritional skin diseases are much more common in these regions.

Conclusions

Transmissible ectoparasitic skin diseases frequently are more common in tropical and subtropical locales. The incidence of infectious skin diseases such as pyoderma, dermatophytosis, dermatophilosis, and infections with less common bacterial, fungal, and protozoan organisms varies greatly with global region. In general, infectious skin diseases are more common and more severe in regions of the world with elevated humidity and temperature.

The understanding of global variations in veterinary dermatology is in its infancy but will increase as more data are gathered and information is shared through international congresses and cooperating regional organizations. Combining this knowledge with information from human medicine should allow a better understanding of the processes of disease and the impact of such factors as climate, geography, genetics, and culture on disease in humans and domestic and nondomestic animals.

References

1. Muller GH, Kirk RW, Scott DW: Small Animal Dermatology, 4th ed. Philadelphia: WB Saunders, 1989:1–1007.
2. Scott DW: Large Animal Dermatology. Philadelphia: WB Saunders, 1988:1–487.
3. Von Tscharner C, Halliwell REW, eds., Advances in Veterinary Dermatology. London: Bailliere Tindall, 1990:1–500.
4. Willemse T: Clinical Dermatology of Dogs and Cats: A Guide to Diagnosis and Therapy. Philadelphia: Lea & Febiger, 1991:1–141.
5. Gross TL, Ihrke PJ, Walder EJ: Veterinary Dermatopathology: A Macroscopic and Microscopic Evaluation of Canine and Feline Skin Disease. St. Louis: Mosby-Yearbook, 1992.

6. Sischo WM, Ihrke PJ, Franti CE: Regional distribution of ten common skin diseases in dogs. *J Am Vet Med Assoc* 1989;**195**:752–756.

7. Kral F, Novak BJ: Veterinary Dermatology. Philadelphia: JB Lippincott, 1953:viii–ix.

8. Schwartzman RM, Orkin MA: A Comparative Study of Skin Disease in Dogs and Man. Springfield, MA: Charles C. Thomas, 1982:5–7.

9. Halliwell REW: Flea B Dermatitis. *Compend Contin Educ Pract Vet* 1979;**1**: 367–371.

10. Kwochka KW, Bevier DE: Flea dermatitis. In: Nesbitt GW, ed. Dermatology. New York: Churchill Livingstone, 1987:21–55.

11. Ihrke PJ, Franti CE. Breed as a risk factor associated with skin diseases in dogs seen in northern California. *Calif Vet* 1985; **39**(5):13–16.

12. Fadok VA: Parasitic skin diseases of large animals. *Vet Clin North Am* (*Large Anim Pract*) 1984;**6**(1):3–26.

13. Pascoe RR: Infectious skin diseases of horses. *Vet Clin North Am* (*Large Anim Pract*) 1984;**6**(1): 27–46.

14. Mullowney PC, Hall RF: Skin diseases of swine. *Vet Clin North Am* (*Large Anim Pract*) 1984;**6**(1): 107–129.

15. Mullowney PC: Skin diseases of sheep. *Vet Clin North Am* (*Large Anim Pract*) 1984;**6**(1):131–142.

16. Hunt E: Infectious skin diseases of cattle. *Vet Clin North Am* (*Large Anim Pract*) 1984;**6**(1):155–174.

17. Allaker RP, Lloyd DH, Lamport AI: Bacterial interference in the control of exudative epidermitis of pigs. In: Tscharner CV, Halliwell REW, eds. Advances in Veterinary Dermatology. London: Bailliere Tindall, 1990:327–334.

18. Allaker RP, Lloyd DH, Smith IM: Prevention of exudative epidermitis in gnotobiotic piglets by bacterial interference. *Vet Rec* 1988;**123**:597–598.

19. How SJ, Lloyd DH, Sanders AB: *Dermatophilus congolensis* infection in ruminants: Prospects for control. In: Tscharner CV, Halliwell REW, eds. Advances in Veterinary Dermatology. London: Bailliere Tindall, 1990:465.

20. Barre N, Woodman S: Workshop on dermatophilus. In: Tscharner CV, Halliwell REW, eds. Advances in Veterinary Dermatology. London: Bailliere Tindall, 1990:407–411.

21. Burrell DH: The bacteriology and pathogenesis of fleece rot and associated myiasis; Control of these diseases with *Pseudomonas aeruginosa* vaccines. In: Tscharner CV, Halliwell REW, eds. Advances in Veterinary Dermatology. London: Bailliere Tindall, 1990:347–358.

22. Stewart DJ, Kortt AA, Lilley GG: New approaches to footrot vaccination and diagnosis utilizing the proteases of *Bacteriodes nodosus.* In: Tscharner CV, Halliwell REW, eds. Advances in Veterinary Dermatology. London: Bailliere Tindall, 1990:359–369.

23. Foil CS: Cutaneous fungal diseases. In: Nesbitt GH, ed. Dermatology: Contemporary Issues in Small Animal Practice. New York: Churchill Livingstone, 1987:146–155.

24. Foil CS: Dermatophytosis. In: Greene CE, ed. Infectious Diseases of the Dog and Cat. Philadelphia: WB Saunders, 1990:659–668.

25. Moriello KA: Management of dermatophyte infections in catteries and multiple-cat households. *Vet Clin North Am* (*Large Anim Pract*) 1990;**20**:1457–1474.

26. Blackford J: Superficial and deep mycoses of horses. *Vet Clin North Am* (*Large Anim Pract*) 1984;**6**(1):47–58.

27. Selby LA, Becker SV, Hayes HW: Epidemiologic risk factors associated with canine systemic mycoses. *Am J Epidemiol* 1991;**113**:133–139.

28. Wolf AM: Histoplasmosis. In: Greene CE, ed. Infectious Diseases of the Dog and Cat. Philadelphia: WB Saunders, 1990:679–686.

29. Legendre AM: Blastomycosis. In: Greene CE, ed. Infectious Diseases of the Dog and Cat. Philadelphia: WB Saunders, 1990:669–678.

30. Barsanti JA, Jeffery KL: Coccidioidomycosis. In: Greene CE, ed. Infectious Diseases of the Dog and Cat. Philadelphia: WB Saunders, 1990:696–706.

31. Medleau L, Barsanti JA: Cryptococcosis. In: Greene CE, ed. Infectious Diseases of the Dog and Cat. Philadelphia: WB Saunders, 1990:687–695.

32. Foil CS: Miscellaneous fungal infections. In: Greene CE, ed. Infectious Diseases of the Dog and Cat. Philadelphia: WB Saunders, 1990: 731–741.

33. Dunstan RW, Reimann KA, Langham RF: Feline sporotrichosis. *J Am Vet Med Assoc* 1986;**189**: 880–883.

34. Rosser EJ, Dunstan RW: Sporotrichosis. In: Greene CE, ed. Infectious Diseases of the Dog and Cat. Philadelphia: WB Saunders, 1990:707–710.

35. Nesbitt GH, Schmitz JA: Fleabite allergic dermatitis: A review and survey of 330 cases. *J Am Vet Med Assoc* 1978;**173**:282–288.

36. Halliwell REW, Gorman NT: Veterinary clinical immunology. Philadelphia: WB Saunders, 1989: 264–267.

Part IV
Anthropologic Dermatology

20

Comments

Sidney N. Klaus

Anthropology—physical and cultural—is the study of biological diversity. Because global dermatology is concerned with patterns of dermatologic disease among diverse peoples in all parts of the world, the importance of an anthropologic approach in studies related to global dermatology cannot be underestimated. We know, of course, that certain features of human skin differ among ethnic groups, that these features have been influenced by the evolutionary process, and that genetic differences between ethnic groups have a profound influence on many types of inherited skin disorders. But up to now, we have paid scant attention to other types of ethically related differences; for example, differences involving climate, nutrition, religious practices, ethical beliefs, medical lore, and local customs (such as those related to child rearing, dress, hygiene, etc.). We are now learning that all of these differences may have a profound effect on the prevalence and appearance of skin lesions. By carefully observing and recording the patterns of skin disease from diverse locations around the globe, we are beginning to recognize more clearly the role of ethnic influences. In the near future, using this approach, we may be able to illuminate more exactly not only the role of inheritance but also the role played by toxins, pollutants, and infectious agents in dermatologic disease. In addition, we should be able to develop new insights into how the diseases themselves evolved.

Of course, "anthropologic dermatology" is a relatively new discipline, and further developments are expected. I am certain that new and more exacting types of analyses will be developed, along with more precise definitions of what constitutes a "people."

The current decade (the 1990s) has witnessed a wave of political self-determination, unprecedented since the 1920s, and many groups with common cultural and religious values, and with shared ethnicity, are now seeking political autonomy. This trend, if it continues, is bound to impact on the patterns of skin disease in the same way that the patterns were altered by famines, forced population migrations, and the great world wars.

The chapters in this section are focused on skin diseases found among five ethnically diverse peoples: Arabs, Australian aborigines, blacks, Jews, and native Americans. As we pay more attention to the role of physical and cultural anthropology and as we refine the methods for analyzing these roles, we can anticipate that the benefits of viewing skin diseases from this perspective will also continue to grow.

21

Diseases Among Arab People

Mohamed Amer

The wide geographic variation in the incidence of skin diseases presumably is influenced by social, ethnological, climatic, socioeconomic, and environmental factors. Arab countries are located in Asia and Africa and share nearly the same climate and environmental factors. These countries differ to an extent in their socioeconomic state and certain habits that may lead to variations in their pattern of skin diseases. They are included in the group of countries collectively known as developing countries.

Socioeconomic State

The picture of skin diseases in developing countries mirrors to a great extent the socioeconomic state in these countries. Skin infection and parasitic infestations dominate the clinical picture due to the poor socioeconomic situation in Africa, Asia, and South and Central America. Approximately 12 million people are still suffering from leprosy, which is a most fascinating disease with its great variations in clinical and immunological manifestations. Up to now, this disease has not been under control and the number of patients suffering from leprosy has not been reduced in the developing countries. This is closely associated with socioeconomic underdevelopment.[1]

The incidence of skin diseases in the United Arab Emirates (UAE) constitutes 9.3% of the total number of patients attending the outpatient clinic departments during a period of 2 years.[2] It is almost similar to that reported in Scotland[3] and Bristol,[4] where it was 8.3% and 10.5% respectively, whereas a much higher incidence was reported from Calcutta, India (20%).[5] This not only reflects the influence of climate but also the effects of socioeconomic and environmental factors. It is known that in developing countries the majority of the population belongs to the low-income group, with inadequate hygienic environments, poor nutritional standards, and insufficient facilities for healthy living. This explains the low incidence of bacterial and superficial fungal infections in countries with high standards of living, such as the UAE, which plays a major role in limiting chances for spread of infections regardless of climate, as illustrated in Table 21.1.

Amer,[6] in a 1-year survey on the pattern of skin diseases in Sharkia (a governorate in Egypt), showed that skin infections were the most common skin diseases. He concluded that socioeconomic standards rather than climatic factors seem to be responsible for the pattern of skin diseases. This was confirmed in a similar survey done by Amer et al. in 1987.[7]

Decreased incidence of certain infectious diseases may suggest slight improvement of family and personal hygiene; however, this improvement is not significant and socioeconomic conditions are still playing the most important role in the high incidence of these infections. The group of eczemas (dermatitis) was the most common noninfectious skin diseases. Lack of modern in-house equipment and certain occupations as well may be a factor

TABLE 21.1. Comparative incidence in percentage of common dermatoses among different countries.

Skin diseases	Ethiopia	Zambia	UK	Mexico	India	UAE
Eczema	23.0	14.7	35.6	8–12	15–20	20.98
Acne vulgaris	5.0	2.1	5.6	3	3.5	9.07
Superficial mycosis	7.8	10.8	3.2	13	15–20	8.5
Pyoderma	7.1	20.3	4.6	6.5	30–40	2.55

Source: After Ref. 2.

of importance responsible for the high incidence of contact dermatitis.

Mycoses constitute public health and economic problems, and are common in tropical countries. In the past decade, the World Health Organization has acknowledged the importance of mycoses as an important sociomedical problem. Dermatophytoses are, therefore, encountered frequently in the tropics and subtropics where, in addition to poverty and inadequate hygiene, warmth and humidity favor the growth of fungi.

Environment

Certain general aspects of particular epidemiologic, clinical prophylactic, and therapeutic importance must be underlined. For example, the incidence of fungal infections has increased considerably in the last decades, whereas that of bacterial infections has decreased. Greater cases of travel, working in the tropics and other areas where certain skin diseases are endemic, wars, promiscuity in large urban centers, and the incorrect use of pharmaceutical substances are all factors that explain the changes of the epidemiologic map of fungal infections in all continents as well as the increasingly frequent modifications in their clinical manifestations and their increased resistance to topical therapy alone.[8]

Dermatophytoses are encountered frequently in the tropics where, in addition to poverty and inadequate hygiene, warmth and humidity favor the growth of fungi. The species of dermatophytes encountered in the tropics (arranged in order of decreasing occurrence) include: *Trichopytoa violaceum, Microsporum audouinii, T. soudanense, M. ferrugineum, M. canis, T. rubrum, T. tonsurans, T. schoenleinii, T. mentagrophytes,* and *Epidermophyton floccosum.*[9] Geographical distribution of the principal causes of scalp ringworm (*Tinea capitis*), *Tinea corporis,* and *Tinea pedis* are indicated in Table 21.2.

TABLE 21.2. Geographical distribution of dermatophytes.

Clinical variety	Africa	Asia	South America
T. capitis	*T. violaceum*	*T. violaceum*	*T. tonsurans*
	T. audouini	*M. canis*	*M. canis*
	T. ferrugineum	*M. ferrugineum*	
	T. soudanense	*T. schoenleinii*	
T. corporis	*T. soudanense*	*T. rubrum*	*M. canis*
	T. ferrugineum	*M. canis*	*T. rubrum*
	M. canis	*T. mentagrophytes*	*T. tonsurans*
	T. rubrum		
	T. mentagrophytes		
T. pedis	*T. rubrum*	*T. rubrum*	
	T. mentagrophytes	*T. mentagrophytes*	*T. rubrum*

Source: After Ref. 10.

In a study done in the UAE, *M. canis* was by far the most common organism isolated (68.8%). *T. mentagrophytes* was the next most common organism found (9.4%). Another zoophilic species, *T. verrucosum*, was isolated in a percentage of 3%. Cats are common in the locality; dogs, for religious reasons, are not approved of as domestic animals. Pet rabbits would appear to have been the source of *M. canis* infection, whereas camels may be a reservoir for some zoophilic species because many inhabitants keep camels, which are valued for their milk and for racing purposes. *T. violaceum* is the most common causative agent of *T. capitis* in India (54.7%) as reported by Khosa et al.[12] and in Egypt (52%) as reported by Amer et al.[13] This may explain the frequent isolation of *T. violaceum* in the UAE during the last 2 years where there are large expatriate Indian and Egyptian communities in the UAE.

In Kuwait, dermatophytoses are most frequently found in children under 10 years of age. *Tinea capitis* is the form most often represented clinically (71%) and is caused by *M. canis* in 76% of cases. This agent accounts for 60.7% of all dermatophytoses.[14] In Greece and at the other extreme of the Mediterranean, in Spain, there has been an almost identical picture in the reduction of anthropophilic and an increase in the zoophilic dermatophytes.[15]

Reports on deep mycoses as an imported pathology are increasingly frequent outside their endemic area. Chromonycosis was a particularly diffuse subcutaneous mycosis in Latin America and Africa and that sporotrichosis, particularly the pulmonary form, was typical of temperate and tropical regions with a high incidence in Mexico.[16]

There is no doubt that psoriasis is multifactorial in origin in that both genetic and environmental factors play important roles. Saudi patients with psoriasis differ from both white Caucasians and Orientals in not showing strong association either with B17 (which is a feature in Caucasians) or B37 and DR7 (which is more frequent in Orientals). This study shows that in psoriasis, the most frequent association in Saudi patients was HLA-CW 6.

A school survey of pediculosis capitis in Ben-ghazi, Libya, revealed an alarmingly high prevalence of 78.6%. It was more frequent in schools located in rural areas (85.55%) than in urban areas (44.28%). Several factors have been suggested for the current high prevalence of head lice including, among others, extensive tourism and reports of resistance of lice to the widely used pediculicides. In addition, the lack of health education of family members may play a crucial role in transference and louse infestation.[18]

Scabies continues to pose a major public health problem and there continues to be considerable morbidity in the current epidemic that began in 1982. The peak of the epidemic, however, appears to have occurred. The epidemiology of the disease is still not entirely clear. The transmission of the disease does not always appear to follow the expected pattern. The occurrence of epidemics probably results from a complex interaction of various factors, including the immune status, behavior of the population, and seasonal factors.[19]

In Egypt, scabies was reported to constitute 93.44% of parasitic skin disease presented at Zagazig University Medical Center, in a 1-year survey.[6] A figure of 87.67% was reported 9 years later (1987) in a similar survey done at the same center.[7] Although the two studies were done during two different epidemics of scabies, these figures may reflect improvement of personal and family hygiene.

The most important cause of failure to cure scabies is intimate contact with untreated cases, as in overcrowded houses, camps, or boarding schools. Improvement of the water supply, sewage disposal, and well-constructed sanitary houses may be a factor in decreasing the incidence of the disease. Conditions of war tend to produce an environment that encourages the spread of the disease (movement of populations, crowding, and deterioration of personal hygiene).

Friedman[20] maintained that in all extended wars, scabies has been a major problem. The two previous pandemics appeared to be associated with the world wars. This may, in part, explain the decrease of the incidence of scabies in 1987 following the cessation of the Egypto-Israeli state of war (1948–1973).

Geographic Locations

A group of diseases can be named after a place for various reasons. The disease can be endemic in the area after which it is named, or it can be a condition that was described in a particular location but whose geographic distribution extends beyond that location.[21] For example, Baghdad boil or Oriental sore, an ulcerating nodule and a form of cutaneous leishmaniasis, was discovered in Baghdad, the capital of Iraq. In addition, it is present in Africa, the Middle East, and northwest India. Another example is Dum-Dum fever or Kala-Azar, visceral leishmaniasis which was discovered in Dum-Dum, a town in India. It is also present in Africa, the Mediterranean coast, and Latin America.[22]

Ebola virus disease is a disease that was discovered in Ebola, a river in Zaire. It is characterized by severe hemorrhagic illness with maculopapular eruption, ulcerative enanthem, cough, and chest pain with an etiologic agent closely related to Marburg virus. It also occurs in Sudan.[23]

Familial Mediterranean fever is a genetic disorder affecting predominantly Jews, Arabs, Turks, and Armenians, especially those from the Middle East and North African countries that enclose the Mediterranean Sea. It is characterized by episodic fever and an erysipelaslike eruption on the lower extremities.[24]

Sowda is the name given to onchocerciasis endemic in Yemen and southern Saudi Arabia. In contrast to the generalized symmetrical type of onchocercal dermatitis in Africa, Sowda is a localized type, limited with striking asymmetry to one limb, rarely involving both legs.[25] The name Sowda, meaning black in Arabic, describes the clinical presentation of a dark hyperpigmented lichenified lesion. The fact that only one limb is involved and the parasitic load is very small can be explained on the basis of immunological studies done on other strains of *onchocerca volvulus*. Immune mechanisms keep the population of microfilaria small and restrict their migration.[26]

Selim et al.[27] reported that there was a sudden outbreak of a pruritic eruption in patients reporting to the skin clinics in Kuwait. The cause was suspected to be a new invader previously not known to attack humans. Arthrop is a hemipteran insect, which usually feeds on plant saps called *Leptodemus minutus*. The clinical presentations were unusual for both patients and physicians. The lesions were sometimes severe and the patients gave no clue to the history of exposure to insects, probably because such an eruption may follow the insult 24–48 h later. The persistence of some lesions and the poor response to steroids added more to the diagnostic confusion. The distribution of lesions over the site of exposure to insect bite and the isolation of the causative factor, which was identified as *Leptodemus minutus*, can help in the diagnosis.

Guineaworm was discovered in Guinea, a country in western Africa. It is common in India and the Middle East, especially in Saudi Arabia. It is a chronic infestation caused by *Dracuncula medinensis* (after Medina in Saudi Arabia) with the presence of a worm under the skin. It causes intense inflammation that subsides when the worm penetrates the skin and discharges larvae.[22]

Immigration

Some countries have experienced large-scale immigration. There are many socioeconomic differences between the majority population and such immigrant communities. Most of the immigrant groups are poorer and have moved to find work. There are generally widely different cultural backgrounds. There may be different religious allegiances and differences of skin color also. There is often poor communication between the majority population and newer ethnic groups. It is clear from common experience that there are disease differences between immigrant groups and the majority population, most notably "imported" infectious diseases such as tuberculosis and leprosy.[28] There has been little attempt to quantify or qualify this in the dermatologic field.

One study done by Mahmoud and Ben Azadeh[29] in Qatar showed that leprosy is not endemic in this country, and as in some other parts of that world, it occurs almost exclusively in expatriate workers coming from the endemic areas such as India, which represent the main source of transmission of leprosy. Out of 104 proven leprosy cases, 103 were expatriates and only 1 patient was a Qatari. Indian expatriates formed the largest group (60.6%), followed by Bangladeshi (6.7%) and Pakistani (5.8%). Some of the patients were not diagnosed on their arrival and were incubating the disease; it appeared later during their residence in Qatar, thus forming a potential public health hazard. Hence, there is a need both for periodic expatriate checkups, especially for those coming from endemic countries, and for periodic examination of children who are in contact with expatriate domestic helpers.

The number of leprosy patients among the Saudi population in the eastern province suggests the extreme rarity of this disease in this part of the world. There were 114 non-Saudi patients detected, suggesting a serious problem in the eastern province due to imported leprosy. Most of these people came from areas with a high endemicity of leprosy. The Saudi population has unusual age and sex structure (more men than women and predominantly aged 20–50 years). The male population is more exposed to leprosy because it is much more mobile and exposed to the external environment than women, who may also be protected from droplet infection by the masks with which they cover their faces. Tuberculoid lesions (TT) were significantly more common among the Saudis than the non-Saudis. Imported leprosy is a significant threat to this country. Active case finding and treatment of positive cases appear to be rewarding in the control of leprosy, but the management of leprosy in foreign workers while they are living in Saudi Arabia is still a controversial matter.[30]

During the last decade, all forms of leishmaniasis have been more prevalent than had been suspected. Improved health care coverage has accounted for more frequent diagnoses. Better communication and reporting systems have contributed to an apparent increase in the number of cases. There is no doubt that there also has been a real increase in both prevalence and geographic distribution, primarily resulting from the opening of forest lands to new agricultural development. Population pressures throughout the world and in the Arab countries,

are pushing humans into new lands where the infection is endemic and, thus, are bringing many more humans into contact with the natural vectors. This results in the increased infection rates.[31]

References

1. Lommolt G: Conditions for dermatological treatment in a developing country. *Int J Dermatol* 1990;**29**:511–514.
2. Abushare'ah AM, Abdel Dayem H: The incidence of skin of diseases in Abu Dhabi (United Arab Emirates). *Int J Dermatol* 1991;**30**:121–124.
3. Ratzer MA: Incidence of skin diseases in the west of Scotland. *Br J Dermatol* 1969;**81**:456–461.
4. Warin RP: The incidence of skin diseases in man. In: Rook AJ, Walton GS, eds. Comparative Physiology and Pathology of the Skin. Philadelphia: FA Davis, 1965:21–32.
5. Banerjee BN, Datta AK: Prevalence and incidence pattern of skin diseases in Calcutta. *Int J Dermatol* 1973;**12**:41–47.
6. Amer MA: Pattern of skin diseases in Sharkia Governorate. Proceeding of the first Ain Shams Medical Congress. *Ain Shams Med J* 1977;5–77.
7. Amer MA, El-Garf AK, Salem AA, et al: Incidence of common skin diseases in Sharkia during 1989. A comparative study with the same skin diseases during 1976. *N Egypt J Med* 1989;**3**:1863–1868.
8. Binazzi M, Papini M, Simonetti S: Skin mycoses—geographic distribution and present-day pathomorphosis. *Int J Dermatol* 1983;**2**:92–97.
9. Philpot CM: Geographical distribution of the dermatophytes. A review. *J Hyg Camb* 1978;**80**:301.
10. Mahgoub El-S, ed: Dermatophytosis in Tropical Mycoses. Janssen Research Council, 1989:9–24.
11. Lestringant GG, Qayed K, Blayney B: Tinea capitis in the United Arab Emirates. *Int J Dermatol* 1991;**30**:127–129.
12. Khosa RK, Girgla HS, Hajini GH, et al: Study of dermatomycoses (in India). *Int J Dermatol* 1981;**20**:130–132.
13. Amer M, Taha M, Tosson Z, et al: Frequency of causative dermatophytes in Egypt. *Int J Dermatol* 1981;**20**:431–434.
14. Karaoui R, Selim M, Mousa A: Incidence of dermatophytosis in Kuwait. *Sabouraudia* 1979;**17**:131.
15. Marcelou-Kinti O, Papa geogroiu S, Papa

vassiliou I, Capetanakis L: Los dermatofitosy su ecologia en Grecia. *Dermatol Rev Mex* 1973; **17**:184.

16. Beneke ES: Geographic distribution and epidemiology of mycoses. *Mykosen Suppl* 1978;**I**:17.

17. Al-Sogair SM, Rahi A, Mathur M, et al: Histocompatibility antigen (HLA) and psoriasis in Saudi Arabia. *J Pan-Arab League Dermatol* 1990;**1**:11–14.

18. Bharija SM, Kanwar AJ, Singh G, Belhaj MS: Pediculosis capitis in Benghazi, Libya, A school survey. *Int J Dermatol* 1988;**27**:165–166.

19. Kimchi N, Green MS, David S: Epidemiologic characteristic of scabies in the Israel Defence Force. *Int J Dermatol* 1989;**28**:180–182.

20. Friedman R: The Story of Scabies, Vol. 1. New York: Froben Press, 1947:1–3.

21. Lin AN, Imaeda S: A dermatologic Gazetteer. *Int J Dermatol* 1990;**7**:468–417.

22. Beaver PC, Jung RC, Cupp EW: Clinical Parasitology. Philadelphia: Lea & Febiger, 1984:70–77, 335–367.

23. Manson-Bahr PEC, Apted FIC: Manson's Tropical Diseases. London: Balliere, Tindall, 1982:288, 453–483.

24. Eliakim M, Rechmilewit AM: Recurrent polyserositis (familial Mediterranean fever, periodic disease). In: Weatherall DJ, Ledingham JGG, Warrell DA, eds. Oxford Text Book of Medicine. Oxford, Oxford Univ Press 1987:24.4–24.6.

25. Connor, DH, Gibson DW, Taylor HR, et al: Onchocerciasis. In: Strickland GT, ed. Hunter's Textbook of Tropical Medicine. Philadelphia: WB Saunders, 1984:667–680.

26. Yarzabal L: Immunology of onchocerciasis. *Int J Dermatol* 1985;**24**:349–358.

27. Selim MM, Dvorak R, Khalifa T, et al: Insect bite lesion in Kuwait. Possibly due to leptodemus minutus. *Int J Dermatol* 1990;**29**:507–510.

28. Jackson SIID, Bannan LT, Beevers DG: Ethnic differences in respiratory diseases. *Postgrad Med J* 1981;**57**:777–778.

29. Mahmoud SF, Ben Azadeh: Leprosy in Qatar. *Int J Dermatol* 1991;**30**:125–126.

30. Al-Sogiar SM, Ellahbadi SL, Namnyak SS: Leprosy in the eastern province of Saudi Arabia. *Saudi Med J* 1989;**10**:48–53.

31. World Health Organization. The Leishmaniases. Technical Report Series 701. Geneva: World Health Organization, 1984:1–140.

22

Diseases Among Australian Aborigines

Allen C. Green

The Australian Population

In December 1991, the Australian population was about 17.35 million. It is cosmopolitan and multicultural.

The indigenous people are the Australian and Tasmanian Aborigines and the Torres Strait Islanders. They are distinct racial and cultural groups and live in separate geographic areas. In 1986, they numbered 227,465, about 1.45% of the population. The numbers of full-bloods and of mixed race were not given.[1]

The non-Aboriginal population is mainly Caucasian and white. Nowadays, besides the people born there, others and their descendents have come from Britain, European countries especially Greece and Italy, the Middle East, Southeast Asia and India, the Americas, and some from Africa. The majority live in the capital cities and in towns along or near the coast on the east, southeast, and southwest of Australia.

The genetic inheritances, cultures, environments and lifestyles of the indigenous people show remarkable differences from the non-Aboriginal population. These differences explain many of the diverse patterns of disease found in these two groups. With continuing migration, residents returning from overseas, foreign students, and visitors coming to Australia, exotic diseases need to be considered as diagnostic possibilities.

The Australian Aborigines

For about 40,000 years, the Aborigines lived in isolation from the rest of the world. Before white settlement in 1788, their estimated numbers were around 300,000, divided into about 500 tribes of 100–1500 people with an average of 500–600.[2]

The Aborigines were nomadic hunters and gatherers of food. They lived in temporary camps, made shelters from branches, bark, and bushes, had few and simple possessions, planted no crops, and dogs were the only animals they kept. They had complex concepts of religion, fundamental links with land and all living things, and strict systems of tribal law and behavior.

Many accounts of the Aborigines before, when, and after the "outsiders" came are available. Some are listed and most give additional references.[2-14]

The "Outsiders"

European explorers visited Australia from the sixteenth century onward. Macassans, who fished for trepang and sought other commodities, came to northern Australia from about 1700 to 1906.[15]

The first British soldiers, convicts, and settlers arrived in January 1788 to begin what became Sydney. Later came more convicts, and settlers, inland explorers, pastoralists, squatters, farmers, miners, Christian missionaries, "developers," and others.

The Chinese arrived after the discovery of gold in the 1850s. Kanakas from islands in the southwest Pacific were brought, virtually as slaves, first in 1847 and up to 1901.[12]

Endemic Diseases

The Aborigines were relatively free from disease before the "outsiders" came. Diseases believed to have been endemic include yaws, donovanosis (granuloma inguinale), pediculosis capitis, Q fever in northern Queensland, and trachoma.[15] Wounds apparently healed rapidly and without infection.

Introduced Diseases

Excepting the explorers, the "outsiders" introduced many diseases to the Aborigines.

Dermatophytoses, due to *Trichophyton rubrum* (granular variant), was brought by the Macassans to the Aborigines of tropical, high rainfall, coastal, northern Australia. In about 20 Aboriginal languages spoken in this region the words for ringworm are based on the old Macassarese word for ringworm *poera*, nowadays written as *pura'*. Isolates of this dermatophyte from Aborigines in northern Australia and from Macassans in Ujong Pandang in Sulawesi (previously Macassar in the Celebes) were indistinguishable (unpublished personal observations).

Hookworm was probably brought by the Chinese and perhaps by the Macassans and the Kanakas.[5,12]

Smallpox, syphilis, gonorrhea, measles, tuberculosis, other respiratory infections, poliomyelitis, and possibly infections with pyogenic cocci were introduced mainly by Caucasians.

Leprosy is believed to have been introduced to the Aborigines of the Northern Territory by Chinese laborers. They came in relatively large numbers after 1874 when gold was discovered in the Territory. "The Big Sickness" is a name used by some Aborigines for leprosy, which is still endemic. Unlike most people, Aborigines do not ostracize sufferers from this disease.[16,17]

Aboriginal Skin

Knowledge of the normal appearances of the skin, its appendages, and mucous membranes is important in understanding the changes seen in disease.[6] In dark skins, these changes often look different from those seen in light skins and can be confusing to inexperienced observers.

Aborigines, and other dark-skinned people, show several differences from people with light skin. These include color; considerable protection from sun damage, photoaging and skin cancer; liability to keloid and hypertrophic scars (see Fig. 22.1); body odor; and, apparently, a reduced liability to allergic sensitivity reactions.

Patterns of Skin Conditions in Aborigines

Genetically Related

Mongolian spots, single or multiple, are seen in most Aboriginal infants at birth.

Blonde hair is a striking sight in some Aboriginal children in central Australia. Girls may stay fair up to early adult life. In boys, the hair usually darkens about the eighth year. Their fair hair is not due to malnutrition (see Fig. 22.2). Madarosis, mainly in women, and hairy ears in men, affect members of some families.

Gyrate or folded skin on the forehead, and sometimes on the scalp, occurs mainly in men of some families. When well developed, it can suggest the changes seen on the forehead in lepromatous leprosy (see Fig. 22.3). Pseudoacanthosis nigricans occurs in the body folds of most obese Aborigines.

Dermatosis papulosa nigra (DPN) is prevalent in both sexes but more so in women. The condition appears after puberty, usually in the malar regions, and extends over several years

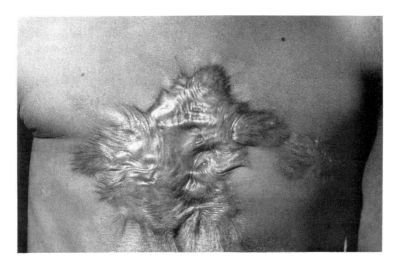

FIGURE 22.1 Keloid after burn in presternal region of a part-Aboriginal boy aged 9.

(see Fig. 22.4). Some Aborigines relate DPN to their "Dreamtime," a time of their spiritual origins. Removal of the lesions may leave hypopigmented areas or keloidal scars.

Albinism has been seen in two related girls, one of whom was reported.[18] Some members of a family with multiple neurofibromatosis and two unrelated individuals with neurofibromas are known to the writer. Pseudo-hermaphroditism was reported in one family.[19]

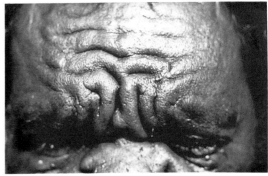

FIGURE 22.3 Gyrate (folded) skin on forehead of adult Aboriginal male.

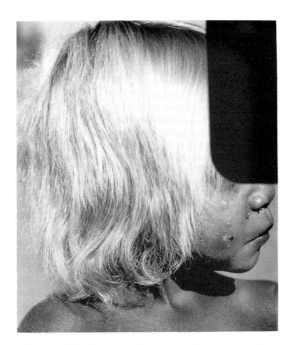

FIGURE 22.2 Blonde hair of an Aboriginal girl in central Australia.

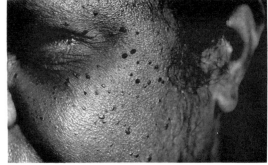

FIGURE 22.4 Dermatosis papulosa nigra and sparse eyebrow in Aboriginal woman.

Developmental Anomalies

Traditionally, Aboriginal infants born with deformities and the weaker of twins were killed or allowed to die. An impression is that developmental anomalies are less common in full-blood Aborigines than in Caucasians.

Common nevi include hyperpigmented and hypopigmented macules and patches, hairy pigmented moles, blue nevi, and, warty, linear epidermal nevi. Other anomalies are accessory thumbs, bifurcated little toes, accessory nipples and areolae, preauricular nodules, and webbed and malformed fingers. Harelips, cleft palates, and pilonidal sinuses occur occasionally. Strawberry and capillary nevi are rarely seen. The latter can be overlooked.

Culturally Related Conditions

Scars and mutilations result from various cultural practices of Aborigines.

Among children and adolescents, examples are burns in patterns on the dorsum of the hands and forearms, usually self-inflicted by adolescent females who think they result in "nice marks" (see Fig. 22.5); in both sexes, tattoos are made with plants and seeds with caustic properties, matches, razor blades, and other means (see Fig. 22.6); application of ochres and decorations used in adult ceremonies; and, pierced ear lobes that may result in a keloidal reaction. At puberty and adolescence and in adults, various tribal practices leave lifelong signs. Circumcision and penile subincision are done by central Australian tribes. Subincision is exteriorization of the urethra to the ventral surface of the penis to make a hypospadias, commonly called "whistle-cock" (see Fig. 22.7).

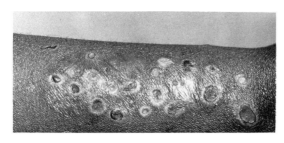

FIGURE 22.5 Self-inflicted burns to make "nice marks" on forearm of an Aboriginal woman aged 19.

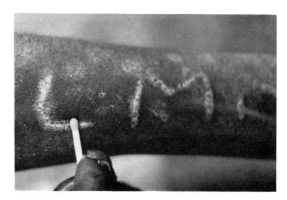

FIGURE 22.6 Self-inflicted tattoo on forearm done by an Aboriginal boy aged 12.

Young men in central Australia consider that they "look good" after an upper incisor has been avulsed. Lacerations on the chest, upper abdominal wall, and upper arms, usually filled with ashes and ochres to encourage keloidal scars, were of traditional tribal significance. Such lacerations are now less often seen (see Fig. 22.8).

Western-style tattoos, usually crudely done, are seen in both sexes. In men, such tattoos are often done when in jail. "Sorry-cuts" are wounds that are self-inflicted at the time of death or burial of a relative or friend. Women beat their scalp with a stone, club, bottle, or some other blunt instrument. An area of alopecia on the vertex with scarring often results. Men make deep cuts on the lateral surface of the arms or thighs (see Figs. 22.9 and 22.10).

Scars result from fire, spears, clubs, knives, and injuries made by other means to punish offenders for tribal transgressions. Venesection produces blood needed for ceremonial purposes. Scars and fibrous nodules over veins, usually in the forearm, are seen in some elderly males.

Aboriginal Environments

The majority of full-blood Aborigines live in remote parts of Australia on settlements, church missions, cattle stations, or in bush camps. Some live in, or on the fringes of, small towns. Part-Aborigines tend to live in localized areas

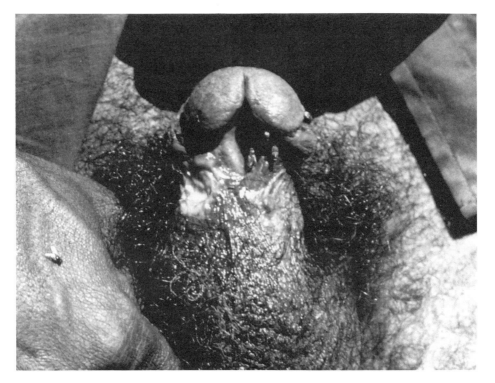

FIGURE 22.7 Subincised penis and primary chancre to right of the midline.

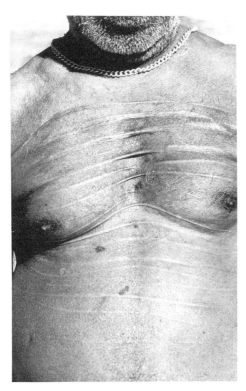

FIGURE 22.8 Traditional tribal scars.

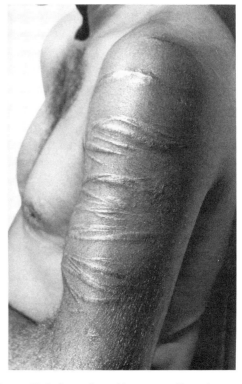

FIGURE 22.9 Scars from "sorry cuts" on the arm of an Aboriginal man.

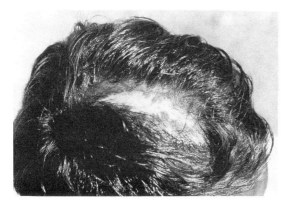

FIGURE 22.10 Scar and permanent alopecia from "sorry cuts" on scalp of Aboriginal woman.

in the cities and larger towns. Within such places the environmental conditions are poor and well below those in which most non-Aborigines live.

Some of the depressing features of Aboriginal environments are poor housing and primitive shelters, close personal contact, little privacy, often limited personal hygiene, ground living, water supplies either insufficient, polluted, or both, inadequate facilities for storage and preparation of food, unsuitable food, and improper nutrition. Few in remote areas have the benefits of electricity. Disposal of garbage and excreta is often inadequate or dangerous. Aboriginal camps have other hazards: old iron, barbed wire, broken glass, fires on the ground, work tools, weapons (clubs, spears, boomerangs, knives), and numerous dogs. Hunting in the bush and "walkabout" remains popular in remote places. Conditions and activities such as these predispose to injuries, burns, bites, and stings, the spread of infections and infestations, and exposure to environmental risks.

Other problems include petrol sniffing among children, excessive use of alcohol, smoking, gambling, fighting, road crashes, unemployment, high rates of imprisonment, unsuitable systems of education, and the continuing struggle for land rights.

Politicians, government employees, and those with vested interests, such as property owners, miners, missionaries, "developers" and promoters of tourism, have often been responsible for disastrous results on Aboriginal health, welfare, and culture.

Aboriginal Health

Compared with non-Aborigines, the health of Aborigines remains appalling.[1,20]

In infants and children, common causes of ill-health are malnutrition, repeated gastroenteritis, chronic rhinitis with persistent nasal discharge, otitis media with perforated ear drums and deafness, pneumonia, infestations with intestinal worms, acute exanthems (measles, chickenpox), numerous traumatic injuries, burns, and petrol sniffing.

In adolescents and adults, common causes of ill-health are alcoholism, smoking, sexually transmitted diseases, and hepatitis B. Obesity affects about 55% of adult females and 22% of males. Hypertension, diabetes, respiratory disease, tuberculosis, trachoma and blindness, chronic renal disease, and mental illness are particularly prevalent.

Aboriginal Influences

In the background of such problems are Aboriginal systems, laws, beliefs, teachings, and practices and a culture struggling to survive. Aboriginal concepts of disease, the place of tribal doctors and traditional treatments, Aboriginal fears, and superstitions are understood by few non-Aborigines.

Persistence of the predisposing and precipitating causes of ill-health means that improvements toward good health will inevitably be slow. Until Aborigines can be trained in sufficient numbers to manage successfully their own affairs, solutions to their problems seem a long way into the future.

General medical, specialist, and nursing services have been and are provided within the cultural and environmental backgrounds outlined. The place of dermatological services must also be seen in a similar perspective.

Conditions Related to the Environment

Physical Causes

Sunlight causes varying degrees of sunburn in infants and Aborigines with relatively light skin.

Exposed skin becomes darker than covered skin. Photosensitivity appears to be uncommon. Signs of sun damage in older Aborigines are minimal.

Heat, humidity, poor housing, and lack of air conditioning predispose to miliaria in Aboriginal infants.

Trauma results in cutaneous and other injuries of various kinds in children, adolescents, and adults. Sources of trauma include play and other childhood pursuits, falls, work, hunting in the bush, fighting, tribal practices, treatments, and punishments, animal and plant hazards in the natural environment, car crashes, and other misadventures. Injuries range from bruises, blisters, calluses, abrasions, scratches, lacerations, lodgement of foreign bodies, penetrating wounds, fractures, and internal damage. Injuries usually become secondarily infected, often to a gross degree.

Fires on the ground mean burns occur in toddlers, drunks, epileptics, and the blind. Burns are common, often extensive, and may be accidental or due to carelessness. Burns are also deliberately inflicted for decorative, therapeutic, or for punishment purposes.

Keloids can be large and, in sites such as flexures, seriously disabling. Ulceration creates a difficult and additional problem.

Lateral malleolar bursitis develops in some Aborigines from sitting cross-legged on the ground for long periods. In a few, chronic ulcerations occur (see Fig. 22.11). When this happens, leprosy should always be considered and excluded.

Where hookworm is endemic, transmission through the skin often is associated with ground living, bare feet, scanty clothes, and improper disposal of feces.

Licking, sucking, biting, and chewing lips are common habits among many Aborigines. Results include dryness, scaling, excoriation, ulceration, hypopigmentation, and scarring. Similar changes are seen in discoid lupus erythematosus (DLE) of the lips.

"Bush feet" is a name for the hyperkeratotic reaction that occurs on the dorsum of the toes and feet from going barefoot through scrub and sand (see Fig. 22.12). The condition, common in children from about 2 to 15 years, has been

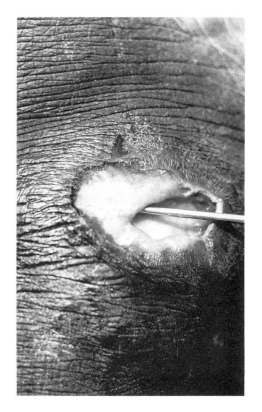

FIGURE 22.11 Lateral malleolar bursitis with ulceration into bursa.

mistaken for dry, cracked mud (sometimes present as well, but mud washes off) and localized ichthyosis.[21]

Dust, dirt, mud, and ochres used for ceremonial body painting, can leave curious

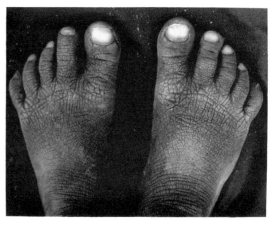

FIGURE 22.12 "Bush feet" of an Aboriginal boy.

patterns on the skin and scalp not related to ring-worm, tinea versicolor, or dandruff.

Chemical Causes

Pitjuri (native tobacco) and tobacco are chewed and sucked. Quids are held on the lower lip, in the mouth, or behind an ear. Cheilitis and buccal mucositis, but not often cancer, may result.

In some areas, high natural levels of fluoride in the drinking water often result in markedly mottled teeth but minimal caries.

Aboriginal children who are put in napkins (diapers) may develop a related rash.

Contact dermatitis, either primary contact or allergic sensitization, seems uncommon among Aborigines. Drug reactions occur but also appear less common than in non-Aborigines.

Biological Causes

Viral Infections

Warts of the usual kinds and molluscum contagiosum are found frequently in Aboriginal children. Cold sores and shingles are less frequent in Aborigines than in non-Aborigines.

Measles has caused considerable morbidity and mortality in the past. Rubella (German measles), other exanthems, and erythematous rashes can be difficult to detect in dark skins. Chickenpox in Aborigines can usually be readily diagnosed and not confused with miliaria.

Coccal and Bacterial Infections

Pyogenic infections with staphylococci and streptococci, either primary or secondary, are prevalent. Cutaneous injuries, burns, bites and stings, and skin conditions such as scabies and pediculosis of the scalp are often masked by secondary infection. Ecthymatous sores are a common result. These sores are usually numerous and persistent especially in Aboriginal children.

Other skin infections include impetigo (see Fig. 22.13), boils, folliculitis, pyogenic granulomas, and, occasionally, carbuncles.

Leprosy in an Aborigine of the Northern Territory was first diagnosed in 1890.[16] Since then, about 1000 Aborigines have been affected.

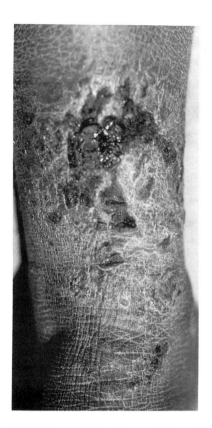

FIGURE 22.13 Crusted impetigo and dry skin on lower leg of an Aboriginal girl.

The disease has come under a good measure of control. However, new cases still occur. Between 1970 and 1989, 100 cases of leprosy were diagnosed in all ethnic groups in the Northern Territory. The male:female ratio was 63:37. The ethnic breakdown was Aborigines 77.7%, mixed race (Aboriginal descent) 9.9%, Europeans 8.6%, Chinese and Southeast Asian 3.3%, others 0.5%. The paucibacillary:multibacillary ratio was 75:25. In 1990, 190 patients were receiving treatment, but many could probably have ceased treatment after review. In 1989, the case detection rate for Aborigines was 0.14/1000 (5 cases in a population of 34,658).[22]

Infections with *Mycobacterium ulcerans* were first described in Australia and may occur in Aborigines. Melioidosis has been described in the past and there has been a recent upsurge of the condition.[23-25]

Neonatal tetanus was reported as an isolated instance.[26] Cutaneous diphtheria either as primary or secondary infection occurs occasionally in central Australia. Yaws, once endemic, appears to have been eradicated, probably due to widespread use of penicillin. A few old Aborigines may still show signs of the tertiary disease.

Trichomycosis axillaris (lepothrix), due to *Corynebacterium tenuis*, is common in adults, especially in hot, humid areas (see Figs. 22.14 and 22.15). Young people may ask about the condition in the mistaken belief that it is due to dried sweat, powder, lice, or other causes.

Sexually transmitted diseases (STDs) prevalent among Aborigines are syphilis, donovanosis (granuloma inguinale) (see Fig. 22.16), and gonorrhea. The acquired immunodeficiency syndrome (AIDS) has yet to penetrate Abor-

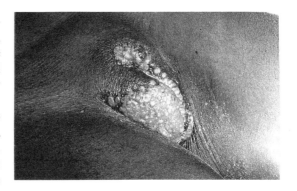

FIGURE 22.16 Donovanosis (granuloma inguinale) in adult Aboriginal female.

iginal communities. Hepatitis B infections are widespread among Aborigines.

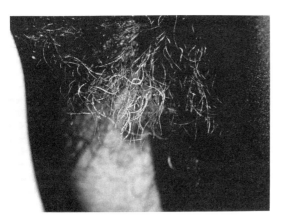

FIGURE 22.14 Trichomycosis axillaris in Aboriginal male.

Fungal Infections

The patterns of fungal infection among Aborigines and the dermatophytes responsible show interesting differences from those in non-Aborigines.[27]

T. rubrum (granular variant) occurs mainly in high rainfall, humid, tropical northern Australia. Both sexes, and children, adolescents, and young adults are affected, but no age is spared. The infection often begins under the usually tight waistbands of clothes. From there, the ringworm extends upward and downward. Failure to inspect the bathing-trunk area will mean that the diagnosis is often missed. The changes seen in the skin are various combinations of scaling, hyperpigmentation, and, rarely, decreased pigment, increased skin markings sometimes ranging to lichenification, papules, and an obvious spreading edge behind which the previously affected skin shows a less distinct margin[28] (see Fig. 22.17).

T. tonsurans and *T. violaceum* affect Aborigines in central and southern Australia.[27]

A new strain of *Microsporum canis* was found at Maningrida some 200 miles east of Darwin. In some children, this dermatophyte resulted in an asymptomatic carrier state.[29]

Tinea versicolor (called "white handkerchief" by some Aborigines) is prevalent. Often widespread on the trunk and upper arms, it is

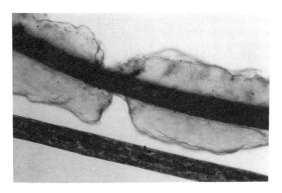

FIGURE 22.15 Trichomycosis axillaris: concretions of *Corynebacterium tenuis*. Magnification × 50.

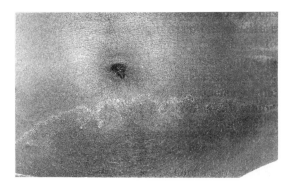

FIGURE 22.17 Ringworm due to *T. rubrum* (granular variant).

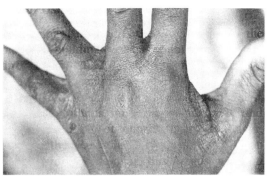

FIGURE 22.19 Scabies

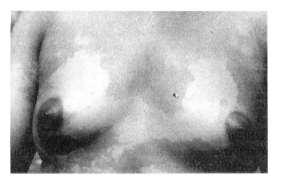

FIGURE 22.18 Tinea versicolor and gynaecomastia in part-Aborigine aged about 16.

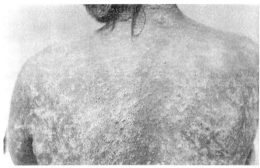

FIGURE 22.20 Crusted scabies in adult Aboriginal female.

sometimes seen on the neck and face (see Fig. 22.18). Superficial scaling forms of pityriasis versicolor and *T. rubrum* infections can be clinically confused. Direct microscopy usually confirms pityriasis versicolor, and culture should yield *T. rubrum*.

Chromoblastomycosis occurs mainly in Queensland. Cryptococcosis, usually systemic, occasionally has cutaneous lesions and occurs in northern Australia and less often elsewhere. Sporotrichosis, nocardiosis, and actinomycosis have been reported in Aborigines and non-Aborigines mainly in tropical Australia; however, these conditions are relatively rare.[30,31]

Parasitic Infestations

Scabies is endemic and sometimes epidemic (see Fig. 22.19). Crusted scabies occurs in Aborigines but the diagnosis is often delayed and the condition recalcitrant (see Fig. 22.20). In central Australia, pediculosis of the scalp is also endemic, particularly among children and less often in adults. Epidemics occur elsewhere in Aboriginal and non-Aboriginal children.

Demodiciosis occurs in Aborigines but no associations with skin conditions have been observed.[32,33]

Hookworm remains endemic in high rainfall, tropical Australia.

Myiasis is seen in neglected wounds and sometimes in children with suppurative otitis media.

Humans sometimes accidentally become hosts to kangaroo ticks, *Amblyomma triguttatum* and *Ornithodorus gurneyi*, and to *Ixodes holocyclus*.[34] Avian schistosomiasis occurs occasionally in different parts of Australia. Aborigines and non-Aborigines may be affected.

Noxious and Harmful Fauna

Terrestrial examples include mosquitoes, biting midges (usually called sandflies), black flies, march flies, biting ants, fleas, hairy caterpillars ("itchy grubs" of *Ochrogaster* and *Euproctis* species found in central Australia), spiders, centipedes, scorpions, lice, snakes such as the taipan, king brown, death adder, and tiger snake (each very venomous), wild pigs, and, in the Northern Territory, buffaloes.[34,35]

Marine examples include the sea wasp or box jellyfish (*Chironex fleckeri*) and the Portuguese Man-o'-War or bluebottle of the genus *Physalia* in northern Australian waters. From October to May sea wasps are present in considerable numbers. Other marine hazards include corals, certain cone shellfish, stone fish (*Synanceja trachynis*), the blue-ringed or banded octopus (*Hapalochlaena maculosa*), stingrays, sea snakes, sharks, and in northern Australia, crocodiles.[35,36]

Noxious and Harmful Flora

Physical and other injuries from plants occur among Aborigines especially during excursions to the bush and in children. Parts of plants responsible include thorns, spikes, hooks, bristles, hairs, sharp cutting edges, irritant saps, and specialized parts such as found in stinging nettles. Types of injuries include abrasions, blisters, lacerations, penetrating wounds, and implantation of plant parts.

Some knowledge of the regional fauna and flora is useful particularly in rural and remote areas. Information can be obtained from local, state, and territory sources.

Miscellaneous Conditions

Acne is more often comedonal than papular, pustular, and cystic, although these forms occur (see Fig. 22.21). Keloidal and hypertrophic scars result particularly in the presternal region. Adolescent Aborigines, mainly women who are concerned about their personal appearance, nowadays seek treatment.

Discoid lupus erythematosus (DLE) is geographically widespread among Aborigines in whom it is much more prevalent than among non-Aborigines living in similar areas. Females are more prone to DLE than males. In Aborigines, the clinical features are modified by their dark skin. On the scalp, scarring alopecia may result. This looks similar to scars from "sorry-cuts" in females. On the face, hypopigmented scars cause considerable embarrassment. A notable feature in Aborigines is the frequent occurrence of DLE on the lips, usually the upper, sometimes the lower, and in a few, on both. Three stages of DLE are seen on the lips. When acute, the lips are red, granular, friable, and may be covered with blood clot and crust. In the subacute stage, superficial ulceration, crusting, and maceration are seen. Hypopigmentation and scarring mark the chronic

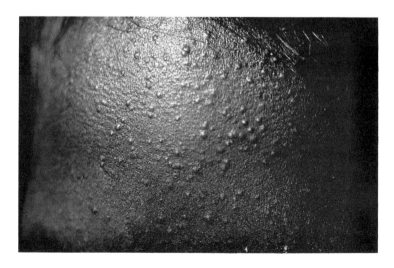

FIGURE 22.21 Comedonal acne in an Aboriginal boy aged 12.

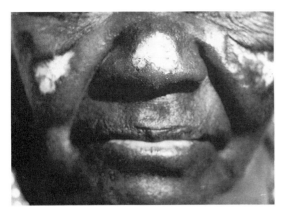

FIGURE 22.22 Discoid lupus erythematosus with scarring in cheeks, plaque on nose, lower lip. In an Aboriginal woman.

stage. Of about 40 cases of DLE among Aborigines known to the author squamous cell cancerous change in the lips has occurred in 3. Biopsy material from the lips should always be examined by both light microscopy and immunofluorescent methods, otherwise the diagnosis of DLE may be missed. Discoid lupus erythematosus, which has striking clinical signs, is probably a fairly recent development among Aborigines as no mention of it was made by earlier writers (see Fig. 22.22).

Other conditions include cradle cap; milium, sebaceous, and other cysts; ganglia; dry skin in varying degrees; gynaecomastia in a few young males; facial hirsutism in elderly females; halo nevi; different pigmentary patterns and focal epithelial hyperplasia in the mouth; skin tags; punctate keratosis of the palms and soles; angular stomatitis; trichotillomania (see Fig. 22.23); and isolated cases of epulis, ameloblastoma, melanoma on the feet, and multiple xanthomata. Vitiligo, especially when on exposed surfaces, causes considerable embarrassment and concern.

Conditions Not Observed, Rare, Or Apparently Absent in Full-Blood Aborigines

Examples of these conditions include alopecia areata, atopic dermatitis, pityriasis rosea, pompholyx, psoriasis,[37] solar-related basal and

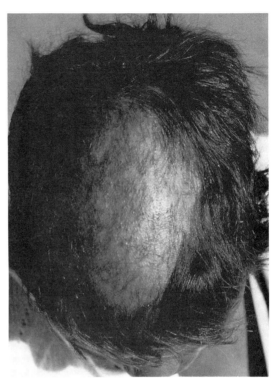

FIGURE 22.23 Trichotillomania in an Aboriginal woman aged 21.

squamous cell skin cancer, strawberry nevi, stucco keratoses, varicose veins (see Fig. 22.24) and related conditions such as eczema and ulceration. Part-Aborigines are sometimes affected by alopecia areata, atopic dermatitis, and psoriasis. However, the prevalence is much less than in non-Aborigines.

Other conditions, which seem rare or apparently absent, include lichen planus, morphea, pityriasis lichenoides, dermatomyositis, pityriasis rubra pilaris, sarcoidosis, scleroderma, and a number of others.

Skin Conditions Among Non-Aborigines

Among the non-Aboriginal people in Australia the skin conditions found are generally similar to those in comparable, cosmopolitan communities in the Western world. A notable exception in Australia is the incidence and prevalence of

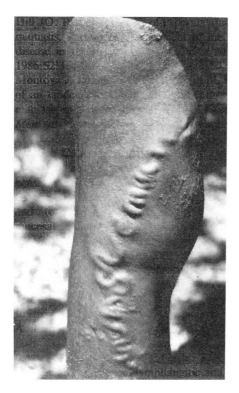

FIGURE 22.24 Varicose veins are rare in Aborigines. The two plaques are ringworm due to *T. rubrum* (granular variant).

sun-damaged skin and its sequelae including skin cancers.

Sun-Damaged Skin and Skin Cancer

Australia has wide open spaces, abundant sunshine, and beautiful beaches. Many Australians spend their plentiful leisure time in sporting and other outdoor activities, often with scant regard for the results on their skin. Relatively few children, especially teenagers, regularly wear hats and other protective clothing when outside. Many people believe that a suntan is fashionable, sexu-ally attractive, a sign of good health, and of superior social status. Tourist brochures invite people to "Come for fun in the sun" and make claims such as "...climate allows for year-round outdoor dining." Added to sun-seekers such as these are the thousands whose occupations expose them to the sun.

A predominantly white, fair-skinned, Caucasian population, many people with a Celtic genetic inheritance, the Australian climate and geographic features and the popular outdoor lifestyles in vogue have combined to make sun-damaged skin and skin cancer a national problem.[38,39]

Australians have the doubtful distinction of having the highest rates of skin cancer in the world. Estimates are that 2 out of 3 people will develop one nonmelanotic skin cancer and 1 in 60 will develop a melanoma during the course of an average life span.[40–43]

In recent years, increasing numbers of people are seeking advice about moles and possible early skin cancers. Each November, "Skin Cancer Awareness Week," under the aegis of the Australasian College of Dermatologists and anticancer organizations, attracts a reasonable measure of interest and publicity.

Three Groups of Skin Conditions

The skin conditions seen among non-Aborigines in Australia are listed in three groups that relate broadly to their frequency and ease of diagnosis.

Group 1

The conditions in Group 1 are common and most have sufficient features to enable a diagnosis on careful clinical examination depending on the presentation and the experience of the observer.

For other conditions, the history and clinical findings should raise sufficient diagnostic suspicions so that selected laboratory studies may clarify the diagnosis and direct appropriate treatment. Obvious examples are bacteriological, mycological, and histolological investigations.

Group 1 conditions include:

- Epidermal, vascular, pigmented, and other nevi present at birth or later.
- Atopic dermatitis (eczema), napkin (diaper) dermatitis, occupational, "hand" and "housewive's" dermatitis, and pompholyx are prevalent. In Aborigines, such conditions are uncommon, rare, or practically unknown.
- Skin damage from trauma and fire resulting

in injuries such as abrasions, lacerations, penetrating wounds, and burns are relatively less common than among Aborigines.

- Sun-damaged skin and its sequelae are evident in most fair-skinned people over 40; however, in those with particularly susceptible skins, such signs may be found from the age of 10 onward.
- Viral infections occur, such as warts of various kinds, herpes simplex, herpes zoster, molluscum contagiosum, occasionally hand-foot-and-mouth disease and, sometimes, orf in those who work with sheep.
- Acute and chronic coccal, bacterial, and other infections are moderately common but generally less so than in Aborigines.
- Scabies and pediculosis of the scalp occur sporadically and occasionally as epidemics. Among non-Aboriginal school children, these two conditions usually evoke considerable public and press concern but pass with little or no comment when Aboriginal children are affected. Pubic pediculosis is usually sexually transmitted. Pediculosis of the body is less often seen than in the first half of the 1900s. The main dermatophytes cultured from non-Aborigines, in distinction from those usually found in Aborigines, are *T. rubrum*, *M. canis*, *E. floccosum*, and *T. mentagrophytes*. *T. rubrum* is now probably the most frequently isolated dermatophyte. Many people, pharmacists, and practitioners mistakenly believe that ringworm (tinea) can be diagnosed simply on clinical inspection. Accordingly, a variety of topical applications are used and griseofulvin is taken for conditions other than ringworm. Many do not realize that ringworm and tinea are different names for the same condition and that precise diagnosis depends on isolation of a dermatophyte in culture.
- *Candida* species, usually *C. albicans*, infections are seen most commonly in children usually as a primary or secondary cause of napkin rash, in paronychia affecting housewives and workers in wet occupations, in angular stomatitis, in females especially those who have taken antibiotics, and in some elderly people.
- Tinea versicolor in its usual clinical forms is prevalent but less so than among Aborigines.
- Acne, in greater or lesser severity, occurs in up to 85% of adolescents. Delays in seeking specialist advice, often for several years, are not unusual even in patients with severe acne. Over-the-counter preparations, products from cosmetic companies, and "health" shops, alternative medicines, and traditional remedies are popular despite their limited efficacy in acne.
- Dandruff, seborrheic dermatitis, rosacea, and perioral dermatitis are common in non-Aboriginal people but not in Aborigines.
- Psoriasis affects up to 2% of people at some time in their lives. The condition shows the usual features. Psoriasis has not been reported in full-blood Australian Aborigines.[37]
- The usual types and causes of pruritus are regularly found.
- Dry skin, besides that seen in atopic subjects and inherited ichthyotic conditions, is frequently related to common Australian bathroom habits. These include long hot showers or baths, excessive rubbing of soap into the skin, scrubbing the skin with washcloths, sponges, brushes, loofahs, and the like, and vigorous and "thorough" drying with a towel. Generous applications of body colognes and talcum powders are popular particularly among elderly people.
- Urticaria is an annoyance to many people and the cause often perplexing to practitioners and patients.
- Miliaria is seen mainly in infants living in hot, humid environments without the benefits of air conditioning.
- Granuloma annulare, pityriasis rosea, erythema multiforme, aphthous ulcers, angular stomatitis, corns and calluses, lichen planus, ichthyosis, hyperhidrosis, keloids, and hypertrophic scars are regularly seen and should be diagnosed on clinical grounds.
- Campbell de Morgan spots, seborrheic keratoses, skin tags, stretch marks, milia, stucco keratoses, trichomycosis axillaris, and small dermatofibromas are continuing causes of patients' inquiries and concern. Explanation, advice, and reassurance should be given to patients about these harmless conditions.

- Varicose eczema and ulceration can cause a prolonged need for medical and nursing care. Varicose veins are rare in full-blood Aborigines.
- Vitiligo is a cosmetic problem especially when it occurs on exposed skin. There is some doubt whether the time, trouble, and expense of long-term treatment justify the ultimate results.
- Discoid lupus erythematosus is less frequently seen and less evident in Caucasians than Aborigines.
- Baldness in males, androgenic hair loss and hirsutism in females, alopecia areata in both sexes, trichotillomania and ringworm of the scalp, and various disorders of the nails result in a range of reactions by patients and mixed therapeutic responses.
- Tattoos, done well by most professionals and crudely by amateurs, are popular among some social groups. Infection with hepatitis B and human immunodeficiency virus (HIV) are risks of tattooing.

Group 2

When the diagnosis is not quickly evident, the following conditions should be considered:

- Drug eruptions and reactions, which have long superseded syphilis as great imitators.
- Atypical presentations of common conditions can be sources of diagnostic confusion.
- Scratching, rubbing, and picking; trauma from towels, brushes, loofahs, and "back-scratchers"; secondary eczematous changes and infection; and reactions to topical applications can alter clinical appearances and mask the original condition. Atopic dermatitis, scabies, and tinea are examples of conditions that may be so changed.
- Bites, stings, and injuries from harmful terrestrial and marine fauna and injuries from potentially harmful plants produce a range of cutaneous changes. Knowledge of the distribution of the fauna and flora and their reactions in exposed individuals can lead to correct diagnosis and treatment.

Neurodermatitis, cutaneous behavioral disorders, for example, factitious dermatitis, neurotic excoriations, delusions of parasitosis, and neurocutaneous dermatoses, such as glossodynia, hyperesthesia, and causalgia can be difficult to diagnose and manage. Dermatological diagnoses such as "an allergy" and "a nerve rash" are not helpful and indicate the need for another opinion.

Sexually transmitted diseases (STDs) are no respecters of persons. Among the non-Aboriginal people of Australia, the common STDs are infections caused by *Neisseria gonorrhoeae*, *Chlamydia trachomatis*, and the human papilloma virus, genital herpes, scabies, pubic pediculosis, and molluscum contagiosum. Infections with HIV, syphilis, and hepatitis B occur mainly, but by no means exclusively, in homosexual males and drug users who share needles and syringes.

Exotic diseases can be acquired and spread rapidly by people who move from one country to another often over a few days or weeks. Tourists and business people are at particular risk. Migrants are the source of exotic diseases and cultural practices unknown to most Australians. Exotic diseases should be considered when diagnostic doubt exists. The diagnosis may well be missed unless certain questions are asked: Where do you come from? Where have you been? When were you there? What did you do? These days in Australia, exotic diseases are increasingly recognized. Examples include leprosy, cutaneous leishmaniasis, STDs, and malaria.

Group 3

Uncommon and rare disorders can cause diagnostic difficulties and delays depending on the clinician's training and experience. A few examples are the less common vesiculo-bullous diseases such as dermatitis herpetiformis and pemphigus, the porphyrias, pyoderma gangrenosum, and conditions usually shown at clinical meetings or reported as rare and interesting cases.

Cutaneous Manifestations of Systemic Diseases

The skin and its appendages are meeting places for dermatology and general medicine. As was once said, "Nature is neither husk nor kernel; she is all in one."

The cutaneous manifestations of systemic diseases are innumerable but important in diagnosis and management. A few examples are alterations in skin color and texture, the exanthemata, particular infections such as leprosy, syphilis, tuberculosis, and with HIV, the skin signs of internal malignancy, and auto-immune, metabolic, and endocrine diseases.

Conclusions

The patterns of skin conditions in the Aboriginal and non-Aboriginal people of Australia have been outlined and the remarkable differences emphasized.

The dermatological needs of the Aborigines are much less well served than those of the non-Aborigines. Prevention and management measures, improved dermatological education, and clinical services for Aborigines could be developed through the National Health Strategy.[1] Prevention of solar damage and skin cancer in non-Aboriginal Australians needs a national program funded ideally by the Commonwealth Government and implemented in all schools.

Research should be directed to reasons why conditions such as psoriasis and atopic dermatitis are rare or absent in full-blood Australian Aborigines and to why others, such as DLE, are relatively prevalent.

References

1. National Aboriginal Health Strategy Working Party: A national Aboriginal health strategy. March 1989.
2. Elkin AP: The Australian Aborigines: how to understand them. Sydney: Angus and Robertson, 1948.
3. Nind S: Description of the natives of King George's Sound (Swan River colony) and adjoining country. *J Roy Geog Soc Lond* 1832;**1**:21–49.
4. Board for Anthropological Research, University of Adelaide: Aboriginal man in South and Central Australia. Part 1. Cotton BC, ed. Adelaide: Government Printer, 1966.
5. Cook CE: Medicine and the Australian Abor-
iginal: a century of contact in the Northern Territory. *Med J Aust* 1966;**1**:559–565.
6. Moodie PM, Pederson EB: The health of Australian Aborigines: an annotated bibliography. Commonwealth Department of Health, School of Public Health and Tropical Medicine, University of Sydney. Service publication No. 9. Canberra: Australian Government Publishing Service, 1971.
7. Rowley CD: The destruction of Aboriginal society. Victoria: Penguin Books Australia, 1972.
8. Davies D: The Last of the Tasmanians. Sydney: Shakespeare Head Press, 1973.
9. Abbie AA: The Original Australians, rev. ed. Seal Books, 1976.
10. Lofgren ME: Patterns of life: the story of the Aboriginal people of Western Australia. Western Australian Museum Information Series No. 6, Perth, Western Australia, 1980.
11. Flood J: Archaeology of the Dreamtime. Sydney: Collins, 1983.
12. Cumpston JHL: Health and disease in Australia. Lewis MJ, ed. Canberra: Australian Government Publishing Service, 1989.
13. Aboriginal and Torres Strait Islander Commission: Aboriginal Australia: Aboriginal people of New South Wales. Canberra: Australian Government Publishing Service, 1990.
14. Pybus C: Community of thieves. Port Melbourne, Victoria: William Heinemann Australia, 1991.
15. Macknight CC: The voyage to Marege: Macassan trepangers in northern Australia. Carlton, Victoria: Melbourne University Press, 1976.
16. Cook CE: The epidemiology of leprosy in Australia. Commonwealth of Australia, Department of Health. Service Publication No. 38. Canberra: Government Printer, 1927.
17. Northern Territory Medical Service of the Australian Department of Health: Leprosy in Northern Territory Aborigines: a short guide for field staff in the diagnosis and management of leprosy in Aborigines. Canberra: Australian Department of Health, 1970.
18. Walker AC: Albinism in a full-blood Aboriginal child. *Med J Aust* 1969;**2**:1105.
19. Ford E: Congenital abnormalities of the genitalia in related Bathurst Island natives. *Med J Aust* 1941;**1**:450.
20. Moodie PM: Aboriginal health. Canberra: Australian National University Press, 1973.
21. Ford E: Medical conditions on Bathurst and Melville Islands. *Med J Aust* 1942;**2**:235–238.
22. Hargrave JC: Northern Territory Department of Health and Community Services. *Communicable Diseases Intelligence* 1990;**24**:(Oct);4–8.

23. Crotty JM, Bromwich AF, Quinn JV, Brotherton J: Melioidosis in the Northern Territory: a report of two cases. *Med J Aust* 1963;**1**:274–275.

24. Bayliss P: Rare disease kills eight. *Med Observer* 1991 (Mar 1):4.

25. Ashdown L: Epidemiological aspects of melioidosis in Australia. *Commun Dis Intell* 1991;**15**: (Aug);272–273.

26. Blake GP: Neonatal tetanus in a Northern Territory Aboriginal child. *Med J Aust* 1980;**12**:9.

27. Green AC, Kaminski GW: Australian Aborigines and their dermatophytes. *Australas J Dermatol* 1977;**18**:132–136.

28. Green AC, Kaminiski GW: *Trichophyton rubrum* infections in Northern Territory Aborigines. *Australas J Dermatol* 1973;**14**:101–120.

29. Kaminski GW, Green AC: Tinea capitis in Aboriginal children at Maningrida, Northern Territory, Australia: a variant of *Microsporum canis*. *Australas J Dermatol* 1977;**18**:88–97.

30. Barrack BB: Mycotic granulomata in Australia. *Med J Aust* 1957;**7**:189–192.

31. Crotty JM: Systemic mycotic infections in Northern Territory Aborigines. *Med J Aust* 1965;**1**:184–186.

32. Nutting WB, Green AC: Hair follicle mites (Acari: Demodicidae) from Australian Aborigines. *Australas J Dermatol* 1974;**15**:10–14.

33. Nutting WB, Green AC: Pathogenesis associated with hair follicle mites (*Demodex* spp.) in Australian Aborigines. *Br J Dermatol* 1976;**94**: 307–312.

34. Lee DJ: Arthropod bites and stings and other injurious effects. Sydney: School of Public Health and Tropical Medicine, University of Sydney, 1975.

35. Commonwealth Serum Laboratories: Venomous Australian animals dangerous to man. Garnet JR. ed. Parkville, Victoria: Commonwealth Serum Laboratories, 1968.

36. Cleland JB, Southcott RV: Injuries to man from marine invertebrates in the Australian region. In: Lee DJ, Bennett I, eds. National Health and Medical Research Council, Special Report Series No. 12. Canberra ACT: Commonwealth of Australia, 1965.

37. Green AC: Australian Aborigines and psoriasis. *Australas J Dermatol* 1984;**25**:18–24.

38. McCarthy WH, Shaw HM: Skin cancer in Australia. *Med J Aust* 1989;**150**:469–470.

39. Marks R: Skin cancer control in the 1990's, from Slip! Slop! Slap! to Sun Smart. *Australas J Dermatol* 1990;**31**:1–4.

40. Marks R, Jolley D, Dorevitch AP, Selwood TS: The incidence of non-melanotic skin cancers in an Australian population: results of a five-year prospective study. *Med J Aust* 1989;**150**:475–478.

41. Marks R: Skin cancer—childhood protection affords lifetime protection. *Med J Aust* 1987;**147**: 476.

42. Cockburn J, Hennrikus D, Scott R, Sanson-Fisher R: Adolescent use of sun-protection measures. *Med J Aust* 1989;**136**:140.

43. Emmett A: The bare facts—the effect of sun on skin. Artarmon, New South Wales: MacLennan and Petty, 1989.

23

Diseases Among Black People

K. Erik Kostelnik and Chérie M. Ditre

The dermatologic literature, while limited, has recognized the various presentations of skin disorders in black, white, and Asian skin. Although dermatologists rely on clinical appearance (i.e., the lesion's morphology, color, location, etc.) to make a diagnosis, racial variations do exist. For example, unique skin disorders afflicting black skin have been documented both clinically and histologically. The diagnostic challenge, then, is in recognizing these unique diseases as well as the variations of the "classic" morphology of common maladies. In this chapter, we discuss (1) the normal histology of black skin, (2) the presentations of common skin diseases, (3) the normal variants seen, and (4) dermatoses more commonly seen in black skin.

A clarifying point about the term "black" must be made at the outset. This term can be confusing as there are actually three black races (the Capoid, the Negroid, and the Australoid), and these have all been diluted with genes from other races.[1] Therefore, in this chapter, "black" shall refer to skin with a dark hue in a person with ancestry in one of the three black races.

Histology

Histologically, the hue of black skin is due to the production and distribution of melanin pigment. Although the melanocytes are larger and have more dendritic branching in black skin, it is the larger and more melanized melanosomes that give the skin a deeper pigment. These melanosomes are produced at a greater rate and have a slower rate of degradation, as well as having a higher degree of dispersion in all layers of keratinocytes. It has been reported in the literature that the epidermis is thicker in black skin,[2] but recent literature does not support this.[3] In the work of Montagna and Carlisle, the dermis shows an increased number of hypertrophied and multinucleated fibroblasts and macrophages. Interestingly, compared to the sun-exposed Caucasian, the dermis of black skin does not have as much elastotic material, presumably because the melanocytes act as an umbrella to protect the underlying dermis.[3] Some authors believe the increased skin turgor of black skin is due to the numerous glycoprotein molecules in the matrix.[3]

Eccrine ducts are distributed similarly on black and white skin,[4] but Montagna and Carlisle found more apoeccrine glands on facial skin of blacks.[3] Apocrine and sebaceous glands are larger, but they are no more numerous when compared with aged-matched white subjects.[4] Finally, although pigment is the most pronounced racial difference, it appears that it is only part of a histologic mosaic.

Common Skin Presentations in Blacks

The presentation of the same dermatologic disorders in black and white skin can vary dramatically. The deeper hue of the skin and the

137

reaction of melanocytes to inflammation make particular dermatoses more or less prominent. For example, deeper pigment may obscure erythema to the untrained eye. Additionally, postinflammatory hyperpigmentation and hypopigmentation are more apparent, and frequently are the chief complaint of the patient. Black skin may respond with different morphologic patterns in certain diseases, namely, with follicular accentuation, annular configurations, and granulomatous presentations.

Pigmentary Disorders

Pigmentation contributes to over one-half of all dermatologic conditions in blacks.[5] Surprisingly, the incidence of vitiligo in blacks is the same as it is in other races,[6] however, the sharp color contrast against dark skin makes it more striking. Vitiligo is an acquired melanocytopenic disease clinically manifested as well-demarcated, depigmented white macules (Fig. 23.1). There

may be associated endocrine disorders, or ocular abnormalities. Trichrome vitiligo, displaying areas of depigmentation, hypopigmentation, and normal pigment, may represent the development of vitiligo in stages. Vitiligo is more challenging in black skin because it is more disfiguring, and is felt to be more difficult to treat both medically and cosmetically. Furthermore, the question of pharmacologic complete depigmentation for extensive vitiligo is a momentous decision for both patient and physician.

Similarly, pityriasis alba is another hypopigmenting dermatologic condition more striking in blacks. The lesions are superficial, slightly scaly, hypopigmented patches on the face, chest, and upper limbs. It occurs predominantly in children and is found with equal incidence on dark- and light-skinned individuals.[7] The etiology is unknown, but has been related to eczema[8-10] and impaired transfer of pigment from melanocytes to keratinocytes.[11]

On the other hand, hyperpigmentation can be just as disfiguring. Melasma, an irregular acquired hypermelanosis of the face, can appear more sharply defined when compared to its presentation in fair-skinned individuals (Fig. 23.2). This brown pigmentation is usually seen in women, especially when pregnant or while taking oral contraceptives, but has been described in men as well. Melanin is deposited either in the dermis or the epidermis and can be very distressing to lighter-skinned blacks.

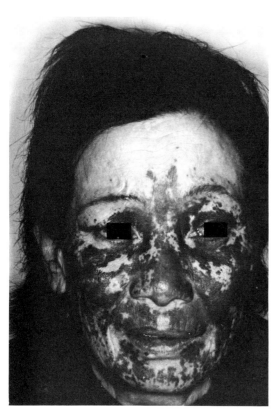

FIGURE 23.1. Vitiligo in a black woman.

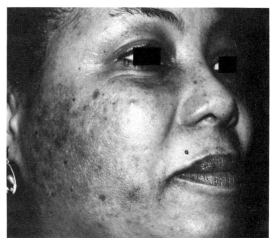

FIGURE 23.2. Melasma.

Postinflammatory hyperpigmentation or hypopigmentation is not unique to the black race, but is of greater concern because of its greater intensity and tendency to last longer. The list of dermatoses resulting in secondary pigmentary changes is lengthy. Simply put, physical trauma or other irritation to melanocytes can have varied responses, from destruction of these cells, to stimulation of melanin production. For example, eczema and tinea versicolor present on black skin with both hyperpigmentation and hypopigmentation. Prediction of the response is difficult. Hypopigmentation may result from allergic, atopic, and contact dermatitides; sarcoidosis; secondary syphilis; seborrheic dermatitis; and other diseases, as well as treatments with cryotherapy, fluorinated steroids, and dermabrasion (Figs. 23.3–23.6). Hyperpigmentation is common following lichen planus, acne vulgaris, pityriasis rosea, psoriasis, and lupus erythematosus among others. Keratolytic therapy and occasionally bleaching creams such as hydroquinones may also result in hyperpigmentation.

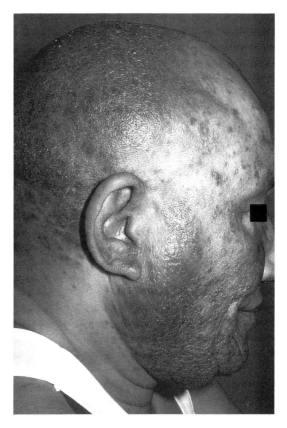

FIGURE 23.3. Atopic dermatitis.

Morphologic Variants

Certain common diseases tend to have a follicular component in blacks. Eczema, especially in children, frequently exhibits tiny papules at the hair follicle, and tinea versicolor, lichen simplex chronicus, lichen planus, secondary syphilis, and pityriasis rosea may also display this morphology (Fig. 23.7). The "inverse" presentation of pityriasis rosea, affecting the face, lower abdomen, and extremities, is more

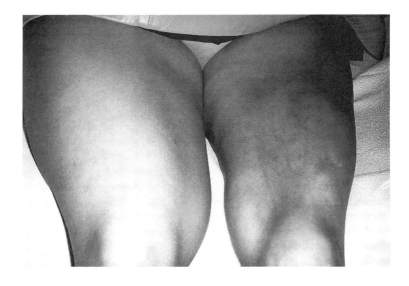

FIGURE 23.4. Linear scleroderma and fibrosing sarcoidosis in a black woman 40 years old

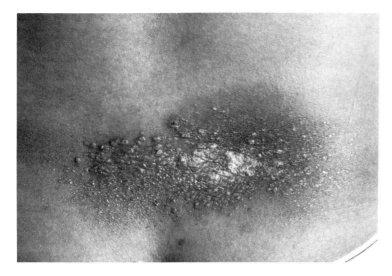

FIGURE 23.5. Cutaneous sarcoidosis.

common in this papular variety.[12] The papules of lichen nitidus are more apparent on black skin, and although it has not been shown to be more prominent in any racial group, it is associated more commonly with black skin[11] (Fig. 23.8). Discrete papules in sarcoidosis are commonly seen in blacks. A follicular pattern is also seen in uncommon dermatoses that are unique to blacks, such as hamartoma moniliformis and disseminate and recurrent infundibulofolliculitis.

Secondary syphilis occasionally presents in blacks with an annular configuration, typically not seen in whites. Less commonly, one may see an annular component to seborrheic dermatitis, lupus erythematosus, and lichen planus. Sarcoidosis can be annular (Fig. 23.9), and other

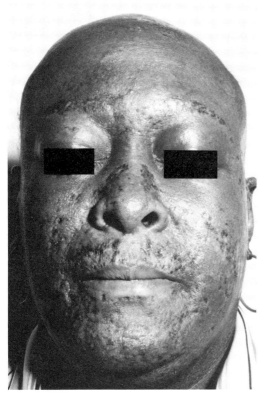

(a)

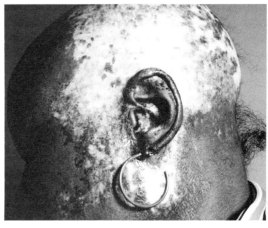

(b)

FIGURE 23.6. Discoid lupus erythematosus.

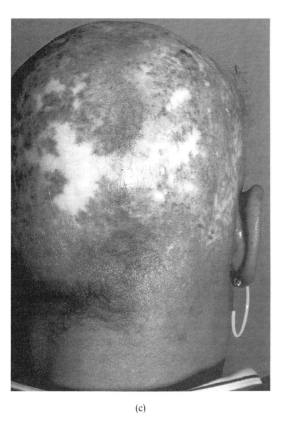

(c)

FIGURE 23.6. Continued.

FIGURE 23.8. Lichen nitidus.

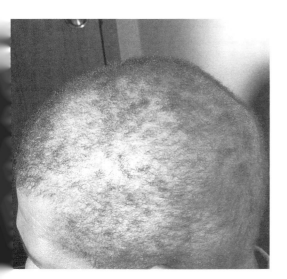

FIGURE 23.7. Patchy alopecia associated with secondary syphilis.

forms (ulcerative, alopetic, ichthyosiform, and verrucous) have been seen exclusively in blacks.[1]

Normal Variants

Futcher's (Voigt's) Lines

Pigmentary demarcation lines are common normal skin markings in darker-skinned people. The most common of these is a symmetric pair of lines occurring on the upper arms, Futcher's lines (Fig. 23.10). Futcher's lines are lines of abrupt pigmentary change on the anterolateral surface of the upper limbs, described as running along the lateral edge of the biceps or along the course of the cephalic vein. When they occur, they are usually bilateral, and the anterolateral aspect is darker than the anteromedial. They have been noted at birth or shortly thereafter and do not change in incidence over time. These lines are most common in blacks (17.5%–44%),

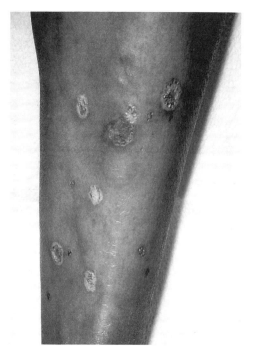

FIGURE 23.9. Fibrosing sarcoidosis.

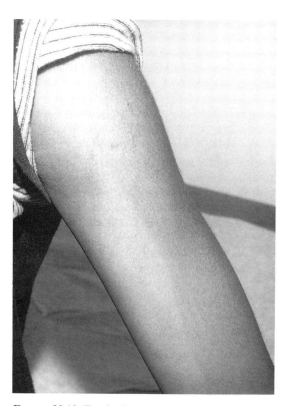

FIGURE 23.10. Futcher's or Voigt's lines.

less common in Asians (4%), only sporadically reported in Caucasians,[5,13,14] and have a higher prevalence in women. Similar pigmentary demarcation lines have been described on the lower limbs by Matzumoto,[14] and these have been observed to be more intense during pregnancy.[5]

Futcher's lines had been noticed for hundreds of years, but they were first postulated by Voigt, a 19th-century Viennese anatomist, to follow the distribution of spinal nerves. Futcher drew attention to these lines in blacks in 1938, and since then, its relationship to the dermatomes has been questioned.

Hair and Nails

Black hair shafts and follicles are curved with a tendency to grow back toward the skin. This hair is referred to as spiral or helical hair. These hairs are also a flattened elliptical shape in cross section when compared to a nearly circular shape in Mongoloids and an intermediate shape in Caucasians.[1] Hair also differs in a more sparse body distribution and a slower beard growth in blacks.[1] Canities (graying) occurs a decade later in blacks, and balding at the vertex is four times more common in whites.[1]

The nails of blacks clinically differ from those of lighter-skinned races in a number of ways: the nail plate is usually longer and angular and there may be lateral and/or posterior nail fold pigmentation. Diffuse pigmentation of the nail plate is seen in darker blacks, and there is a higher incidence of pigmented longitudinal stripes.[1,15] Pigmented longitudinal stripes are the most striking of these, and they show a definite increase in incidence with increasing age. They are not present at birth and have been reported in 53% of all blacks 30 years of age and older.[1] These linear dark bands vary in width and number and show no sexual predilection. The melanonychia striata seen here (Fig. 23.11) vary with intensity of skin pigment, for example, the incidence in light-skinned blacks is 4%, whereas in darker-skinned blacks is 76%.[15] Histologically, these represent melanin deposits in the nail bed, and it has been suggested that it is a result of trauma. It is

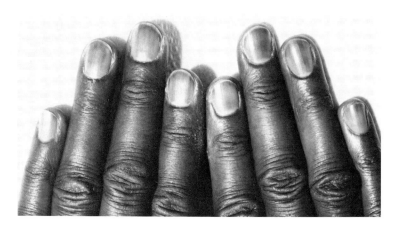

FIGURE 23.11. Melanonychia.

important to recognize this normal variant and to differentiate it from subungual melanoma, postirradiation melanonychia, Addison's disease, or Peutz-Jegher's disease.

Keratotic Pits of the Palmar Creases

The incidence of keratotic pits of the palmar creases (KPPC) has been reported ranging from 0.05% to 58%. The true incidence in blacks is probably between 3% and 8%,[16–18] whereas it is much less common in Caucasians. KPPC are 1–4 mm hyperkeratotic plugs in sharply marginated "cup-like depressions of the epidermis,"[18] located on the larger palmar creases (proximal interphalangeal and distal and medial transpalmar creases) (Fig. 23.12). They are generally bilateral and rarely affect the soles. KPPC has been reported to be associated with manual labor but is also seen in many blacks without this history. There is no sex predilection, and they are almost always asymptomatic. Tenderness and pain have been reported in a few cases and may require surgical intervention. Keratolytics and retinoids have been attempted, but only provide temporary relief. Histologically, these lesions show compact hyperkeratosis with a normal dermis in an epidermal depression. Sweat ducts are also seen, some with apical occlusion.

KPPC are distinguished from punctate keratoses distributed throughout the palmar surface, which has an autosomal dominant inheritance pattern.

Midline Hypopigmentation

The anterior chest of blacks may show areas of hypopigmentation that are normal variants. The more common of these is a mediosternal vertically oriented hypopigmented patch. These hypomelanotic bands may bend away from the midline and/or extend onto the abdomen overlying the linea alba. These markings have been noted to be inherited in an autosomal dominant pattern in some cases.[5,19] Midline hypopigmentation is most evident in prepubescent children (66–69% incidence) and fades over time (27% incidence in blacks over 13 years old).[19,20] Another type of hypopigmentation is characterized by discrete oval macules over the anterior chest, especially the infraclavicular and periareolar areas. Their incidence also shows a preponderance of cases prepubertally when compared to postpubescent (46% vs. 5%).[19] Both of these are asymptomatic and otherwise unremarkable. These macules and patches should be differentiated from the depigmented lesions of vitiligo and nevus depigmentosus, and the hypopigmented lesions of tuberous sclerosis, pityriasis alba, and nevus anemicus.

Mongolian Spot

The mongolian spot is a cutaneous finding more common in blacks than in many other races (Fig. 23.13). This blue/gray macule appears most

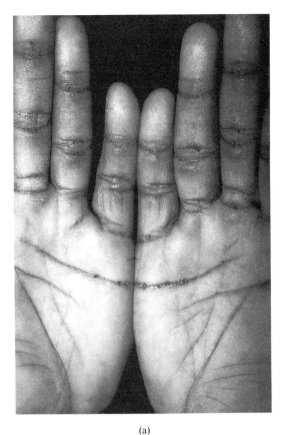

(a)

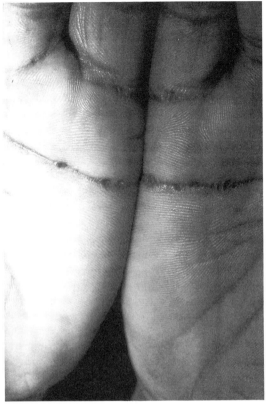

(b)

FIGURE 23.12. Palmar pits.

commonly in the sacrogluteal region in infants, but it can also be found on the shoulders, back, and the extensor surfaces of extremities. There is no sexual predilection, and often it is multiple. It can vary in size from a few millimeters to 6 centimeters or more, and its borders are irregular, gradually blending into the pigment of the surrounding skin. Clinically, this macule has been reported in 70–96% of black newborns, greater than 90% of Orientals, 46% of Hispanics, and 4%–9% of Caucasians.[21,22] Certain ethnic groups have higher incidence as well, such as the Yemenite Jews, with a 90% occurrence.[21] Histologically, this marking is made up of dermal melanocytes distributed between collagen fibers.[23]

The mongolian spot is a benign finding that usually spontaneously fades during the first or second year of life. One study showed a 95% incidence of mongolian spots in black infants less than 1 year old, compared to a 3% incidence in 10-year-olds,[22] however, no prospective study has been done. The spot's significance is unknown. There is no reported malignant potential in this spot, and the differential should include a blue nevus, the Nevus of Ota, and the Nevus of Ito.

Oral Pigmentation and Leukoederma

Examination of the oral mucosa in blacks is likely to show two normal variants: oral pigmentation and oral leukoederma. Oral pigmentation, ranging in color from brown/black to purple/blue macules, is most prominent on the gums (89%) but is also seen on bucca

FIGURE 23.13. Mongolian spot in an adult.

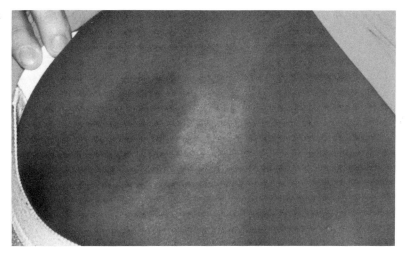

mucosa, hard palate, tongue, lips, and soft palate. When the floor of the mouth is affected, pigment is seen around the orifices of the salivary ducts. With the exception of the tongue, this pigmentation is almost always symmetric. Monash noted that the darker skinned the individual, the deeper the color and the more extensive the oral pigmentation;[24] however, recent literature does not confirm this.[5] The extensive pigmentation can even form a complete band around the gum line. If the pigment is present at birth, it is slight and it develops over the first two decades of life. After this time, the pigmentation persists, and any additional pigment can usually be found to have a nonphysiologic cause. A differential diagnosis includes heavy metal exposure, amalgam tattoos, antimalarials or phenothiazines, tobacco exposure, Addison's disease, hemochromatosis, neurofibromatosis, Peutz-Jegher's disease, black hairy tongue, oral melanomas, and pigmented tumors.

The other condition, oral leukoederma—first described in 1953 by Sandstead and Lowe[25]—is an asymptomatic, opalescent, pearly, whitish-gray, thickened plaque on the buccal mucosa that can be coarsely granular or shaggy and wet. It has been described in up to 90% of Negro adults (compared to 43% of Caucasians) and 51% of Negro children with no sex predilection.[26,27] As with oral pigment, this lesion tends to be symmetric. There is a direct relationship of severity of leukoederma to melanin pigment of the buccal mucosa such that a group with slight buccal pigmentation had a 16% incidence of leukoederma, whereas a heavily pigmented group had a 88% incidence.[27] Although the cause is still unknown, it has been linked to poor oral hygiene and cigarette smoking. It is not believed to be premalignant.

Palmar and Plantar Pigmentation

The palms and soles of blacks are generally less pigmented than the rest of their skin; however, these areas have more hyperpigmented markings when compared to palms and soles of lighter-skinned races. The palms show increased pigmentation of skin creases as well as a greater incidence of melanocytic nevi. Melanocytic nevi are also common on the soles of blacks as is pigmentary mottling. All of these findings are more common in darker-skinned blacks than in lighter. Lesions from secondary syphilis appear similar; however, their border is usually smoother and they are more prominent on the arch of the foot, whereas physiologic pigmentation generally spares this area. Premalignant tumors and acral lentiginous melanomas must also be considered in the differential.

Dermatoses More Commonly Seen in Blacks

Dermatosis Papulosa Nigra

Dermatosis papulosa nigra is seen almost exclusively in adult blacks with an incidence

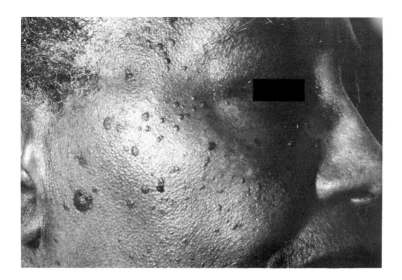

FIGURE 23.14. Dermatosis papulosa nigra.

reported between 10% and 77%.[28] Multiple small hyperpigmented pedunculated, sessile, or verrucous papules appear on the malar areas of the face, and are also seen on the neck, chest, and back (Fig. 23.14). They are rarely seen before puberty and increase in number over time. Women are affected more commonly than men, and a positive family history has been reported in more than 50% of patients in one study.[28] Histologically, these lesions are indistinguishable from seborrheic keratoses (Fig. 23.15) even though they clinically differ from these greasy lusterless lesions. The lesions probably are variants of seborrheic keratoses and display no spontaneous regression or malignant potential.

Treatment for these is cosmetic, and removal can be accomplished by electrodessication, cryotherapy, or light abrasive curettage.[29]

Keloids

Keloids are benign, nodular dermal growths resulting from proliferation of fibrous connective tissue. Ranging in consistency from soft and doughy to hard and rubbery, their surface is usually shiny, smooth, and hairless. Initially red or brown, they become pale over time. Keloids may occur on any site of the body, even the tongue, but are commonly found on the presternal area, the back and shoulders, the

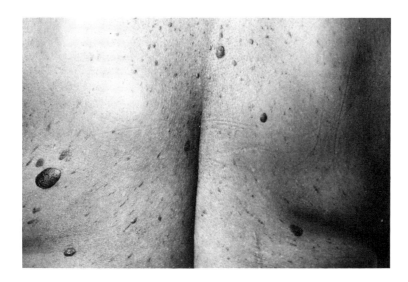

FIGURE 23.15. Seborrheic keratosis.

lateral cheek overlying the mandible, and the helix and lobe of the ear (Fig. 23.16). Patients often complain of tenderness, pruritus, and pain in the keloids. Rarely, they involute or ulcerate. Keloids differ from hypertrophic scars by their extension beyond the margins of the injury.

Although keloids have been noted in many races, blacks have a greater tendency toward keloid formation than whites; ratios of 2:1 to 19:1 have been reported.[1] Younger blacks (age 15–30) have the greatest incidence, and men and women are affected equally. Familial predisposition, especially in blacks, has been seen, and both autosomal dominant and recessive inheritance patterns have been reported.[30] Trauma (thermal burns and surgical incisions) initiate keloid formation; however, patients may not remember the prior trauma as this may have been slight and unnoticed. Endocrine dysfunction, skin tension, and intradermal sebum secretion have all also been cited as possible causes.[31,32]

Disorganized whorls of collagen, rarely extending into the underlying subcutaneous tissue, characterize the histologic appearance. This fibrous proliferation disrupts the normal architecture of the skin appendages and stretches the overlying epidermis. Fibroplasia continues beyond the normal peak of 3 weeks of wound healing. Treatment consists of either single use or a combination of modalities,[31] including intralesional and tropical corticosteroids, cryosurgery, surgery, lasers, ligatures, radiotherapy, pressure gradient garments, topical tretinoin, and oral or parenteral methotrexate.[33]

Pediatric Diseases

Acropustulosis of Infancy

Acropustulosis of infancy was first described in the 1970s as a recurrent pustular dermatosis that was recalcitrant to most therapies. It primarily affects black male infants between 2 and 10 months of age (rarely at birth) and is characterized by crops of intensely pruritic papules that enlarge into vesicopustules in 24 h. The lesions are distributed on the palms, soles, and dorsa of hands and feet, with sporadic involvement of wrists, ankles, scalp, and face. The crops last 7–14 days, and recur 2–3 weeks after the resolution of the previous lesions. As the infant gets older, the vesicopustules resolve in less time, and there is a longer hiatus between outbreaks. Spontaneous resolution occurs by 2–3 years of age, and no residual effects have been reported. Peripheral eosinophilia has been reported on laboratory examination.[34] Histological examination reveals an intraepidermal or

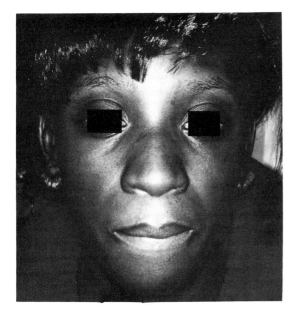

(a)

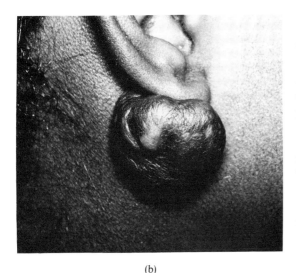

(b)

FIGURE 23.16. (a) Bilateral earlobe keloids. (b) Keloid in ear-piercing site.

subcorneal pustule filled with polymorpho-nuclear leukocytes.

Treatments with topical and systemic steroids, and topical and systemic antibiotics have been unsuccessful. Soporific doses of antihistamines have been used to control the itching, and in one case report, dapsone (2 mg/kg/day) has aided in the resolution of lesions.[35] The cause is unknown. The differential diagnosis should include scabies, transient neonatal pustular melanosis, impetigo, pompholyx, toxic erythema of the newborn, subcorneal pustular dermatosis, pustular psoriasis, and tinea.

Transient Neonatal Pustular Melanosis

Another disease predominantly affecting black infants is transient neonatal pustular melanosis. It is reported in 4–5% of black infants, males and females afflicted equally, compared to an incidence of 0.6% in white infants.[36] It presents at birth with clusters of sterile superficial vesicopustules with no surrounding erythema. Within 24 h, these rupture leaving a collarette of fine scale surrounding a hyperpigmented tan macule. The macule can persist, but usually fades in 3–12 weeks. These vesicopustules and pigmented macules appear on the face, chin, forehead, nape of the neck, and anterior shins. Bullae have been reported on the scalp, palms, and soles.

The etiology is unknown; there is no correlation with maternal infection or drug use. Biopsy will show an intracorneal or subcorneal blister with neutrophils, few eosinophils, and cellular debris. The pigmented macules show focal basilar hyperpigmentation. This disease can be distinguished from erythema toxicum neonatorum by examination of lesional contents for eosinophils characteristic of the latter. Other diseases it should be differentiated from are viral infections, impetigo, and herpes simplex.

Hair and Scalp Diseases

Dermatitis Papillaris Capillitii

Dermatitis papillaris capillitii has been called acne keloidalis nuchae for many years, which is erroneous because this disease has no relation-ship to acne vulgaris or keloidal formation. It is almost only seen in black men after puberty; however, it has been reported to have a male to female ratio of 3:1.[1] Dermatitis papillaris capillitii is a chronic folliculitis and peri-folliculitis of the occipital scalp and nape of the neck that can progress to infections and large fibrotic scars. At the onset, there are isolated flesh-colored papules and occasional pustules around hair follicles, representing inflammation of follicles at the general area of attachment of the sebaceous gland. There are no comedones or ingrown hairs. Eventually, this portion of the follicle is destroyed, and the lower hair follicle continues to grow, causing a foreign-body reaction with much fibroplasia. Clinically, this corresponds to coalescing of the papules into a keloidlike scar with patchy alopecia and polytrichea. Infrequent symptoms are itching, pain, and malodorous draining infections; however, the main concern is cosmetic as these lesions can become very large.

The cause of this entity is uncertain. Speculation has included mechanical factors (short thick necks, starched collars, and baseball caps), shaving, comb injuries, pomades, auto-immunity, and a transepithelial elimination disorder akin to the perforating skin diseases.[37,38] The majority of these lesions are resistant to treatment, which consists of moist compresses, manual epilation, corticosteroid injections, systemic antibiotics, topical corti-costeroids and antibiotics, and surgery with destruction of the hair follicle.

Follicular Degeneration Syndrome

Formerly known as hot-comb alopecia, the follicular degeneration syndrome is a disorder seen predominantly in black women in their second, third, and fourth decades (Fig. 23.17). This irreversible, diffuse alopecia begins on the crown and spreads laterally and frontally, sometimes reaching the frontal hairline. The lateral and posterior hairlines are spared. The involvement is diffuse, not patchy, and appar-ently normal hairs can remain in these areas. There is a decreased density of follicular orifices, evidence of polytrichea, and no inflammatory or pigmentary changes. Some patients report a dysesthesia (pins and needles) at the onset or

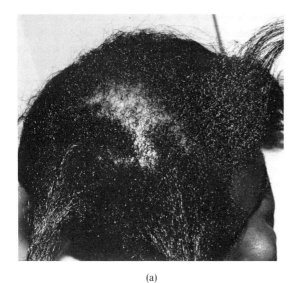

(a)

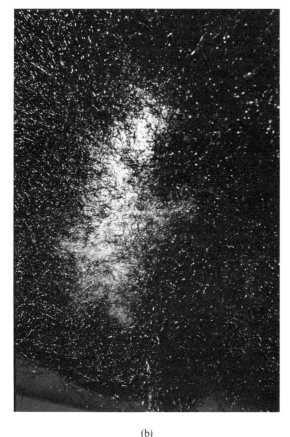

(b)

FIGURE 23.17. (a) Follicular degeneration syndrome. (b) Follicular degeneration syndrome of vertex scalp in black female.

progression of alopecia. Histologically, there is a chronic inflammation around the upper hair follicle with disruption of the internal and external root sheaths, and replacement of the follicle by a fibrous cord. Other forms of scarring alopecia are in the differential diagnosis: lupus erythematosus, lichen planopilaris, scleroderma, and pseudopalade of Broque.

Recently, the theory of follicular destruction by hot petrolatum from the process of hot-comb hair straightening originally postulated by LoPresti[39] has been doubted. Sperling and Sau noted a poor correlation between onset/progression of alopecia and usage of a hot comb, as well as cases of follicular degeneration syndrome in patients who never used a hot comb.[40] Their hypothesis is that there may be a predisposed population (blacks) to desquamation of the inner root sheath, and coupled with the innate tight curl of the hair, plus mechanical and cultural factors, degeneration of the follicle ensues.

Another disorder of the scalp, lipedematous alopecia, has only been reported in four black women aged 28–75.[41] The patients complained of pruritus and pain at the vertex, and examination revealed an area of short hairs and generalized hair loss. The scalp also felt thick and boggy.[42] This correlates with the histologic picture of hyperkeratosis, follicular plugging, atrophy, and an increase in normal-appearing subcutaneous fat. This fat extended into the dermis. The pressure from this subcutaneous fat has been implicated in the cause of this disease by not allowing adequate nutrition of the hair follicles.[43] Oral prednisone improved one patient's condition.[44] It is possible that this disease is follicular degeneration syndrome overlying thickened subcutaneous fat, and it would be interesting to further examine these cases histologically.

Perifolliculitis Capitis Abscedens et Suffodiens

Another scalp disorder affecting predominantly black men is perifolliculitis capitis abscedens et suffodiens (dissecting cellulitis of the scalp, Hoffman's disease). The terms abscedens and suffodiens mean suppurating and undermining, respectively, and true to the name, this chronic disease consists of sterile, boggy abscesses with sinus tracts and burrows of the vertex and occiput. Beginning with large comedones and multiple firm and fluctuant nodules, as the undermining cellulitis progresses, patients have minimal pain, lymphadenopathy, and systemic symptoms. Overlying hairs loosen and exfoliate, leading to a scarring alopecia, and sausage-shaped ridges on the scalp may become apparent. Secondary bacterial infection often occurs, and sinus tracts may drain purulent material. Although the etiology is uncertain, keratin plugging of follicles and a granulomatous reaction to the keratin has been implicated.

There is often an association with acne conglobata and hidradenitis suppurativa, which has been termed the follicular occlusion triad. Treatment is disappointing, as oral antibiotics and intralesional steroids provide only temporary relief. Incision and drainage of lesions may help with early lesions. More severe or resistant cases have been treated with zinc,[45] dapsone,[46] x-ray epilation (Adamson-Keinbock technique), and scalp excision with split thickness grafting. A single report of a squamous cell carcinoma arising in a long-standing case of perifolliculitis capitis abscedens et suffodiens has appeared in the literature.[47]

Pomade Acne

Many emollient creams and oils (pomades) are used by blacks on their hair scalps, and sometimes faces for grooming. This common practice can lead to pomade acne, a variant of acne cosmetica. The clinical picture is one of closely set open and closed comedones on the forehead and temples. The eruption may appear papular; however, inflammation, pustules, and cystic nodules are not usually seen. All age groups are susceptible to the disorder. As in acne vulgaris, postinflammatory hyperpigmentation may follow pomade acne. The cause is the application of the comedogenic substances, either directly to the areas or from transfer from the scalp and hair. It has been shown in one study that black skin responds to ointment under occlusion with comedone formation, whereas white skin more frequently responds with an inflammatory acneform reaction.[1]

However, this observed distinction has not been widely accepted as a predisposing factor to pomade acne.[48] Treatment is discontinuation of the inciting agents.

A disease that may be a variant of this, dermatitis cruris pustulosa et atrophica, is seen in Africa and Trinidad. A pustular folliculitis and scaling of the skin occurs between the knee and the ankle, and is correlated with the use of palm oils and emollients on these areas.[1,48]

Pseudofolliculitis Barbae

Pseudofolliculitis barbae is seen in 45–83% of black men who shave.[1,49] Commonly seen on the anterior neckline, mandibular areas, cheeks, and chin, this disease is characterized by small flesh-colored or hyperpigmented papules that occur due to ingrown hairs with foreign-body reaction. Pustules are only seen when lesions become secondarily infected. There are two mechanisms by which hairs become ingrown: extrafollicular and transfollicular, and both are related to the innate curvature of black hair follicles and shafts. Extrafollicular refers to hairs that have been sharpened from shaving, growing back toward the epidermis, and reentering the skin 1–2 mm from where it originally exited. The hair penetrates through the epidermis to the dermis where it incites a foreign-body reaction. The transfollicular mechanism occurs when shaving against the grain of the hair when the skin is taut. These hairs are cut too short and are sharp, and they have a tendency because of the curved follicle to pierce the follicular wall and cause a foreign-body reaction. Both mechanisms cause the characteristic papules that can be traumatized further by shaving.

Treatment of this condition is to allow the hairs to grow for 1 month, during which time most of the lesions resolve (most hairs grow out). When shaving resumes, one should keep hairs at a length of 0.5–1 mm. Electric clippers, razors with safety guards, manual freeing of ingrown hairs, chemical depilatories (barium sulfide, calcium thioglycolate), complete epilation, and topical antibiotics have also been advocated.

Traction Alopecia

Most alopecias in blacks are found to have a traumatic origin. The shape of black hair makes it more susceptible to fracture, and with concomitant use of hair relaxers, which reduce disulfide bonds and weaken the hair, black hair breaks much easier than hairs of other races. Both frequent combing, especially with a metal-toothed comb, and friction from hats causes these hairs to fracture. Traction alopecia is traumatic as well, but results from tension put on the hair follicle by tight braiding. Early in the disease follicular erythema and pustules may be evident. The hair loss then occurs at the margin of the individual tufts and temporal and frontal regions of the scalp as hairs become loosened from the follicles and follicular inflammation and atrophy ensue. The atrophic follicles can only produce thin short hairs. There may be a thin patch of hair at the distal margin representing hair that was too short to be incorporated into the hair style.

Although not unique to blacks, the process is very common due to tight plaits in children and cornrow patterns in adults (Fig. 23.18). Early recognition of traction alopecia and changing of hair styles is the treatment of choice, but punch

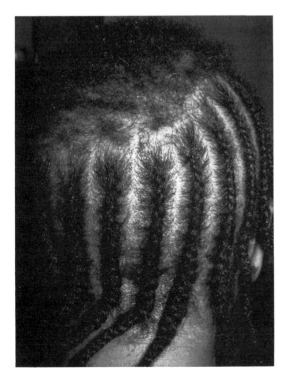

FIGURE 23.18. Cornrowing alopecia.

grafting and flap rotation surgery have been used for more severe cases.

Sickle Cell Peculiarities

Although only 0.2% of blacks in the United States are homozygous for sickle cell disease, it is worth mentioning a few cutaneous manifestations of this disease. The first and most common is jaundice. This occurs in up to 95% of patients at some time in their lives and may be mild and difficult to see. The next, dactylitis (hand–foot syndrome), has been reported as the most common finding in children, with 45% of children affected by 2 years of age in one study.[34,50] This febrile condition of painful, erythematous non-pitting edema affecting the hands and sometimes the feet represents microinfarctions in the small bones in the hands and feet. It is seen more in the winter months, like other painful crises, and is associated with minor infections (gastroenteritis and upper respiratory tract infections).

Sickle cell leg ulcers occur in 25–75% of patients in their lifetime,[1] generally when they are over 15 years of age. If there is any prior trauma, the ulcer is out of proportion to the severity of the injury. One sees sharply marginated ulcers with an indurated gray base, which are unilaterally found above the medial malleolus. They are also seen on the elbows, dorsa of feet, and anterior thighs.

The fourth condition, the extra transverse digital crease, is an anatomic sign seen in 28–90% of homozygous sickle cell patients.[51,52] This crease is found on the palmar surface of the fingers, distal to the normal distal interphalangeal crease, and separated from it by two or more epidermal ridges. The extra crease must not connect with the normal crease to be considered a true extra crease. Present at birth, the third finger is the most common location, and occasionally it is bilateral. To date, it has not been seen in patients with sickle cell trait, and it must be kept in mind that it has occurred in 10% of a normal control population.[52]

Finally, a rare type of alopecia has been reported in three patients with sickle cell anemia. Resembling ophiasis, there is alopecia extending from the temple to the occiput in symmetric bands. This was correlated in one patient to a sickle cell crisis.[53]

Conclusions

A discussion of variations of dermatoses of African-Americans, African blacks, and other black races, as well as the literature concerning all black skin disorders is beyond the scope of this chapter. Instead, it is our hope that this chapter has enlightened its reader to a better understanding and appreciation of problems and normal variants encountered in black skin.

References

1. Brauner GJ: Cutaneous Disease in Black Races. In: Moschella SL, Hurley HJ, eds. Dermatology, 2nd ed. Philadelphia: WB Saunders, 1985:1904–1945.
2. Weigand DA, Haygood C, Gaylor J: Cell layers and density of negro and caucasian stratum corneum. *J Invest Dermatol* 1974;**62**:563–568.
3. Montagna W, Carlisle K: The architecture of black and white facial skin. *J Am Acad Dermatol* 1991;**24**:929–937.
4. Andersen KE, Maibach HI. Black and white human skin differences. *J Am Acad Dermatol* 1979;**1**:276–282.
5. McLaurin CI: Cutaneous reaction patterns in blacks. *Dermatol Clin* 1988;**6**:353–362.
6. Kenney JA, Jr: Vitiligo. *Dermatol Clin* 1988;**6**: 425–434.
7. O'Farrell NM: Pityriasis alba. *AMA Arch Dermatol* 1956;**73**:376–377.
8. Martin RF, Lugo-Somolinos A, Sanchez JL: Clinicopathologic conference study on pityriasis alba. *Bol Asoc Med PR* 1990;**82**:463–465.
9. McDonald CJ: Dermatologic problems in black skin. *Prog Dermatol* 1973;**7**:15–20.
10. Wentzell JM, Baughman RD: Pityriasis alba. In: Demis DJ, chief editor. *Clinical Dermatology.* Philadelphia: JB Lippincott, 1990: Unit 13–5.
11. McDonald CJ, Kelly AP: Dermatology of black skin. In: Demis DJ, chief editor. *Clinical Dermatology.* Philadelphia: Harper and Row, 1987: Unit 30–1.
12. Parsons JM: Pityriasis rosea update: 1986. *J Am Acad Dermatol* 1986;**15**:159–167.
13. Futcher PH: A peculiarity of pigmentation of the upper arm of negroes [letter]. *Science* 1938;**88**: 570–571.
14. James WD, Carter JM, Rodman OG. Pigmentary demarcation lines: a population survey. *J Am Acad Dermatol* 1987;16:584–590.
15. Monash S: Normal pigmentation in the nails of the Negro. *Arch Dermatol Syphilol* 1932;**25**:876–878.
16. Brauner GJ: Keratosis puncta [letter]. *Arch Dermatol* 1981;**117**:66.
17. Rustad OJ, Vance JC: Punctate keratoses of the palms and soles and keratotic pits of the palmar creases. *J Am Acad Dermatol* 1990;**22**:468–476.
18. Weiss RM, Rasmussen JE: Karatosis punctata of the palmar creases. *Arch Dermatol* 1980;**116**:669–671.
19. Selmanowitz VJ, Krivo JM: Hypopigmented markings in Negros. *Int J Dermatol* 1973;**12**:229–235.
20. Brauner GJ: Cutaneous disease in black children. *Am J Dis Child* 1983;**137**:488–496.
21. Cordova A: The mongolian spot; A study of ethnic differences and a literature review. *Clin Pediatr* 1981;**20**:714–719.
22. Vollum DI: Skin markings in children from the West Indies. *Br J Dermatol* 1971;**85**:260–263.
23. Kikuchi I: The biological significance of the mongolian spot. *Int J Dermatol* 1989;**28**:513–514.
24. Monash S: Normal pigmentation of the oral mucosa. *Arch Dermatol Syphilol* 1933;**26**:139–147.
25. Sandstead HR, Lowe JW: Leukoedema and keratosis in relation to leukoplakia of the buccal mucosa. *J Natl Cancer Inst* 1953;**14**:423–437.
26. Archard HO, Carlson KP, Stanley HR: Leukoedema of the human oral mucosa. *Oral Surg Oral Med Oral Pathol* 1968;**25**:717–728.
27. Martin JL, Crump EP: Leukoedema of the buccal mucosa in Negro children and youth. *Oral Surg Oral Med Oral Pathol* 1972;**34**:49–58.
28. Grimes PE, Arora S, Minus HR, Kenney JA, Jr: Dermatosis papulosa nigra. *Cutis* 1983;**32**:385–386, 392.
29. Kauh YC, McDonald JW, Rapaport JA, et al: Surgical approach for dermatosis papulosa nigra. *Int J Dermatol* 1983;**22**:590–592.
30. Knox JM, Knox JM: Keloids. In: Demis DJ, chief editor. *Clinical Dermatology.* Philadelphia: JB Lippincott, 1990: Unit 4–15.
31. Kelly AP: Keloids. *Dermatol Clin* 1988;**6**:413–424.
32. Osman AAA, Gumma KA, Satir AA: Highlights on the etiology of the keloid. *Int Surg* 1978;**63**:33–37.
33. Onwukwe MF: Surgery and methotrexate for keloids [letter]. *Schoch Letter* 1978;**28**:4.

34. McLaurin CI: Pediatric dermatology in black patients. *Dermatol Clin* 1988;**6**:457–473.
35. Kahn G, Rywlin AM: Acropustulosis of infancy. *Arch Dermatol* 1979;**115**:831–833.
36. Ramamurthy RS, Reveri M, Esterly NB, Fretzin DF, Pildes RS: Transient neonatal pustular melanosis. *J Pediatr* 1976;**88**:831–815.
37. Dinehart SM, Herzberg AJ, Kerns BJ, Pollack SV: Acne keloidalis: A review. *J Dermatol Surg Oncol* 1989;**15**:642–647.
38. Goette DK, Berger TG: Acne keloidalis nuchae. A transepithelial elimination disorder. *Int J Dermatol* 1987;**26**:442–444.
39. LoPresti P, Papa CM, Kligman AM: Hot comb alopecia. *Arch Dermatol* 1968;**98**:234–238.
40. Sperling LC, Sau P: Follicular degeneration syndrome. *Arch Dermatol* 1992;**128**:68–74.
41. Crounse RG: Lipedematous alopecia. In: Demis DJ, chief editor. *Clinical Dermatology.* Philadelphia: JB Lippincott, 1990: Unit 2–38.
42. Scott DA: Disorders of the hair and scalp in blacks. *Dermatol Clin* 1988;**6**:387–395.
43. Curtis JW, Heising NA: Lipedematous alopecia associated with skin hyperelasticity. *Arch Dermatol* 1964;**89**:819–820.
44. Coskey RJ, Fosnaugh RP, Fine G: Lipedematous alopecia. *Arch Dermatol* 1961;**84**:135–138.
45. Berne B, Venge P, Ohman S: Perifolliculitis capitis abscedens et suffodiens (Hoffman): Complete healing with oral zinc therapy. *Arch Dermatol* 1985;**121**:1028–1030.
46. Halder RM: Hair and scalp disorders in blacks. *Cutis* 1983;**32**:378–380.
47. Curry SS, Gaither DH, King LE, Jr: Squamous cell carcinoma arising in dissecting perifolliculitis of the scalp. *J Am Acad Dermatol* 1981;**4**:673–678.
48. Rosen T, Martin S: Atlas of black dermatology. Boston: Little, Brown and Company, 1981.
49. Brown LA, Jr: Pathogenesis and treatment of pseudofolliculitis barbae. *Cutis* 1983;**32**:373–375.
50. Stevens MC, Padwick M, Serjeant GR: Observations on the natural history of dactylitis in homozygous sickle cell disease. *Clin Pediatr* 1981;**20**:311–317.
51. DeJong R, Platou RV: Sickle cell hemoglobinopathy: An anatomic sign *Am J Dis Child* 1967;**113**:271–272.
52. Zizmor J: The extra transverse digital crease. A skin sign found in sickle cell disease. *Cutis* 1973;**11**:447–449.
53. Cornbleet T, Schorr HC, Barsky S: Pseudo-ophiasis and sickle cell anemia. *AMA Arch Dermatol* 1959;**59**:519–521.

24

Diseases Among Jewish People

Abraham Feinstein

The Jewish people includes various ethnic groups that are unified by virtue of a common religion, language, history, and culture. The history of the Jewish people can be traced back to 1800 B.CE., when Abraham, who is considered to be the first Jew, emigrated from Mesopotamia (Iraq today) to Canaan (Israel today). Indeed, most of the Jews living today are considered to be his descendants. In 583 B.CE., Babylon conquered the country and expelled the majority of the population to the land that is now Iraq. With the passage of time, the Jewish people moved and resided in other countries. Today, Jewish people can be found in almost every country in the world, with their number estimated at approximately 14 million.

The main groupings of Jews include the following.

1. *Oriental Jews* are those who settled mainly in the countries of Asia. They lived under Islamic rule and represent the original gene pool of the Jewish people.
2. *Sephardi Jews* initially lived in Spain (the word Spharad means Spain in Hebrew) but later emigrated in the main to countries bordering the Mediterranean Sea. They lived under Turkish Islam rule and had a specific language, Ladino, which is Spanish intermixed with Hebrew, Arabic, and Slavic.
3. *Ashkenazi Jews* resided in Germany (the word Ashkenaz means Germany in Hebrew), from where they migrated to other European lands, mainly Poland and Russia. They lived under Christianity and spoke a common

language, Yiddish, which is basically German with sprinklings of Hebrew, Polish, and Russian.

Over the years, mass migration of the Jewish people brought changes in the settlement of different ethnic groups. In the 16th century, a large Sephardi community moved to the Netherlands, and over the past century, many Sephardi Jews moved from countries of North Africa to France. Many Jews, most of them Ashkenazi, sought new lives in the United States, Canada, South America, and South Africa. Over the past decades, mass immigrations of Ashkenazi, as well as Sephardi and Oriental Jews, firmly established these communities in Israel.

Many scientific studies that utilized genetic markers and other similar criteria have shown that there is a strong homogeneity among the Jewish people, regardless of which of the three major groupings to which they may belong. These findings are not surprising given the fact that they share a common ancestry, even though this extends back 4000 years. A certain degree of heterogeneity has been found among the groups, however, due probably to conversions and mixed marriages, which brought new genes into the original Jewish gene pool. In addition, environmental factors such as climate, diet, and so on had significant influence on the development of diseases and other genetic traits.

Homogeneity was found to be more characteristic of the Ashkenazi Jews than of the Sephardi or Oriental Jews. Many investigators, therefore,

TABLE 24.1. The major ethnic groups of the Jewish People and their main resident countries.

Non-Ashkenazi Jews		Ashkenazi Jews
Oriental Jews	Sephardi Jews	
Afghanistan	Algeria	Australia
Ethiopia	Bulgaria	Austria
India	Egypt	Czechoslovakia
Iran	France	England
Iraq	Greece	France
Israel	Israel	Germany
Lebanon	Italy	Hungary
Pakistan	Libya	Israel
Syria	Morocco	Netherlands
Yemen	Netherlands	South Africa
	Spain	North America
	Turkey	Poland
	Yugoslavia	Russia
		South America

use the defining terms Ashkenazi and non-Ashkenazi Jews, the latter including Oriental and Sephardi Jews, who may be further distinguished by their country of origin. The ethnic groupings of the Jewish People are listed in Table 24.1.

Although the diseases that are reported for the Jewish people are not different in their manifestations from those that are noted for the general population, some variations may be found in prevalence figures, both for the Jewish people as a population and for specific ethnic communities within this people. This accords with the usual findings in isolated ethnic and racial groups. These considerations underlie the discussion that follows. In addition, isolated and rare syndromes that have been found among Jews will be described.[1-5]

Diseases or Conditions with Cutaneous Manifestations

Stub Thumb[6]

Main findings: The presence of short and broad terminal phalanges of the thumb and the big toes. In many cases, it appears with an absence of the proximal phalanx of the fourth toe.

Dermatologic manifestations: The above findings.

The inheritance is autosomal dominance, and it is found to occur in 1.6% of the Jewish population, compared to 0.1–0.4% in other population groups.

Hairy Ears[7]

Main findings are the dermatologic manifestations.

Dermatologic manifestations: Coarse hair on the pinna of the ear.

Controversy exists as to whether this trait is Y-linked, autosomal dominance, or both. This condition is relatively common among Jews. In Ashkenazi Jews, the hair grows more commonly on the top of the ear, whereas in Iraqi and Iranian Jews, the hair tends to grow out of the side of the ear.

Down's Syndrome (Mongolism)[8]

Main findings: Mental retardation is the rule. The subject is usually short and broad with thick legs and trunk. The arms are short, the hands are broad, and the fingers are thick. The eyes have inner and outer epicanthal folds. The mouth is small and is usually open.

Dermatologic manifestations: The tongue is thick and furrowed by deep folds; scalp hair is usually absent.

Its incidence among Jews is found to be higher than in the general population.

Werner's Syndrome[9]

Main findings: Small size and thin limbs, prematurely aged face, arteriosclerosis in early age, diabetes mellitus, cataracts, subcutaneous calcification, hypogonadism, and typical skin changes. The face shows beaked nose, taut lips, protuberant teeth and recessive chin. The voice is high pitched.

Skin manifestations: The skin is poikilodermic, typically atrophic, with pigmentary changes and scaliness and, in some cases, telangiectasia. Sclerodermoid changes may also develop, and deformed digits are also seen.

Thick keratoses develop over points of pressure. The hair becomes gray and thin at an early age.

This is a rare autosomal recessive disease, which to date has been described in less than 200 cases. Its occurrence among Jews, especially Ashkenazi Jews, is relatively very high.

Pemphigus Vulgaris[10,11]

Main findings are the dermatologic manifestations.

Dermatologic manifestations: Flaccid, easily ruptured bullae on the skin and mucous membranes, especially the mouth, are the hallmark of the disease. Unless properly treated, the bullae spread and the disease may be fatal.

It is relatively more common among Ashkenazi Jews than in the general population. It is associated with HLA A26, Bw38, and, especially, DRw4.

Bloom's Syndrome (Congenital Telangiectatic Erythema and Stunted Growth)[12]

Main findings: Growth retardation, telangiectatic erythema on the face, and photosensitivity.

Dermatologic manifestations: Telangiectatic erythema, which affects mainly the forehead, nose, cheeks, and ears. Cafe au lait spots are noted in half of the cases. Other skin manifestations that have been described and are probably coincidental are keratosis pilaris, ichthyotic skin, acanthosis nigricans, hypertrichosis, syndactyly, absence of a toe, supernumerary digit, clinodactyly, absence of upper lateral incisors, and prominent ears.

The disease, which is transmitted by an autosomal recessive inheritance, is very rare and less than 150 cases have been described to date, half of them in Ashkenazi Jews.

Kaposi's Sarcoma (Multiple Idiopathic Hemorrhagic Sarcoma)[5]

Main findings: This is a multifocal proliferative neoplasm, which in its classic form involves the vascular tissue and primarily affects the

skin, lymph nodes, or gastrointestinal tract, and may spread to other visceral areas.

Dermatologic manifestations: Reddened macules appear on the skin, mostly on the legs and feet of adult persons. These macules progress to form plaques or tumors.

The classic disease is not considered to be genetically determined, but familial occurrence has been described in a few cases. The disease is probably more frequent among Ashkenazi Jews and Italians.

Hereditary Hemorrhagic Telangiectasia (Osler-Weber-Rendu's Syndrome)[13]

Main findings: The most consistent finding of this disorder is the appearance of cutaneous, mucosal, and visceral telangiectases with recurrent bleeding, most commonly in the second or third decades. In addition, arterovenous malformations of the lung and other organs may occur. Cyanosis, clubbing of the nails, and dyspnea may be manifested as well as neurologic abnormalities. Cerebrovascular accidents, brain abscess, and high-output heart failure can also be found.

Dermatologic manifestations: Most typical are telangiectasia of the hands and feet as well as the oral cavity.

The disease is transmitted in an autosomal dominant inheritance and is probably more frequent among Ashkenazi Jews.

Familial Dysautonomia, Type II[14]

Main findings: The appearance during infancy of feeding problems due to dysphagia, recurrent pneumonia, and hypotonia due to neuropathy is typical. The facial appearance is characteristic and is described as being sad and frightened.

Dermatologic manifestations: An absence of fungiform papilla of the tongue is a pathognemonic feature.

The transmission is autosomal recessive, and the vast majority of cases occur in Ashkenazi Jews.

Selective Vitamin B$_{12}$ Malabsorption[15]

Main findings: Weakness, failure to thrive, GI symptoms (anorexia, vomiting, diarrhea), mild hepatosplenomegaly.
Dermatologic manifestations: Pallor, glossitis.

Most of the reported cases are either Scandinavian or Sephardi Jews.

Familial Mediterranean Fever[16,17]

Main findings: Attacks of fever accompanied by abdominal and joint pain. The attack subsides in 1–3 days and recurs weeks or months later. In up to 25% of cases, amyloid is accumulated in various tissues, mainly along blood vessel walls. When kidneys are involved, the condition is usually fatal.
Skin manifestations: Erysipelaslike erythema of the leg is a typical accompanying sign. It may also be the only feature of the disease.

The disease is found almost exclusively among North African Sephardi communities. The occurrence among other Jews and in non-Jews is rather rare.

Ataxia Telangiectasia (Louis-Bar's Syndrome)[18]

Main findings: Progressive cerebellar ataxia and oculocutaneous telangiectasia.
Dermatologic manifestations: Telangiectasia of the conjunctivae appear at age 3, and on the skin at the age of 6, mainly on the ears, eyelids, butterfly area, necklace, dorsa of the hands and feet, antecubital and popliteal fossae, and palate. Other skin changes include pigmented nevi, cafe au lait spots, vitiligo, seborrhea, xerosis, keratosis pilaris, atopic dermatitis, and sclerodermalike changes. In addition, progeric changes, such as premature graying of the hair, loss of subcutaneous fat, the appearance of atrophic scars and poikiloderma may occur. Actinic keratoses and basal cell carcinomas may appear at an early age.

The transmission is autosomal recessive, and its frequency is higher among the Moroccan Jewish community (at least 1:8000) compared to the general population (1:40,000).

Phenylketonuria (Folling's Disease, Phenylpyruvic Oligophrenia)[19]

Main findings: Retardation, seizures, tumors, and microcephalus.
Dermatologic manifestations: Hypopigmentation of the skin, hair, and eyes is the rule. In 10–60% of cases, atopic dermatitis is also found. Sclerodermalike changes have also been reported in a few cases.

Its transmission is autosomal recessive, and it has been found more frequently among non-Ashkenazi Jews, particularly in Yemenite Jews.

Ichthyosis[20]

Ichthyosis vulgaris, which is transmitted as an autosomal dominance inheritance, and X-linked ichthyosis are the two more-frequent groups of the ichthyotic disease.

Main findings: A variable degree of scaling that covers most of the body skin is the main feature of these diseases.
Dermatologic manifestations: In the X-linked ichthyosis, large, dark scales cover most of the trunk and limbs. In the ichthyosis vulgaris variety, the legs are mainly involved with the upper extremities being affected to a lesser degree. The antecubital and the popliteal fossae are not affected and the disease is more severe during the winter months. Follicular keratosis and prominent creases of palms are found in ichthyosis vulgaris. Atopic dermatitis is frequently found in patients with this variant.

Whereas the prevalence of the ichthyotic diseases among Jews is the same as in the general population, there is a substantial difference in its frequency among specific ethnic groups. In Iraqi Jews, one finds only X-linked ichthyosis, whereas Indian Jews suffer only from ichthyosis vulgaris.

Hyperbilirubinemia (Dubin-Johnson's Syndrome)[21]

Main findings: Chronic or intermittent jaundice, deposit of melanin or melaninlike substance in liver cells, and, in some cases, hepatomegaly and abdominal pain.

Dermatologic manifestations: Yellow skin.

Transmission is autosomal recessive, and it is found mostly in Iranian Jews (minimum frequency of 1:1300) compared to 1:40,000 in Sephardi Jews and 1:100,000 in Ashkenazi Jews. It is much rarer among the non-Jewish population.

Isolated Syndromes with Skin Manifestations

The diseases described here are usually reported in one or a few families. They are usually autosomal recessive in their inheritance and most of them described in the non-Ashkenazi Jewish population, due to a relatively high frequency of consanguineous marriages among these ethnic groups. The main reasons for their inclusion are as follows:

1. Not all of them are present in only one family and an awareness of this may help their recognition in other families.
2. The study of rare genetic diseases frequently advances medical knowledge that is applicable to more common diseases.
3. Their recognition is important for genetic counseling.

Aldolase A Deficiency[22]

A disorder characterized by hepatosplenomegaly, physical and mental retardation, and peculiar facial appearance with flat nose, epicanthic folds, strabismus, and short neck without webbing. The skin is pale and lax. The disease was found in an Ashkenzi Jewish family.

Leprechaunism[23]

The patients have a typical facial appearance with widely spaced eyes, large and low-set ears, broad nose, large mouth and thick lips. Enlargement of the breast, clitoris, or penis is usually noted at birth. The hands and feet appear large. In some cases, mild jaundice with slight hepatomegaly is noted. Such patients have facial hirsutism with generalized increase in body hair. In many cases, acanthosis nigricans

is present. The disease has been described in a few Sephardi Jewish families although it is also known among non-Jewish families.

Skin Mastocytosis with Short Stature, Conductive Hearing Loss, and Microdontia[24]

This syndrome was described in a Sephardi Jewish girl whose parents were consanguineously related. It includes short stature, microcephaly, conductive hearing loss, skin mastocytosis, and microtia.

Congenital Deafness and Onychodystrophy[25]

In this syndrome, an association between congenital deafness with onychodystrophy of the nails of all fingers and toes was found. This syndrome was described only in Sephardi Jews.

Congenital Deafness with Total Albinism[26]

This disease, which includes congenital deafness with total albinism, was described in four children of two consanguineous Moroccan Sephardi Jews.

Albinism–Deafness Syndrome (Ziprkowski's Syndrome)[27,28]

The characteristic clinical findings are piebaldism with total sensorineural deafness, marked vestibular hypofunction, and occasionally, heterochromia of the iris. The disease is transmitted in an X-linked pattern and it was described in a large Sephardic Jewish family of Moroccan origin. The gene responsible for this disorder was recently found to be located at Xq26.3-q27.1.

Tel-Hashomer Campodactyly Syndrome[29]

The syndrome includes short stature, peculiar facial appearance (ocular hypertelerism, small mouth, asymmetry, high arched palate), thoracic scoliosis, campodactyly, syndactyly, clinodactyly, dislocated radii, club feet, and hypoplasia of muscles. This order was described in two siblings of Jewish Moroccan ancestry and later in two Bedouin sisters.

Wrinkly Skin Syndrome[30,31]

In this syndrome, the skin of all the body except the face is dry, with easily formed wrinkles. In addition, the skin on the chest and the dorsal surface of the hands and feet show a prominent venous pattern. The disease was described in consanguineous Iraqi and Moroccan Jewish families.

Blue Sclera and Keratoconus[32]

Keratoconus and blue sclerae are the hallmarks of this syndrome. In addition, some of the cases displayed hyperextensible joints, corneal fragility, decreased hearing, dry skin and hair, poor dental development, dislocated hips, red hair, umbilicated hernia, arachnodactyly, spondylolisthesis, and mental retardation. The syndrome is very rare and most of the cases were Tunisian or Iraqi Jews.

Inherited Progressive Cone-Rod Dystrophy and Alopecia[33]

Progressive alopecia of the scalp and eyebrows with cone-rod dystrophy was described in four individuals belonging to a Yemenite Jewish family. The disease is inherited in an autosomal recessive fashion.

Hereditary Hypotrichosis Simplex of the Scalp[34]

This is a rare trait with onset in early childhood that was described in 51 individuals of a Yemenite Jewish community. Transmission is autosomal dominance.

Congenital Ichthyosis with Atrophy, Mental Retardation, Dwarfism, and Generalized Aminoaciduria[35]

The clinical features include ichthyosiform erythroderma, atrophy over the skin of the dorsa of hands and feet, and bullae over the exposed areas of the body. Neurological examination revealed weakness of the legs, spasticity, and increased reflexes. Generalized aminoaciduria s additionally demonstrated. This syndrome s described in an Iraqi Jewish family.

Familial Leg Ulcers of Juvenile Onset[36]

Chronic ulcerations of the legs with juvenile onset was found in 11 male relatives of an Iraqi Jewish family. Transmission was probably in an autosomal dominant sex-limited inheritance.

Camptodactyly with Fibrous Tissue Hyperplasia and Skeletal Dysplasia[37]

In this syndrome marfanoid appearance, broad nose, camptodactyly, knuckle pads, hammer toes, and a thoracic scoliosis are noted. It was described in an Iranian Jewish family.

Cutis Laxa: A New Variant[5]

This syndrome includes marked wrinkling and laxity of the skin. Facial findings include small mouth, micrognathia, blue sclerae, ocular hypertelorism, and high arched eyebrows. The skull shows brachycephaly, prominent veins about the forehead, and fine scalp hair. Other findings include marked hyperextensibility of the joints, hypospadias, and cryptochidism. The disease was described in an Iranian Jewish family.

Berlin Syndrome[38]

This syndrome includes hypohidrosis and a facial appearance that resembles that of anhidrotic ectodermal dysplasia. Physical and mental development are retarded and the eruption of teeth is delayed. Skin changes include generalized mottled pigmentation, dry skin, and hyperkeratosis of palms and soles. Pubic and axillary hair is sparse. The disease was described in four siblings of an Iranian Jewish family.

Hydropic Ectodermal Dysplasia[39]

The syndrome was described in a Karaite family in which short and dark brown scalp hair and scanty eyebrows were found in addition to the existence of prominent chin and lips and the absence of lateral incisors in the upper and lower jaws.

Acrocephalopolysyndactyly Type IV[40]

An autosomal recessive syndrome characterized by the presence of clinodactyly, campodactyly, and ulnar deviation. It was described in an Indian Jewish family.

Conclusions

Most of the Jewish people can be considered to a certain extent to be genetically interrelated. They can be divided into Ashkenazi and non-Ashkenazi Jews, the latter category being classified further as those of Oriental or

---

Diseases or Disorders Without Skin Manifestations

Conditions More Common Among Jews

- Neoplastic diseases: Carcinoma of colon (carcinoma of the cervix and of the penis relatively rare)
- Lactose intolerance
- Left-handedness

The following diseases are believed to be most frequent and typical of Jewish community; however, this belief has not been confirmed by any controlled study:

- Diabetes mellitus
- Hemorrhoids
- Inguinal hernia
- Mental illness
- Mental retardation
- Polycythemia vera
- Buerger's, disease—Ashkenazi Jews
- Familial iminoglycinuria—Ashkenazi Jews

Conditions More Common Among Ashkenazi Jews

- Abetalipoproteinemia
- Absense of permanent upper canines and lack of wisdom teeth
- Acute hemolytic anemia with familial ultrastructural abnormalities of the red-cell membrane
- Color blindness
- Coronary heart diseases
- Essential pentosuria
- Familial hyperglycinuria
- Gaucher's disease type I
- Gilles de la Tourette syndrome
- Glycinuria with urolithiasis
- Kallman's syndrome
- Legg-Calve-Perthes' disease
- Mucolipidosis type IV
- Multiple sclerosis
- Myopia
- Neurologic syndrome simulating familial dysautonomia
- Nieman-Pick's disease
- Obesity
- Oculopharyngeal muscular dystrophy
- Ovoid pupils
- Primary torsion dystonia
- PTA deficiency
- Regional enteritis
- Spongy degeneration of the central nervous system
- Tay–Sachs' disease
- Tyrosinosis
- Ulcerative colitis
- Upper limb–cardiovascular syndromes
- Wilson's disease
- X-linked gout caused by mutant feedback-resistant phosphoribosylpyrophosphate synthetase

Continued

Diseases More Common Among Non-Ashkenazi Jews

Non-Ashkenazi
- Benign familial hematuria
- Glycogen-storage disease type III
- Persistent mild hyperphenylalaninemia
- Takayasu arteritis

Sephardi
- Combined factor V and factor VIII deficiency

Mediterranean countries
- Glucose 6 phosphate dehydrogenase deficiency

North African and Asian
- Alcoholism, which is very low in Jews but is twice as common among Asian and North African Jews than among Ashkenazi Jews
- Peroxidase and phospholipid deficiency in eosinophils

North African and Yemen
- Celiac disease

North African
- Congenital adrenal hyperplasia III
- Cystinosis

Moroccan
- Bronchial asthma—high in Iraqi Jews in relation to other ethnic Jews
- Cerebrotendinous xanthomatosis
- Familial deafness
- Radioulnar synostosis and craniosynostosis
- Spondyloenchondrodysplasia
- X-linked recessive retinal dysplasia

Libyan
- Creutzfeldt-Jakob's disease
- Cystinuria

Asian
- Congenital malformations

- Cystic lung diseases
- Pituitary dwarfism II

Iran and Iraq
- Pseudocholinesterase deficiency

Iraq and Yemen
- Meckel's syndrome
- Thalassemia

Iraq
- Cleidocranial dysplasia
- Congenital hepatic fibrosis and nephronophthisis
- Familial infantile renal tubular acidosis with congenital sensorineural deafness
- Glanzmann thrombasthenia
- Glycoproteinuria, osteopetrosis, and dwarfism

Iran
- Acrocephalopolysyndactyly type IV
- Pyloric atresia
- Selective hypoaldosteronism
- Wolman's disease

Saudi Arabia
- Metachromatic leukodystrophy

Karaite
- Werding-Hoffmann

Samaritan
- Chronic airway disease

Yemen
- Familial neutropenia
- Familial syndrome of the central nervous system and ocular malformations

Indian
- Metachromatic luekodystrophy: a new variant

Sephardic origin. Although the diseases described here have the same clinical manifestations in the Jewish people as in the population at large, they are noteworthy owing to their relatively high prevalence among Jews in general and, usually, among certain ethnic groups in particular. Furthermore, rare syndromes that have been described only in a single or a few families are detailed. Finally, a short list of conditions without dermatological manifestations that are found more commonly among the Jewish people are listed.

References

1. McKusick VA: Mendelian inheritance in man, 9th ed. Baltimore and London: The Johns Hopkins University Press, 1990.
2. Ramot B, Adam A, Bonne B, et al. Genetic Polymorphism and Diseases in Man. New York and London: Academic Press, 1974.

3. Mourant AE, Kopec AC, Domaniewska-Sobczak K: Research Monograph on Human Population Biology. The Genetics of the Jews. Oxford: Clarendon Press, 1978.

4. Bonne-Tamir B, Adam A, eds. Genetic Diversity Among Jews. Diseases and Markers at the DNA Level. Oxford: Oxford University Press, 1992.

5. Goodman RM. Genetic Disorders Among the Jewish People. Baltimore and London: The Johns Hopkins University Press, 1979.

6. Goodman RM, Adam A, Sheba C: A genetic study of stub thumbs among various ethnic groups in Israel. *J Med Genet* 1965;**2**:116–121.

7. Slatis HM, Apelbaum A: Hairy pinna of the ear in Israeli population. *Am J Hum Genet* 1963;**15**: 74–85.

8. Wahrman J, Fried K: The Jerusalem prospective newborn survey of mongolism. *Ann NY Acad Sci* 1970;**171**:341–348.

9. Epstein CJ, Martin GM, Schultz AL, Motulsky AG: Werner's syndrome: a review of its symptomatology, natural history, pathologic features, genetics and relationship to the natural aging process. *Medicine (Baltimore)* 1966;**45**: 177–221.

10. Simon DG, Krutchkoff D, Kaslow RA, Zarbo R: Pemphigus in Hartford County, Connecticut, from 1972 to 1977. *Arch Dermatol* 1980;**116**: 1035–1037.

11. Feinstein A, Yorav S, Movshovitz M, Schewach-Millet M: Pemphigus in families. *Int J Dermatol* 1991;**30**:347–351.

12. German J, Bloom D, Passarge E, et al: Bloom's syndrome. VI: The disorder in Israel, and an estimation of the gene frequency in the Ashkenazim. *Am J Hum Genet* 1977;**29**:553–562.

13. Garland HG, Anning ST: Hereditary haemorrhagic telangiectasia: a genetic and bibliographic study. *Br J Dermatol* 1950;**62**:289–310.

14. Brunt PW, McKusick VA: Familial dysautonomia: a report of genetic and clinical studies, with a review of the literature. *Medicine (Baltimore)* 1970;**49**:343–374.

15. Ben Bassat I, Feinstein A, Ramot B: Selective vitamin B$_{12}$ malabsorption with proteinuria in Israel: clinical and genetic aspects. *Isr J Med Sci* 1969;**5**:62–68.

16. Sohar E, Gafni J, Pras M, Heller H: Familial Mediterranean fever; a survey of 470 cases and review of the literature. *Am J Med* 1967;**43**: 227–253.

17. Azizi E, Fisher BK: Cutaneous manifestations of familial Mediterranean fever. *Arch Dermatol* 1976;**112**:364–366.

18. Levin S, Perlov S: Ataxia-telangiectasia in Israel. *Isr J Med Sci* 1971;**7**:1535–1542.

19. Cohen BE, Szeinberg A, Pollak S, et al: The hyperphenylalaninemias in Israel. *Isr J Med Sci* 1973;**9**:1393–1395.

20. Ziprkowski L, Feinstein A: A survey of ichthyosis vulgaris in Israel. *Br J Dermatol* 1972;**86**:1–8.

21. Shani M, Seligsohn V, Gilon E, et al: Dubin-Johnson syndrome in Israel. I: Clinical, laboratory and genetic aspects of 101 cases. *Q J Med* 1970;**39**:549–567.

22. Beutler E, Scott S, Bishop A, et al: Red cell aldolase deficiency and hemolytic anemia: a new syndrome. *Trans Assoc Am Phys* 1973;**86**: 154–166.

23. David R, Goodman RM: Leprechaunism in 4 sibs: new pathologic and electron microscopic observations. *Hum Hered* 1977;**27**:172.

24. Wolach B, Raas-Rothschild A, Metzker A, et al: Skin mastocytosis with short stature, conductive hearing loss and microtia: a new syndrome. *Clin Genet* 1990;**37**:64–68.

25. Feinmesser M, Zelig S: Congenital deafness associated with onchodystrophy. *Arch Otolaryngol* 1961;**74**:507.

26. Ziprkowski L, Adam A: Recessive total albinism and congenital deaf-mutism. *Arch Dermatol* 1964;**89**:151–155.

27. Ziprkowski L, Krakowski A, Adam A, et al: Partial albinism and deaf-mutism due to a recessive sex-linked gene. *Arch Dermatol* 1962;**86**: 530–539.

28. Shiloh Y, Litvak G, Ziv Y, et al: Genetic mapping of X-linked albinism-deafness syndrome (ADFM) to Zq26. 3-q27.I. *Am J Hum Genet* 1990;**47**: 20–27.

30. Gazit E, Goodman RM, Bat-Miriam Katznelson M, Rotem Y: The wrinkly skin syndrome: a new heritable disorder of connective tissue. *Clin Genet* 1973;**4**:186–192.

31. Hurvitz SA, Baumgarten A, Goodman RM: The wrinkly skin syndrome: a report of a case and review of the literature. *Clin Genet* 1990;**38**: 307–313.

32. Greenfield G, Stein R, Romano A, Goodman RM: Blue sclerae and keratoconus: Key features of a distinct heritable disorder of connective tissue. *Clin Genet* 1973;**4**:8–16.

33. Samra D, Abraham FA, Treister G. Inherited progressive cone-rod dystrophy and alopecia. *Metab Pediatr Syst Ophthalmol* 1988;**11**:83–85.

34. Kohn G, Metzker A: Hereditary hypotrichosis simplex of the scalp. *Clin Genet* 1987;**32**:120–124.

35. Passwell J, Ziprkowski L, Katznelson D, et al: A

syndrome characterized by congenital ichthyosis with atrophy, mental retardation, dwarfism, and generalized aminoaciduria. *J Pediatr* 1973;**82**: 466–471.

36. Winkler E, Levertowsky D, Shovron A, et al: Familial leg ulcers of juvenile onset. *Lancet* 1991;**337**:15–16.

37. Goodman RM, Katznelson Bat-Miriam M, Manor E: Campodactyly: Occurrence in two new genetic syndromes and its relationship to other syndromes. *J Med Genet* 1972;**9**:203–212.

38. Berlin C: Congenital generalized melanoleucoderma associated with hypodontia, hypotrichosis, stunted growth, and mental retardation occurring in two brothers and two sisters. *Dermatologica* 1961;**123**:227–243.

39. Fried K: Autosomal recessive hydrotic ectodermal dysplasia. *J Med Genet* 1977;**14**:137–139.

40. Goodman RM, Sternberg M, Shem-Tov J, et al: Acrocephalopolysyndactyly type IV: a new genetic syndrome in 3 sibs. *Clin Genet* 1979;**15**: 209–214.

25

Diseases Among
Native American People

Dennis A. Weigand

A fundamental problem with our knowledge of skin disease in native Americans (herein also called Indians) is a lack of basic information on the subject. There are at least three reasons for this deficiency: identification, assimilation, and social/cultural factors. These will be discussed briefly.

The question of who is a native American seems straightforward enough but, in fact, has no single answer. Although nearly 7 million Americans claim some Indian ancestry, the U.S. Census Bureau recognizes a much smaller number.[1] To the average person, an Indian is someone who looks like an Indian, as in the movies, old photographs, or in ceremonial events. From this perspective, many members of the Five Civilized Tribes, who number more than 200,000 in Oklahoma alone, do not even exist because their appearance generally blends in with the rest of the population. To the U.S. Government, an Indian is someone within the 307 federally recognized "entities" (tribes, villages, pueblos, etc.) in the lower 48 states, and some 200 tribes in Alaska. These are basically people living in or near reservations, or tribal or individual acreages in 31 "reservation states".[2] To the native Americans, their own may be those who socially and culturally identify with them, or who are on tribal rolls (which are well known to be far from complete in some cases). Therefore, the difficulty of collecting even basic data is obvious.

Assimilation is, of course, related to the first problem. More than most large minority groups,

the native American has blended into the mainstream of society in the United States. In Oklahoma, the state with the largest Indian population, over 80% are members of the Five Civilized Tribes (Choctaw, Chickasaw, Creek, Cherokee, and Seminole). Briefly, from 1816 to the 1840s, these people were removed from the southeastern United States to "Indian Territory" in what is now Oklahoma. They quickly intermarried and otherwise joined society, commerce, and education to the fullest extent. They have historically resisted or ignored government actions that would set them apart from society as a whole. Although many exhibit the facial and pigmentary features characteristic of "full-blood" Indians, many do not, as they may be one-fourth or one-eighth Indian in terms of blood quanta and still be considered as Indian. Many, through intermarriage, no longer have an Indian-sounding name, or their families have adopted an Anglo-Saxon surname.

Social/cultural factors have perhaps been the greatest obstacle to understanding and management of skin disease in native Americans. One must be careful to distinguish between the idealized notion of Indian culture, as depicted in the legendary "noble savage," and today's reality, which is the culture of poverty. Although certain characteristic or even unique elements of native American culture have endured and are nurtured, such as Indian graphic arts, sculpture, dance, and music, these are of mostly recreational and commercial value. Native Americans are for the most part an impoverished minority.

Census figures from 1980, the most recent detailed figures available, reported about 1.5 million Indians in the United States.[2] Of these, 22% lived in cities and 47% were rural. These situations translate largely to inner city poor and destitute isolated, respectively. Unemployment is twice the national overall figure and is commonly 40%, 50%, or even higher, on reservations and "trust lands." About one-fourth of families have no male head of the household. Health problems are enormous: alcoholism is rampant, drug abuse is increasing, as are deaths from accidents, homicides, and suicides. Diabetes and tuberculosis are lingering problems. The only bright spot is a declining infant mortality rate, which reflects a targeted effort by the Indian Health Service in recent years.[1]

The relationship between the U.S. Government and native Americans has been a long and messy affair, which cannot be detailed here, but basically Indians have been lied to, pushed around, exploited, killed, or fed and watered since colonial days. They were not allowed to be citizens of their own country until 1924, even though many had developed sophisticated systems of government, education, and commerce 100 years before that. There has been a gradual trend from centralized to local tribal control in government, but the funds provided by Congress for Indian services are not mandated. They depend rather on the continuing "trust" relationship and are, therefore, subject to changing political influences.[1]

With this perspective, it is easy to see how skin diseases might seem trivial by comparison to the multitude of serious medical and socioeconomic problems, and receive little attention, from either patients or physicians.

Skin Diseases

The following is a brief discussion of the limited information available on dermatologic peculiarities of native Americans.

Hereditary Polymorphic Light Eruption

Hereditary polymorphic light eruption (HPLE) is apparently limited to American Indians, including many tribes in North, Central, and South America, and the Inuits (who are Eskimos) in Canada.[3] North American tribes reportedly affected include Navaho, Choctaw, Delaware, Shawnee, Creek, Cheyenne, Kickapoo, Kiowa, and Chippewa. The prevalence of the disease among the population groups studied has been consistently more than 1%.[4–6]

The relationships of HPLE, nonhereditary polymorphic light eruption (PLE), and actinic prurigo (AP) are controversial and confused by inconsistent terminology. Some authorities consider them to be the same disease, with minor variations.[7] Others regard them as different, citing the high incidence of actinic cheilitis in HPLE and not in the other two.[8] HLA studies have shown increased incidences of A24 and Cw4 and a decreased incidence of A3 in "actinic prurigo" (used synonymously with HPLE) as compared to PLE in non-Indians.[9]

HPLE is dominantly inherited, with variable expressivity and reduced penetrance. A positive family history has been reported in 75% of one large patient group.[8,10] The eliciting spectrum of light apparently includes UVA and UVB, based on clinical observations. Lesions tend to appear in childhood, are confined to sun-exposed areas, and may be papules, erythematous edematous plaques, or eczematoid plaques (Fig. 25.1). Cheilitis is an especially common manifestation and may be the presenting complaint. Streptococcal pyoderma may complicate the disease.[11]

Treatment of HPLE is problematic, as with other photoeruptions. The newer broad spectrum sunscreens are apparently more effective in preventing exacerbations than were those previously used.[12] Oral beta-carotene has also been used effectively. Desensitization to ultraviolet light by treatment with psoralen and sunlight has been helpful only when carefully controlled exposure is possible.[6] Treatment of existing lesions is generally accomplished with appropriate topical corticosteroids and antipruritic measures.

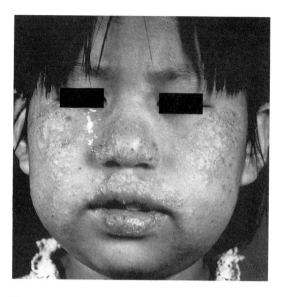

FIGURE 25.1. Hereditary polymorphic light eruption showing photodistributed eczematoid plaques, with characteristic cheilitis.

Other Skin Diseases

Data on the occurrence of individual skin diseases in native Americans are few, partly because of lack of attention to them and partly because of high assimilation into the population at large, as previously discussed. In a survey conducted early in this century, Lain examined 1572 "plains Indians" in western Oklahoma. Notable among the diseases found were keloids in 13 persons, rosacea/rhinophyma in 9, and senile keratoses in 18. Notably absent were any cases of skin cancers, psoriasis, alopecia, or poison ivy dermatitis.[13] In a later survey of Oklahoma plains Indians (predominantly Comanches, Kiowas, and Apaches), Fox found no senile keratoses, cancers, or keloids. Alopecia was seen in only two men, and vitiligo in three individuals. "Prurigo," not further described, was seen in five girls and two women.[14] Brandt's examination of reservation Navahos in the four-corners area was unfortunately reported without figures but indicates that psoriasis was "rare" and skin cancer was "scarce." Vitiligo was seen in an unspecified number of cases. Alopecia was not mentioned.[4]

These three reports suggest what is still generally believed, that is, that keloids occur oftener in dark-skinned races including native Americans than in Caucasians and that psoriasis, androgenic alopecia, and perhaps vitiligo are of low incidence in native Americans. My own experience is similar. Specific information is sketchy, however. In two newer reports, on keloids in "Indians"[15] and psoriasis in "Amerindians,"[16] reports that are sometimes quoted in discussions of these diseases in native Americans, the data really pertain to South American Indians but not North American Indians. The facts may differ between these groups. Skin cancers are understandably less common than in Caucasians. In my experience, where basal cell carcinomas occur, they are frequently of the pigmented variety.

The diagnostic features of these diseases in native Americans do not fundamentally differ from the features as seen in other darkly pigmented persons. The scale of psoriasis is typically more brown and less white or silvery than in most Caucasians. Vitiligo contrasts more sharply with normal skin than in most Caucasians. The translucency of a basal cell carcinoma is harder to discern in dark skin than in pale skin.

The principles and methods of treatment of these diseases in native Americans are also mostly the same as for Caucasians. However, one special consideration is needed in the use of intralesional corticosteroid therapy, whether for keloids, psoriasis, or vitiligo: hypopigmentation secondary to the steroid effect is likely to be more noticeable in the darker skin, and patients should be so advised before treatment is carried out.

The incidence of melanomas is apparently very low in native Americans, and the characteristics of the tumor are similar to those seen in blacks. A recent and very thorough study from the New Mexico Tumor Registry and New Mexico Melanoma Registry identified only 18 native American cases in 20 years, which is only 6% of the incidence in Caucasians living in the same area. Seven of the tumors were subungual and three others were palmar or plantar. Three were mucosal and two were choroidal. This pattern of locations is typical of melanomas in darker-skinned races and correlates with more aggressive behavior: half of the patients in this series died of their melanomas.[17]

Acquired Immune Deficiency Syndrome

There is little information on acquired immune deficiency syndrome (AIDS) in native Americans. Most reviews and periodical updates on the problem report cases in only three racial/ethnic groups: Caucasians, blacks, and Hispanics. Figures from the Centers for Disease Control (CDC) show that through the end of 1988, 0.1% of cases in males and 0.2% of cases in females were in American Indians/Alaskan Natives.[18] The numbers through April 1991 were 0.14% and 0.2%, respectively, a significant increase. The actual numbers are small, but there is an apparently higher incidence in females aged 0–5 and 20–24 among Indians than in other racial/ethnic groups.[19] These figures are well below the representation of American Indians/Alaskan natives in the U.S. population, which is about 0.7%.[20] It is generally believed that the prevalences of both homosexual activity and intravenous drug abuse are lower in Indians than in other groups, but the AIDS figures suggest that one or both are increasing.

Conclusions

If in the future we have generally broader access to dermatologic care in the United States, then native Americans may fare better dermatologically than they have in the past. The outlook regarding the more life-threatening health problems is less promising, with shrinking federal and state dollars devoted to care of the poor. If a national health insurance system evolves, that may change. For the present, we must recognize that native Americans are a growing minority. Their median age, in the 1980 federal census, was 23, compared to 30 for the nation; their birth rate was relatively high, and their infant mortality rate was only slightly higher than the national rate. Most of the Indian

Health Service clinical facilities are located on or near the reservations, leaving the 40% or so of Indians in the cities and suburbs to avail themselves of whatever they can. Although skin diseases among native Americans are now generally neglected, as they are in other impoverished groups, it appears likely that dermatologists, at least those in cities with high Indian populations, will see more "Indian dermatology" in the future.

References

1. US Congress, Office of Technology Assessment: Indian Health Care, Publication No. OTA-H-290. Washington, DC: Government Printing Office, 1986:59.
2. Hoffman MS, ed. The World Almanac and Book of Facts 1991. New York: Pharos Books, 1991:394.
3. Birt AR, Davis RA: Photodermatitis in North American Indians: Familial actinic prurigo. Int J Dermatol 1971;10:107–114.
4. Brandt R: Dermatological observations on the Navaho reservation. Arch Dermatol 1958;77:581–585.
5. Everett MA, Crockett W, Lamb JH, et al: Light-sensitive eruptions in American Indians. Arch Dermatol 1961;83:248–253.
6. Schenck RR: Controlled trial of methoxsalen in solar dermatitis of Chippewa Indians. JAMA 1960;172:1134–1137.
7. Ramsay CA: Cutaneous reactions to actinic and ionizing radiation. In: Rook A, Wilkinson DS, Ebling FJG, et al, eds. Textbook of Dermatology, Vol 1, 4th ed. Oxford: Blackwell Scientific 1986:642–644.
8. Birt AR, Hogg GR: The actinic cheilitis of hereditary polymorphic light eruption. Arch Dermatol 1979;115:699–702.
9. Lane PR, Sheridan DP, Hogan DJ, et al: HLA typing in polymorphous light eruption. J Am Acad Dermatol 1991;24:570–573.
10. Orr PH, Birt AR: Hereditary polymorphic light eruption in Canadian Inuit. Int J Dermatol 1984;23:472–575.
11. Fusaro RM, Johnson JA: Hereditary polymorphic light eruption. JAMA 1980;244:1456–1459.
12. Fusaro RM, Johnson JA: Topical photoprotection for hereditary polymorphic light eruption of American Indians. J Am Acad Dermatol 1991;24:744–746.

13. Lain ES: Skin diseases among full blood Indians of Oklahoma. *JAMA* 1913;**61**:168–171.

14. Fox H: Diseases of the skin in Oklahoma Indians. *Arch Dermatol Syphilol* 1939;**40**:544–546.

15. Bernstein H: Treatment of keloids by steroids, with biochemical tests for diagnosis and treatment. *Angiology* 1964;**15**:253–260.

16. Kerdel-Vegas F: The challenge of tropical dermatology. *Trans St John's Hosp Dermatol Soc* 1974;**59**:1–9.

17. Black WC, Wiggins C: Melanoma among southwestern American Indians. *Cancer* 1985;**55**: 2899–2902.

18. Center for Disease Control: Update: Acquired immunodeficiency syndrome—United States, 1981–1988. *Arch Dermatol* 1989;**125**:749–751.

19. Center for Disease Control: HIV/AIDS surveillance report, May, 1991:12.

20. Hoffman MS, ed. The World Almanac and Book of Facts 1991. New York: Pharos Books, 1991:394, 549.

Part V

Regional Dermatology

26

Comments

Larry E. Millikan

The various presentations of dermatologic disease throughout the world is *raison d'etre* for this book. Other parts have dealt with the approach of genetics, climate, and migration of groups on diseases and their incidence.

Division

In planning for this book, an equally important area of consideration was that of geographical/political region. This section on regional dermatology deals with varying presentations of disease by region. When we speak of region, we look at the broad effects of the influence of microclimates on the natives in the area. Even more important are political considerations in various regions.

Traditionally, the division of the world into the first, second, and third world areas has had many connotations for disease incidence. Presentation of diseases is altered by the availability of expeditious medical care and this relates again to political and socioeconomic factors. Those areas with easy accessibility allow early diagnosis of more typical/classical/presentations for early medical intervention. In many of these diseases, primary treatment results in rapid clinical responses. Individuals in regions where populations are low, distances great, and care often difficult to obtain present with a more complex disease. Often they also present with more secondary complications than the disease seen at first pass through the human host. In some of these remote areas, the patient's overall health and skin symptoms are not modified just by the primary disease but by additional concomitant diseases that take their drain on the host capacity to respond immunologically and nutritionally. Regional characteristics are often as important as vectors, climate, and sanitation. Within geographical or political regions, there are varying races, castes, and social strata that ultimately result in differing access to medical care. The public health standards often change, even in modern countries within certain regions.

Regionally, there is the additional artifact of artificial political boundaries. This often has a dramatic effect in that two neighboring countries within the same environment or life zone can have vastly different cultural, religious, or socioeconomic standards, resulting in extremely variable skin disease presentation and treatment.

Regions

This section continues a most useful summary of (1) variations in common skin diseases by region and (2) unusual skin diseases for these different regions.*

Rhinoscleroma in Poland and the European incidence of acrodermatitis chronica atrophicans are two areas of particular interest. Of even

---

* The editors have selected chapters from several countries worldwide. Not every political entity could be included. In addition, available information is not always uniform from place to place.

greater interest is the geographical difference in *Borrelia*-associated diseases in the United States presenting as Lyme borreliosis, but in Europe a more limited disease, erythema chronica migrans. Here one would assume that regional or genetic variations in the host/pathogen interaction may play an important role. Or perhaps the difference relates to differing vectors between the new and old world.

Many serious viral diseases including most of the retroviruses have been, thus far, traced to origins in Africa. The heretofore unusual African incidence of Kaposi's sarcoma had previously also been a significant regional oddity. In the south of Africa, the genetic stock provided another modifier disease with certain hereditary diseases having particular presentation in different immigrants to that country, including the different genetic porphyrias.

In South America, as many of these countries become more and more urbanized and transportation and communication increase, there is an initial spread of disease prior to the local medical facilities' ability to recognize early and treat. The rural areas also have unusual environmental characteristics as described with the problem of arsenicism in Chile.

Unusual worldwide distribution of another retrovirus, the human T-cell leukemia lymphoma virus, provides a fascinating example. Its incidence in the Orient, as well as in the Caribbean and Mediterranean countries, may point to another regional, political variable, as yet not well understood. In the past, the unusual worldwide distribution of leprosy remained a similar fascinating but poorly understood phenomenon.

Conclusions

All in all, the disease and its presentation in the human host is the result of all of these variables. These multiple etiologies and presentations become more and more clinically relevant with the mobility of modern societies. This approach to skin disease from around the world will become increasingly pertinent and relevant in the practice of dermatology as travel increases and our tools for technique and diagnosis advance.

Caribbean Region

Anthony J. Badame

The Caribbean is a region of tropical islands situated between North and South America near the Gulf of Mexico. The main archipelago is known as the West Indies or the Antilles and separates the Atlantic Ocean from the Caribbean Sea. The islands are further divided into two main groups: the Greater Antilles consisting of Cuba, Jamaica, Hispaniola, and Puerto Rico; and the Lesser Antilles consisting of the Leeward and Windward Islands. Climate is temperate all year with lows near 18°C, and highs approaching 32°C. Humidity is relatively high.

The region supports a population of 28.5 million primarily of African heritage. Other inhabitants include descendents from Spanish, French, Dutch, Chinese, Portuguese, and East Indians. Skin disorders of these people are not well studied. This chapter identifies the more commonly documented skin disorders under the topics of infection, dermatitis, cancer, and other disorders.

Infection

Skin disease of infectious etiology constitutes a major percentage of cutaneous disorders in the Caribbean. In Jamaica, the incidence of cutaneous infections is closely related to socioeconomic status.[1] Poverty, poor hygiene, high humidity, extreme heat, frequent trauma especially from insect bites, and crowded living conditions predispose to infectious skin disease.

These infections may be bacterial, fungal, parasitic, or viral in origin.

Bacterial

Pyoderma is one of the most common skin diseases in the Caribbean. A study from the Dermatology Clinic of the Port of Spain General Hospital in Trinidad revealed *Staphylococcus aureus* as the major cause of single isolate skin infections.[2] In mixed isolate infections, group A beta hemolytic streptococcus was found in conjunction with *Staphylococcus aureus*. Dermatitis was present in almost half of the patients. Primary impetigo accounted for only 10% of cases. A similar percentage of cases had underlying scabies. Nephritogenic strains of streptococci associated with pyodermic skin lesions have been responsible for outbreaks of acute glomerulonephritis in Jamaica and Trinidad.[2,3] Scabies infestation of man and possibly dogs has been implicated in some of these outbreaks.[4]

The *Hippelates* fly has been incriminated in the transmission of streptococci in Trinidad.[5] In addition, *Hippelates* have been blamed for the spread of yaws in Jamaica. These small flies feed on sterile and infected skin lesions. Organisms may survive for more than 24 h on or in the fly and may be passed from human to human, utilizing the fly as a vector.

In Jamaican children, a peculiar disorder termed infective dermatitis has been described.[6] The dermatitis shares features of both impetigo and diffuse impetiginous dermatitis following acute nasopharyngitis. The condition usually begins at about 2 years of age with a rhinitis. The lesions first resemble impetigo near the nostrils and ears. The lesions then progress to a weeping eczematous eruption over the head and neck region and, at times, the inguinal area. Rarely does a history of preceding infantile eczema exist, and it is uncertain whether children later develop atopic dermatitis. Both *Staphylococcus aureus* and beta-hemolytic *Streptococcus* are recovered in the majority of these patients.[7] Long-term antibiotic therapy is necessary, and relapses are common on discontinuance of medication.

In Trinidad, skin infections have been incriminated in the spread of *Corynebacterium diphtheriae*.[8] Natural immunization to *C. diphtheriae* has been thought to result from cutaneous infection with this bacterium.

Fungal

The Caribbean is surrounded by endemic areas for many of the deep mycoses. Cases of chromomycosis and mycetoma have been documented in Puerto Rico, Cuba, Trinidad, and Jamaica. A 20-year analysis of chromomycosis in Jamaica revealed *Fonsecaea* species as the exclusive causative agent in the mycologically confirmed cases.[9] *Histoplasma capsulatum* has been found in the bat and oil bird caves of Trinidad, whereas cases of acute pulmonary histoplasmosis have been recorded in Puerto Rico. Rhinoentomophthoromycosis has been reported from the Grand Cayman Islands. Dolphins infected with *Loboa loboi* have been discovered in the waters of the Caribbean.[10]

Between 1930 and 1949, Carrion studied the prevalence of various dermatophytes in Puerto Rico.[11] *Trichophyton rubrum* accounted for three-fourths of cases of tinea corporis. *T. tonsurans*, *T. mentagrophytes*, *Microsporum gypseum*, *M. canis*, and *Epidermophyton floccosum* were responsible for the remainder of the cases. In patients with tinea pedis, *T. mentagrophytes* was isolated in nearly two-thirds of the cases. *T. rubrum* was found in one-third of these cases. *E. floccosum* was present in only a small number of patients.

A later study in 1982 from the University of Puerto Rico School of Medicine confirmed the finding of *T. rubrum* as the predominant causative agent in tinea corporis;[12] however, *T. rubrum* was also found to be the most common isolate in tinea pedis. This finding was contrary to Carrion's finding of *T. mentagrophytes* as the primary pathogen. In the Dominican Republic, *M. audouini* was cultured most often in cases of tinea capitis, a finding considered rare in other parts of the Caribbean.[13]

Hendersonula toruloidea and *Scytalidium hyalinum* are nondermatophyte molds that cause infections clinically similar to the dermatophyte, *T. rubrum*. *H. toruloidea* produces disease in plants, whereas *S. hyalinum* has not yet been isolated from the environment. In a study from Tobago, West Indies, close to one-third of 45 medical inpatients who were admitted for nondermatologic disorders demonstrated infection with either *S. hyalinum* or *H. toruloidea*.[14] None of these patients complained of symptoms related to the infection.

Parasitic

Cutaneous leishmaniasis is rarely reported in the Caribbean. An autochthonous focus exists in the Dominican Republic.[15] The responsible parasite is similar to the *Leishmania mexicana* complex. The probable vector is the phlebotomine sand fly, *Lutzomyia christophei*. The black rat (*Rattus rattus*) is most likely the main reservoir, although a capromid rodent (*Plagiodontia aedium*) and the mongoose (*Herpestes auropunctatus*) are other possible reservoirs. A few cases presumably caused by *mexicana* are on record in Martinique. In Trinidad and Tobago, no cases of cutaneous leishmaniasis currently exist; however, the disease has occurred sporadically in the past.[16]

Cutaneous larva migrans, also known as creeping eruption, is prevalent in the Caribbean. The disease is most commonly caused by larvae from the dog and cat hookworm, *Ancylostoma braziliense*. Sunbathers from resorts who experience long contact times with moist soils are particularly susceptible to infection. The larvae, which are able to pass through beach towels, penetrate human skin to the level of the epidermis. The disease is self-limiting but creates great distress to vacationers returning from the endemic area.[17,18]

Scabies is a common infestation in Jamaica, especially in the rural areas.[19,20] Almost one-third of all dermatologic diagnoses at a rural clinic in Jamaica involved scabies.[19] In more metropolitan areas, infestation is seen less often due to increased disease control.

Other parasitic infections have been documented in the Caribbean. Filariasis, caused by *Wuchereria bancrofti*, occurs throughout the region. Dracunculosis caused by the guinea worm, *Drancunculus medinensis*, is present in just a few areas. Cercarial dermatitis produced by the cercariae of the nonhuman schistosome is frequent. The intestinal form of schistosomiasis caused by *Shistosoma mansoni* is endemic.[21]

Viral

In 1979, the first case of the acquired immunodeficiency syndrome (AIDS) was encountered in Haiti. An 18-month study between 1983 and 1984 of 134 Haitian AIDS patients revealed a unique, extremely pruritic eruption without an established cause or categorical assignment.[22] Erythematous macules, papules, and nodules first involved the forearms, and progressed in a symmetric distribution to the trunk, legs, and face. A mixed, primarily eosinophilic inflammatory infiltrate was found perivascularly and perifollicularly in the dermis. Nearly 80% of patients with lesions complained of them as the initial manifestation of AIDS. In most cases, the eruption lasted the entire course of illness without response to multiple therapeutic regimens. This eruption has been rarely reported in AIDS patients in the United States or Europe.

Jamaica is endemic for the human T-lymphotropic virus type I (HTLV-I). Adult T-cell leukemia/lymphoma, tropical spastic paraparesis, and possibly polymyositis are associated with HTLV-1. Infective dermatitis, as seen in Jamaican children, is postulated to result from immunosuppression caused by HTLV-1.[23] Obstinate infections of the skin and nasal vestibule caused by nonvirulent *Staphylococcus aureus* or beta-hemolytic streptococci, and concurrent HTLV-1 seropositivity in patients with infective dermatitis provide support for this postulate.

Other Infectious Diseases

Yaws, caused by the nonvenereal spirochete *Treponema pertenue*, was formerly considered a serious public health threat in the Caribbean. Today, only sporadic cases exist on a few islands.[24] Pinta, caused by the nonvenereal spirochete *Treponema carateum*, occurs infrequently in certain regions. Syphilis is common, as is gonorrhea. Granuloma inguinale and lymphogranuloma venereum present without rarity. Leprosy is prevalent.[21]

Dermatitis

One of the most troublesome skin problems in Jamaica and possibly in the other islands is eczema.[20,25] In a study performed at the University of the West Indies, Jamaica, patients with eczema accounted for nearly one-third of all patients with skin disease.[25] Infantile and atopic eczema occurred less frequently in the Jamaican patients as compared to white populations; however, these disorders occurred more frequently when compared to strictly black populations. Likewise, contact dermatitis was seen less often than in the predominantly white-populated British hospitals but more often than in African populations. Modernization and increased industrialization are thought to contribute to the increased incidence of contact dermatitis in Jamaica.

Another study from Jamaica revealed that childhood and adult eczemas had little differences in distribution.[6] The adult pattern maintained extensor accentuation rather than progressing to predominantly flexural involvement. The eczema produced minimal symptoms, and the vicious cycle of European neurodermatitis rarely occurred. Follicular eczema was common in children over 5 years of age. This eczema was difficult to differentiate from keratosis pilaris except for the lack of pruritus in the latter.

Several members of the *Anacardiaceae* (poison ivy family), which are capable of producing delayed contact sensitivity, thrive in the Caribbean.[26] The Brazilian peppertree, *Schinus terebinthifolius*, was introduced into Cuba and Puerto Rico as an ornamental. A delayed dermatitis results from the latex produced by the tree bark and crushed berries. When used as a food seasoning, the berries have been responsible for several outbreaks of diarrhea and perianal dermatitis.

The cashew, *Anacardium occidentale*, was brought into the West Indies from Brazil. Liquid from the nutshell and tree bark is responsible for a vesicant action and dermatitis. The nutshell oil has been used therapeutically for the removal of warts. In the past, vanilla beans were coated with the cashew oil, which produced vanilla bean dermatitis in susceptible dock workers and food handlers. Other sources of contact have included imported jewelry, party favors, and toys made with unroasted nuts.

In 1742, the mango was first introduced into the West Indies. The sensitizing latex is contained within the stem of the fruit. The skin of the fruit may become contaminated with the latex on harvesting. Circumoral dermatitis, cheilitis, and stomatitis core documented in patients who have eaten the unpeeled fruit. Oral desensitization from the constant consumption of mango throughout life is suggested as an explanation of the surprisingly low incidence of mango dermatitis in the tropical areas.

The genus of *Comociadia* is found primarily in the Caribbean. The latex, like the poison ivy sensitizer, turns black on exposure to air. Medical use of the oil includes the treatment of warts and corns. The genus of *Metopium* contains three species and extends throughout the Caribbean. All species are capable of producing dermatitis from the topic catechols found in the exterior parts of the tree.

Cancer

Skin cancer, which develops less commonly in populations of increasing constitutive skin pigment, is present in this region. Basal cell cancer, squamous cell carcinoma, and malignant melanoma comprise the majority of skin cancers seen.[27] Incidences of these cancers vary among the Caribbean islands.

The most common type of cancer in Puerto Rico is skin cancer. Nearly three-fourths of skin cancer cases occur in patients over the age of 50. The overwhelming majority of Puerto Ricans are cognitive of the carcinogenic effects of sunlight and the meaning of the sun protection factor (SPF).[28] Despite knowledge of SPF, only about half of Puerto Rican residents use sunscreens as compared to two-thirds of tourists.

The most common sites for nonmelanoma skin cancer in Purto Ricans are the head and neck. In contrast, close to one-half of melanomas occur on the lower extremities, particularly the foot.[29] Volar melanomas outnumber subungual melanomas by four to one.[30] Melanomas located subungually usually present either on the thumbs or great toes. The course of acral lentiginous melanoma in Puerto Ricans is aggressive with deep invasion and a poor prognosis. These findings correlate with those found in other studies. Walking barefoot has been speculated as a factor in the increased incidence of acrally located melanomas. However, because walking barefoot is not common among native Puerto Ricans, other factors must play a role.

The Netherlands Antilles, which consist of six Caribbean islands, is populated by nearly 75% black inhabitants with the remainder of diverse white heritage. Cancer incidence statistics differ from those calculated in Puerto Rico.[31] In the Netherlands Antilles, skin cancer ranks third in frequency for women and fourth in frequency for men. Similar statistics are found in Jamaica where skin cancer ranks fifth in frequency in both males and females. In Cuba, skin cancer ranks second in frequency in males and fourth in frequency in females. These statistics support the common belief that darker-skinned populations are less susceptible to the development of skin cancer than are lighter-skinned populations.

Other Disorders

A progressive hypomelanosis occurs in blacks of mixed heritage who reside in or who are traveling from the Caribbean region.[32] Progressive macular hypomelanosis of the trunk is the term used to characterize this condition, which is prevalent in women from 18–25 years of age. The macular hypomelanosis advances over the entire trunk with the exception of the dorsolumbar line in a period of 12 months. Resolution occurs gradually with complete clearing in 2–5 years. The lesions are refractory to therapy. Microscopic examination of the hypopigmented macules shows decreased epidermal melanin, whereas ultrastructural analysis reveals a predominance of stage-I–III aggregated melanosomes with few stage-IV single melanosomes. No cause has been determined.

A unique facial eruption in children of African-Caribbean descent has been described, and the acronym FACE (facial Afro-Caribbean childhood eruption), has been proposed.[33] The etiology is unknown. Flesh-colored or hypopigmented papules with a monomorphic appearance are distributed around the mouth, eyelids, and outer helix of the ears. The lesions spontaneously resolve after several months.

Differences in the clinical features of sarcoidosis between West Indians and Caucasians exist.[34] Sarcoidosis with erythema nodosum occurs in nearly one-fourth of Caucasian patients. In contrast, erythema nodosum rarely occurs in patients with sarcoidosis of West Indian origin. Sarcoid involvement of the skin separate from erythema nodosum is suggested to be more common in West Indians. These differences affect prognosis in the course of sarcoidosis. The presence of erythema nodosum in sarcoidosis typically signifies a better long-term outcome, whereas skin sarcoidosis, especially lupus pernio, indicates a less favorable prognosis.

Keloids pose a significant problem in Trinidad where over 50% of the population is of African lineage and a large percentage is of East Indian heritage.[35] The ear lobules are the most common site for keloids followed in decreasing order by the face, hands and forearms, shoulder, sternum, back of neck, and other sites. Ear lobule piercing is the most common cause of keloid formation followed by surgical incisions, vaccinations, violent trauma, and acne. Facial keloids usually result from road accidents or violet trauma, whereas occupational accidents frequently are the cause of hand and forearm keloids. Smallpox or BCG vaccinations are the cause of most shoulder keloids.

Several other skin disorders are present in the Caribbean region. Few have received close examination. As interest develops, more information will emerge and contribute to the growing understanding of cutaneous disease in the tropics.

References

1. Ide A: The epidemiology of pyoderma in Jamaican children. *Cutis* 1989;**44**:321–324.
2. Suite M: Cutaneous infections in Trinidad. *Int J Dermatol* 1990;**29**:31–34.
3. Potter EV, Ortiz JS, Sharrett R, et al: Changing types of nephritogenic streptococci in Trinidad. *J Clin Invest* 1971;**50**:1197–1203.
4. Svartman M, Finklea JF, Potter EV, Poon-King T: Epidemic scabies and acute glomerulonephritis in Trinidad. *Lancet* 1972;**i**:249–251.
5. Bassett DC: Hippelates flies and streptoccal skin infection in Trinidad. *Trans Roy Soc Trop Med Hyg* 1970;**64**:138–147.
6. Sweet RD: A pattern of eczema in Jamaica. *Br J Dermatol* 1966;**78**:93–100.
7. Walshe MM: Infective dermatitis in Jamaican children. *Br J Dermatol* 1967;**79**:229–236.
8. Bray JP, Burt EG, Potter EV, et al: Epidemic diphtheria and skin infections in Trinidad. *J Infect Dis* 1972;**126**:34–40.
9. Bansal AS, Prabhakar P: Chromomycosis: a twenty year analysis of histologically confirmed cases in Jamaica. *Trop Geogr Med* 1989;**41**:222–226.
10. Hay RJ: Mycoses imported from the West Indies. A report of three cases. *Postgrad Med J* 1979;**55**:603–604.
11. Carrion AL: Dermatomycoses in Puerto Rico. *Arch Dermatol* 1965;**91**:431–438.
12. Vazquez M, Sanchez JL: A clinical and mycologic study of tinea corporis and pedis in Puerto Rico. *Int J Dermatol* 1984;**23**:550–551.
13. Bogaert H, Coiscou AA: Superficial mycosis in children of the Dominican Republic. *Mod Probl Paediatr* 1975;**17**:242–247.
14. Allison VY, Hay RJ, Campbell CK: Hendersonula toruloidea and Scytalidium hyalinum infections in Tobago. *Br J Dermatol* 1984;**111**:371–372.
15. Zeledon R, Bogaert-Diaz H, McPherson AB, et

al: Epidemiological observations on cutaneous leishmaniases in the Dominican Republic. *Trans Roy Soc Trop Med Hyg* 1985;**79**:881.

16. Grimaldi G, Tesh RB, McMahon-Pratt D: A review of the geographic distribution and epidemiology of leishmaniasis in the New World. *Am J Trop Med Hyg* 1989;**41**:687–725.

17. Edelglass JW, Douglass MC, Stiefler R, Tessler M: Cutaneous larva migrans in northern climates. A souvenir of your dream vacation. *J Am Acad Dermatol* 1982;**7**:353–358.

18. Lee CP, Bishop LJ: The incidence of cutaneous larva migrans in Montserrat, Leeward Islands, West Indies. *WI Med J* 1988;**37**:22–24.

19. Badame AJ: Incidence of skin disease in rural Jamaica. *Int J Dermatol* 1988;**27**:109–111.

20. Alabi GO, LaGrenade L: The pattern of childhood skin diseases in Jamaica. *WI Med J* 1981;**30**:3–7.

21. Canizares O: A Manual of Dermatology for Developing Countries. Oxford: Oxford University Press, 1982:28–29.

22. Liautaud B, Pape JW, DeHovitz JA, et al: Pruritic skin lesions. A common initial presentation of acquired immunodeficiency syndrome. *Arch Dermatol* 1989;**125**:629–632.

23. LaGrenade L, Hanchard B, Fletcher V, et al: Infective dermatitis of Jamaican children: a marker for HTLV-1 infection. *Lancet* 1990;**336**:1345–1347.

24. Prussia PR, DaSilva PA: Yaws in Barbados. *WI Med J* 1985;**34**:63–65.

25. Walshe MM. Dermatology in Jamaica. Trans St. Johns Hosp Dermatol Soc. 1968;**54**:46–53.

26. Lampe KF: Dermatitis-producing Anacardiaceae of the Caribbean area. *Dermatol Clin* 1986;**4**:171–182.

27. Quintero AL, Torres SM, Sanchez JL: Skin cancer in Puerto Rico. *Bol Assoc Med PR* 1985;**77**:502–503.

28. Ross SA, Sanchez JL: Recreational sun exposure in Puerto Rico: Trends and cancer risk awareness. *J Am Acad Dermatol* 1990;**23**:1090–1092.

29. Pantoja E, Llobet RE, Roswit B: Melanomas of the lower extremity among native Puerto Ricans. *Cancer* 1976;**38**:1420–1423.

30. Vazquez M, Ramos FA, Sanchez JL: Melanomas of volar and subungual skin in Puerto Ricans. A clinicopathologic study. *J Am Acad Dermatol* 1984;**10**:39–45.

31. Freni SC, Freni-Titulaer LWJ: Cancer incidence in the Netherlands Antilles. *Cancer* 1981;**48**:2535–2541.

32. Guillet G, Helenon R, Gauthier Y, et al: Progressive macular hypomelanosis of the trunk: Primary acquired hypopigmentation. *J Cutan Pathol* 1988;**15**:286–289.

33. Williams HC, Ashworth JA, Pembroke AC, Breathnach SM: FACE—Facial Afro-Caribbean childhood eruption. *Clin Exp Dermatol* 1990;**15**:163–166.

34. Honeybourne D: Ethnic differences in the clinical features of sarcoidosis in south-east London. *Br J Dis Chest* 1980;**74**:63–69.

35. Inalsingh CHA: An experience in treating five hundred and one patients with keloids. *Hopkins Med J* 1974;**134**:284–290.

28

Chile

Juan F. Honeyman

Chile, with 14 million people, is the southern-most country of South America. It is 4300 km long and ranges in width from 90 to 900 km. The Andes Mountains with elevations of 22,000 feet stretch the Chilean territory, which is divided from north to south into 12 regions, including the Chilean antarctics. In the middle is Santiago, the capital with 4 million inhabitants. The population is ethnically and culturally homogeneous, and descends from Spaniards mixed with a minority of aborigines and other Europeans, mainly Germans. Low birth and childhood mortality rates, high literacy, and economic and political stability place Chile well above the other countries in Latin America.[1-3]

The skin diseases in Chile are similar to the ones seen in European or North American countries, although a relevant environmental factor for the development of skin cancer and other dermatoses is the presence of high levels of arsenic in drinking water in northern Chile. Since prehispanic periods, there exists an arsenic environment in Regions I through III. Studies in mummified bodies belonging to different epochs show elevated concentration of arsenic in their bodies, especially in skin, nails, liver, and kidney.[4]

Arsenic

The north of Chile is a desert region with few cities on the sea side. There are a few towns and villages up in the mountains dedicated to minerals extractions. The most affected is Region II where the hydric resources show increase of arsenic content due to the geochemical characteristics of this zone because rivers have developed their hydrographic basins in volcanic materials and they originate in the Andes springs. Antofagasta, a city of more than 200,000 inhabitants, Calama with a population of 100,000, and other small towns and villages got their water supplies from As-contaminated sources until 1970. Since then, plants were built for treating water that supplies the larger cities, but the problem still remains in villages and small communities.[5]

Before water treatment plants for As removal were set up, As-induced skin changes were reported in children of Antofagasta; in addition, some severe cardiovascular cases were seen.[6,7] According to available data, the affected population would be about 8000 people. Region II with 3000 inhabitants is the most involved.[5]

The main economic activity of Region II is copper mining. The copper contains different minerals such as sulfurs and arsenic. The extraction tasks and the mineral treatment processes induce changes in the environment, particularly in the air resource. The smoke from the smelting house furnaces has several sub-products such as arsenic trioxide (As_2O_3).[8]

Human health risks due to environmental As exposure have been described in Argentina, Bolivia, Canada, Chile, England, India, Mexico, Taiwan, and the United States among other countries.[9-13] Arsenic is an element present in various compounds identified in ancient times. The Greek alchemist Olympiodorus obtained

179

metallic As by roasting one of its sulfides. Since the 18th century, the arsenical compounds were used in pigments and dyes, in preservatives of animals hides, in glass manufacture, pesticides, and several pharmaceutical substances.[13]

Sources of Organic and Inorganic Arsenic

General Environment

A. The air contains As as inorganic trivalent compounds (As^{3+}) or trioxide. The urban air levels are 0.01–0.02 micrograms (mcg) per cubic meter (m^3).[11] Concentrations greater than 1 mcg/m^3 are found in the neighborhood of smelting furnaces. In mining cities of Region II of Chile, it has been reported at 6 mcg/m^3.[14]

B. Food is the principal source of both organic and inorganic As that are present in varying amounts. Inorganic As is more toxic than organic and is found as either arsenate (As^{5+}) or arsenite (As^{3+}), which is most toxic. Human metabolism of As^{5+} involves reduction to As^{3+} before undergoing detoxification by methylation.[13] The allowed concentration of As in food is 0.05 mgs/kg; human milk contains about 0.003 mg/L. Fish have higher amounts of organic As. The foods with more As in Region II of Chile are fish and seafood (10 mgs of As/kg).[5] Inorganic As may be increased in milk and dairy products, meat (beef and pork), vegetables, and fruits.[11] Bottled mineral water contains arsenic of natural origin, in low concentrations (0.02 mg/ml). Food increases in As content, depending on the source of water and the soil.

C. The normal soil As level averages 10 mcgs/g. In Region II, there are locations with soil As concentrations of 448 mcg/g.[5]

D. Drinking water supplies for the population is the major source of As in northern Chile as well as Argentina, India, Taiwan, and Mexico.[13] The major U.S. drinking water supplies contain As levels lower than 5 mcg/L, but it has been estimated that about 350,000 people drink water containing over 50 mcg/L, the standard for arsenic set by the U.S. Environmental Protection Agency (EPA).[15] In Region II, there are still places with more than 700 mcg/L of As in the drinking water.[5]

E. Other sources are food additives and tobacco. Humans may inhale As through cigarette smoking. The As found in the mainstream smoke of U.S. cigarettes ranges between 40 and 120 ng/cigarette.[17]

Occupational Environment

A. Mining activities, of As or other metals, represent one of the most important risks for the worker. In As mining, dangerous As levels can be observed; the risk increases because the activities are performed in a contaminated environment as occurs in Region II of Chile.[12]

B. Industrial occupational As exposure is seen in persons working in smelting or refining of ores, arsenical insecticides, cattle and sheep dip, arsenical medicaments, ceramics, coloring, tanneries, jewelry, painting, wood preservatives, pyrotechnics, glass, and so on.[16]

C. Agriculture is also a source of As exposure. It occurs in workers who apply or handle herbicides, insecticides, sterilizers, or wood preservatives, mainly in the cultures of cotton, coffee, cacao, vegetables, and grapevine.[11,12]

The arsenic may get into the organism by dust inhalation of polluted air. The lungs absorb 75% of the inhaled As within 4 days. Another means of absorption is gastrointestinal. Depending on the solubility of the compound, ingested As is absorbed in variable amounts (80–90%). The absorption through the skin is poorly known. Arsenite induces skin irritation, increasing As penetration.[12]

Once As has been absorbed, it is spread throughout the body by the blood. After a few hours, high concentrations of the metal are found in the liver, kidney, spleen, bone marrow, lungs, and skin. The As goes through the placental barrier and accumulates inside the fetus.[11,12] With the course of time, it is deposited in the skin, bones, muscles, and nerves. Keratinized structures such as skin, hairs, and nails bind As_3. Normal levels of As are less than 0.1 mg/100 g for hair and nails and less than 0.1 mg/L in the urine.[7]

Inorganic As_3 is detoxified in the liver by enzymatic methylation, reducing to methyl and dimethylarsenic acids. Arsenate must be reduced to As_3 before methylation. Methylation capacity seems to be lower in persons with malnutrition and among individuals with a particular genetic predisposition.[18,19] Ninety percent of the absorbed As is rapidly eliminated within 1 or 2 days. Urinary excretion of dimethylarsenic acid is the most important (60–80%). The feces may eliminate 5% of the As as methylarsenic acid. Arsenic traces are exhaled as trimethylarsine. The average As life in humans has been estimated to be 10 h for inorganic As and 30 h for organic As. It is important to note that industrial As exposures are to As_3, which is more toxic than As_5. Methylated forms are much less toxic than inorganic As.[12,19]

In 1556, the first health effect of arsenical cobalt was reported in *De Re Metallica*.[20] In 1820, J. Ayrton Paris, a physician in Cornwall, England, described the "cancerous disease in tin smelters exposed to arsenical fumes."[16] Jonathan Hutchison associated skin cancer and medicinal inorganic therapy (Fowler's solution) in 1888.[21]

Adverse effects of As are either acute or chronic. Acute toxicity in humans is usually due to homicidal, suicidal, or accidental ingestion. The smallest recorded fatal dose is about 130 mg, but recovery has occurred after much larger doses. Symptoms of poisoning are malaise, abdominal pain, and vomiting, usually within 1 h or ingestion, due to inflammatory changes in the mucous membranes of the stomach and upper gastrointestinal tract. Jaundice usually appears on the second or third day. There may be pyrexia, hemolytic anemia, edema of the lungs, delirium, and coma. In some cases, exfoliative dermatitis and peripheral neuritis follow recovery from the acute symptoms. Death usually occurs from myocardial failure a few days after onset of anuria, indicating kidney damage. With fatal doses, death occurs between 12 and 48 h of ingestion.[22]

Disease States

Chronic exposure to As induces disorders of skin, mucous membranes, and liver as well as diseases of gastrointestinal, nervous, and circula-

tory systems. Chromosomal and teratogenics effects, immunological changes, and cancer may be caused by As salts.[23]

Circulatory disturbances have a clear exposure–response relationship between As levels in drinking water and the frequency of blackfoot disease, a peripheral vascular disease endemic of Taiwan that leads to gangrene of the toes and feet.[24,25] Adverse cardiovascular effects, consisting of myocardial infarction and arterial thickening, have been reported in Chilean children consuming water containing up to 0.8 ml/L of arsenic.[26,27]

Respiratory diseases, such as bronchectasias, pulmonary fibrosis, and pneumonia as well as lung cancer, may be induced by As.[27,28] Gastrointestinal disburbances, such as nausea and vomiting, are observed in patients with chronic hidroarsenicism. Peripheral neuritis of gradual onset, with sensory disturbances in the extremities, numbness, and tingling sensations, is followed by severe weakness in legs and feet.[29]

Chronic As ingestion may cause immunological changes and hematological diseases such as anemia, leukopenia, and thrombocytopenia. Bone marrow changes are also present. Hematological symptoms disappear 3 weeks after cessation of arsenic ingestion.[30] Cell-mediated immunity is diminished with a low proliferative response to antigen stimulation of the T-lymphocytes.[31] A humoral immunity change reported is the increase of IgE synthesis in experimental conditions.[32]

Mucous membranes may be affected by As-containing products. Insecticides can cause conjunctivitis, corneal anesthesia, and ulcers. Arsenic dust coming in contact with the nose may induce chronic rhinitis, pharyngitis, and bronchitis. Necrosis of the nasal septum has occurred among copper-melting workers.[11,22]

Adverse effects on the skin are acute or chronic. Acute lesions observed in industrial poisoning are more frequent than chronic. The dermatitis starts with erythema, associated with burning and itching, giving the skin a mottled appearance. Swelling and papular of vesicular eruptions may also be seen.[22]

Chronic skin lesions seen in hidroarsenicism are hyperkeratoses of palms and soles (Figs.

28.1 and 28.2), hyperhidrosis, hyperpigmentation, and skin cancer. Arsenical melanosis is a common sign and consists of a rather diffuse hyperpigmentation with multiple spots like hypopigmentation, which is called leukomelanodermia. The increased melanin pigment contains no As but derives from epidermal and mainly dermal As-altered cells. The noncancerous skin lesions have been reported to range up to 80% in populations exposed to inorganic As in the general environment. There is a clear exposure–response relationship between As and the frequency of skin lesions. A cross-sectional study of 1277 children in northern Chile confirms this opinion.[5,6,11]

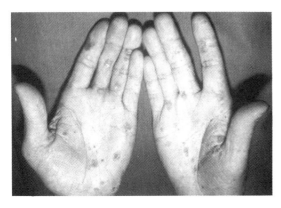

FIGURE 28.1. Hyperkeratoses of palms due to hidroarsenicism.

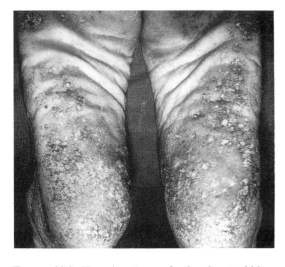

FIGURE 28.2. Hyperkeratoses of soles due to hidroarsenicism.

Chronic As exposure may induce internal and skin cancer. Internal cancers associated with systemic As include leukemia, lung nasorespiratory, gastrointestinal, and genitourinary cancers, and hepatic angiosarcoma. Epidemiological studies show that inorganic As can cause human cancer at several sites. As levels in drinking water over 0.05 mg/L are of potential risks for developing malignancies.[11,13]

As-induced skin cancer is characterized by the development of superficial basal cell carcinomas, Bowen's disease, and squamous cell carinomas. These patients generally have many tumors on both sun- and non-sun exposed skin. A positive correlation exists between the amount of arsenic ingestion and the development of skin cancer. The lifetime risk of skin cancer is 1.3/1000 0.6/1000 per mcg of As per kg of body weight ingested per day for males and females, respectively.[11,13,16,33]

The noncancerous clinical effects of As can be diminished by treatment with 2,3-dimercaptopropanol or BAL (British antilewisite). Arsenic combines with two SH groups and may bind and inhibit biologically active SH-containing substances such as specific enzyme systems. BAL, being a dithiol, forms cyclic dithioarsenites that are more stable than the protein-SH arsenites and are, thus, capable of eliminating excess As from the body. BAL is injected intramuscularly in doses of 1.5–1.6 ml every 6 h. In the treatment of acute chemical dermatitis with BAL, it has been demonstrated that the drug stimulates the urinary excretion of As for the first 3 days.[22]

Reduction of As levels in water supplies is an important measure to prevent hidroarsenicism. Over 2.5 million people are supplied with water containing more than 0.025 mg/L of arsenic. The World Health Organization and several countries are studying the reduction of the allowed As maximal concentration to 0.05 mg/L in drinking water. Arsenic removal from water sources is basically carried out through a process of adsorption with aluminum sulfate or iron hydroxide particles, which can be removed from the water mass. Adsorption takes place due to a physical rather than chemical effect, as a result of attractive forces in surface. After adsorption, the hydroxide precipitate with adhered As is extracted by a flocculation–decantation process followed by filtration. The treatment with chlorine for disinfection ensures a maximal valence state for residual As that would significantly decrease its toxic potential.[34]

Conclusions

Arsenic exposure represents an important environmental risk of cancer in northern Chile. The skin cancer incidence is exacerbated by the increase of ultraviolet radiation that occurs in desert areas as well as in the seaside where people live. Several measures have been taken to reduce arsenic levels in water supplies in cities, although small mining villages are still drinking water with As concentrations over the allowed standard. Educational programs to the community and more plants for As removal are required to prevent this environmental risk.

References

1. Gutierrez F: Geografia fisica. In: Ercilla, ed. Enciclopedia Temática de Chile. Santiago, Chile: Editorial Lord Cochrane Ltd, 1987: 1–175.
2. Jara G, Sanhueza G: Geografia politica. In: Ercilla, ed. Enciclopedia Temática de Chile. Santiago, Chile: Editorial Lord Cochrane Ltd 1987: 1–160.
3. Villagrán JO: Geografia humana. Geografia de la población. In: Ercilla, ed. Enciclopedia Temática de Chile. Santiago, Chile: Editorial Lord Cochrane Ltd, 1987: 1–160.
4. Figueroa L, Razmilic B, González M: Corporal distribution of arsenic in mummied bodies owned to an arsenical habitat. International Seminar Proceedings, Arsenic in the Environment and Its Incidence on Health. Universidad de Chile, Santiago, Chile, 1992: 77–82.
5. Sancha AM, Vega F, Venturino H, et al: The arsenic health problem in northern Chile. Evaluation and control. A case study. Preliminary report. International Seminar Proceedings, Arsenic in the Environment and Its Incidence on Health. Universidad de Chile, Santiago, Chile, 1992: 187–202.
6. Borgoño JM, Greiber R: Estudio epidemiológico en la ciudad de Antofagasta. Rev Med Chile 1971;99:702–709.
7. Borgoño JM, Vincent P, Venturino H, Infante A: Arsenic in the drinking water of Antofagasta: Epidemiological and clinical study before and after the installation of the treatment plant. Environ Health 1980;108:1039–1048.
8. Jamett A, Santander M, Peña L: Arsenic levels in hair samples of inhabitants of the second region of Chile. International Seminar Proceedings, Arsenic in the Environment and Its Incidence on Health. Universidad de Chile, Santiago, Chile, 1992: 87–90.
9. Sastre MSR, Varillas A, Kirschbaum P: Arsenic content in water in the northwest area of Argentina. International Seminar Proceedings, Arsenic in the Environment and Its Incidence on Health. Universidad de Chile, Santiago, Chile, 1992: 91–99.
10. Diaz-Barriga F, Santos MA, Batre L, et al: Health effects in children exposed to arsenic, the San Luis Potosi case. International Seminar Proceedings, Arsenic in the Environment and Its Incidence on Health. Universidad de Chile, Santiago, Chile, 1992: 41–49.
11. Meek ME, Hughes K: Arsenic in the general environment—evaluation of risks to health. International Seminar Proceedings, Arsenic in the Environment and Its Incidence on Health. Universidad de Chile, Santiago, Chile, 1992: 173–181.
12. Quintanilla J: Evaluation of arsenic in bodies of superficial water of the South Lipez of Bolivia (South-West). International Seminar Proceedings, Arsenic in the Environment and Its Incidence on Health. Universidad de Chile, Santiago, Chile, 1992: 109–121.
13. Smith AH, Hopenhayn-Rich C, Bates MN, et al: Cancer risks from arsenic in drinking water. International Seminar Proceedings, Arsenic in the Environment and Its Incidence on Health. Universidad de Chile, Santiago, Chile, 1992: 135–148.
14. Sandoval H, Venturino H: Contaminación ambiental por arsénico en Chile. Cuad Med Soc 1987;28:3–37.
15. Science Applications International Corporation: Estimated national occurrence and exposure to arsenic in public drinking water supplies (revised draft, prepared by EPA, contract No. 68-01-766). Washington DC: Government Printing Office, 1987.
16. Johnson TM, Rowe DE, Bruce R, et al: Squamous cell carcinoma of the skin (excluding lip and oral mucosa). J Am Acad Dermatol 1992;26:467–484.
17. US Department of Health and Human Services: Reducing the Health Consequences of Smoking.

25 years of progress. A report of the Surgeon General, Washington, DC: Government Printing Office, 1989.

18. Johnson LR, Farmer JG: Use of human metabolic studies and urinary arsenic speciation in assessing arsenic exposure. *Bull Environ Contam Toxicol* 1991;**46**:53–61.

19. US Environmental Protection Agency: Special report on ingested inorganic arsenic. Skin cancer, nutritional essentiality. Risk Assessment Forum US Environmental Protection Agency. EPA-625/3-87/0103, 1988.

20. Dibner B: Agricola on Metals. Norwalk, CT: Burndy Library, 1958.

21. Hunter D: The Diseases of Occupations. London: English Universities Press, 1957.

22. Stokinger HE: Industrial hygiene and toxicology. In: Patty S, ed. Toxicology, 3rd ed, Vol IIA. New York: Wiley-Interscience, 1982: 1517–1531.

23. Vergil HF: Arsenic as a teratogenic agent. *Environ Health Perspect* 1977;**19**:215–217.

24. Chen CJ, Wu MM, Lee SS, et al: Atherogenicity and carcinogenicity of high arsenic artesian water multiple risk factors and related malignant neoplasms of blackfoot disease. *Arteriosclerosis* 1988;**8**:452–460.

25. Tseng WP: Effects and dose-response relationship on skin cancer and blackfoot disease with arsenic. *Environ Health Perspect* 1977;**19**: 109–119.

26. Rosenberg H: Systemic arterial disease and chronic arsenicism in infants. *Arch Pathol* 1977;**97**:360–365.

27. Moran S, Maturana G, Rosemberg H, et al.

Occlusions coronariennes liées a une intoxication arsenicale chronique. *Arch Mal Coeur* 1977;**70**: 1115–1120.

28. Schoolmaster WL, White DR: Arsenic poisoning. *South Med J* 1980;**73**:198–207.

29. Feldman RG, Niles CA, Kelly-Hayes M, et al: Peripheral neuropathy in arsenic smelter workers. *Neurology* 1979;**29**:939–944.

30. Kyle RA, Pease GL: Hematologic aspects of arsenic intoxication. *New Engl J Med* 1965;**273**: 18–23.

31. Gosenbatt ME, Vega L, Herrera LA, et al: Arsenite and arsenate inhibit in vitro lymphocyte stimulation and proliferation. International Seminar Proceedings, Arsenic in the Environment and Its Incidence on Health. Universidad de Chile, Santiago, Chile. 1992: 11–14.

32. Cisternas C, Acuña O, Silva G: Chronic ingestion of arsenic and their effect on humoral immune response. International Seminar Proceedings, Arsenic in the Environment and Its Incidence on Health. Universidad de Chile, Santiago, Chile, 1992: 37–40.

33. Everall JD, Dowd PM: Influence of environmental factors excluding ultraviolet radiation on the incidence of skin cancer. *Bull Cancer* 1978;**65**:241–248.

34. Sancha AM, Vega F, Fuentes S: Efficiency in removing arsenic from water supplies for large towns. Salar Carmen plant, Antofagasta, Chile. International Seminar Proceedings. Arsenic in the Environment and Its Incidence on Health. Universidad de Chile, Santiago, Chile, 1992: 159–163.

29

Colombia

Rafael Falabella

Colombia is a tropical country located in the northern part of South America within the equatorial area betwen latitudes 4° south and 12° north, with two oceans, the Caribbean and the Pacific. Two other important geographical characeristics exist in Colombia: the Andes Cordillera with the main ranges and Great Plains area in the southeast part of the country (Fig. 29.1). These geographical attributes provide this nation with a variety of ecological conditions that are unique in the continent.

The country has a population of 32 million inhabitants, primarily with a white Spanish and mestizo ancestry; the latter results from two additional racial groups, blacks and Indians, who are part of approximately 10% and 1% of the total population, respectively. About 70% of the inhabitants are settled in the coastal and Andean urban regions.

Although there is not much variation in the seasons, rainy and dry seasons are clearly defined, due to the low and high lands that play an important role in the environment's temperature and humidity.

Colombia is at present a semi-industrialized country with a steady trend toward development. Although the living standards of its population have improved over the past three decades, much work is needed before ideal conditions and opportunities are equal for everyone; at present, small groups within the largest towns and isolated communities in certain rural areas are affected by poor socioeconomic conditions, predisposing them to disease. Important political and social changes are currently under progress and they will certainly have a favorable outcome with regard to development in the years to come.

Environment and Habitat

The geographical location of Colombia within the tropical area, plus the presence of the Andes, provide a unique situation where all climates and ecological conditions are present all year round. Variations from humid and hot coastal areas, to warm or cool dry valleys, selvatic and isolated jungles, or cold regions make this nation a place where climates have a definite influence on cutaneous illness. In addition, whereas in other tropical nations the desert may be extensive, this is a predominantly green country with much vegetation.

Within this panorama, the inhabitants of Colombia have four options for settling and living: urban (large, medium-sized towns), semirural (small towns and villages), rural (small communities in distant areas), and selvatic (isolated groups within jungle areas). The influence with regard to cutaneous disease is obvious for the last two groups because the geographic/ecologic conditions make vector-transmitted disease probable, and people become more vulnerable to infectious conditions.

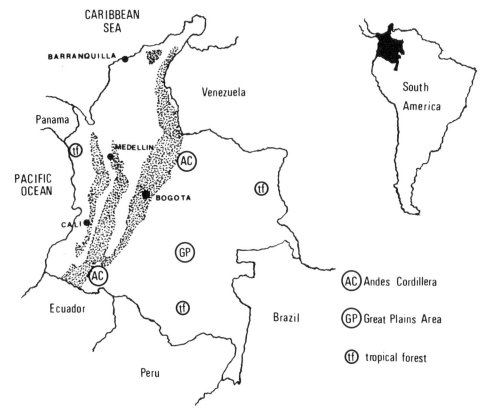

FIGURE 29.1. Map of Colombia.

Development Factors

Much change has occurred during the past 40 years. Although Colombia, as with the other Latin American countries, did not participate directly in the two world wars in the 20th century, these conflicts and others in foreign countries have had a negative impact in the economy and, therefore, an influence in socioeconomic conditions. In addition, the political unrest during this period has interfered with the development process; nevertheless, industrialization and modernization occurred gradually up to the present time. Along with a reduction of the birth rate from 2.8% to 1.7% in the last 20 years, there has been an improvement in the sanitary conditions, a reduction of infant mortality, and a decreased rate of malnutrition, which caused a high number of children to present with skin lesions in the past years. Today, Colombia is experiencing an accelerated rate of development, reflected in better living conditions for a greater number of people.

Dermatologic Background

The Colombian Society of Dermatology was founded in 1958. At that time, a small group of about 12 members initiated periodic meetings, promoted dermatology in the country, and contributed to strengthening university programs. Today, the society has more than 350 members, and dermatology is well established as a specialty.

There are seven dermatology training centers in the country. The specialty requires 3 years of formal education, and in addition to the clinical emphasis, surgery has also been incorporated in the programs. The role of the Colombian Society of Dermatology in the medical care delivered to the general population has been outstanding, as specialized care is offered today to a high percentage of inhabitants in urban centers, a service unavailable before 1958. It has also contributed to the knowledge of cutaneous disease in the country by detecting rates of prevalence and establishing the areas of priority for the future. Postgraduate courses, in well-recognized international dermatologic centers, are taken by a number of Colombian dermatologists after finishing their formal training.

Dermatoses as a Health Problem in Colombia

In general, dermatologic conditions seen in Colombia resemble those in other parts of the world. There are certain variations due to racial factors, socioeconomic status, life expectancy, climatic variations, or geographic and ecological influence.

Racial Factors

Even though the predominant races are the white Spanish and mestizo, other ethnic groups, namely blacks and native Americans, make pigmentary disorders more evident. Also, inflammatory dermatoses may disclose co-existent hyperpigmentation in the darker races as an important component to be considered when making a differential diagnosis.

Socioeconomic Status

Although it has improved in recent years, an important part of the population still belongs to the low-income group, which modulates the living standards. Precarious sanitary conditions at the periphery of large towns and in distant rural areas predispose their residents to scabies, insect bites, prurigo, and impetigo. Superficial fungal infections are more common than in other groups. A low socioeconomic status is frequently also the cause of delayed consultation with regard to skin cancer and inflammatory

dermatoses. AIDS, which is considered a high-risk factor, particularly affects this group.

Life Expectancy

The global life expectancy in this country is 64% (in women, 71%). This difference is at least in part explained because of political violence in the past 40 years, affecting mainly males. This relatively low life-expectancy rate, compared to that of developed countries, may be the explanation for the few diagnoses of dermatological ailments more frequently seen in old age groups, as it occurs with T-cell lymphoma, a condition of increased prevalence in northern latitudes. A similar situation occurs with other skin neoplasia of the elderly and peripheral vascular disease due to arteriosclerosis.

Climate Variations

Although temperature and humidity are fairly steady all year round, the dry and rainy seasons modify these parameters periodically. Superficial fungal infections are influenced by these changes and increase under hot and humid conditions, the most frequent being tinea pedis, tinea cruris, tinea versicolor, and candidiosis.

Mosquitoes and other insects proliferate during the rainy period, and they cause papular urticaria and prurigo simplex. Impetigo and other pyoderma may follow insect bits. Miliaria is a frequent dermatosis among small children or a fair number of adults with an atopic background; dyshidrosis followed by a chronic hand eczema is a very common consultation during the hot and dry season.

Geographic and Ecological Influency

The Andes and the two oceans cause varied ecological conditions; one of the most important is the selvatic environment that has been a reservoir for the insect *Lutzomyia*, the vector for American leishmaniasis. Other tropical ailments, such as paracoccidioidomycosis, chromoblastomycosis, mycetoma, or leprosy, may be associated with other conditions determined by geographic and ecological influence.

Specific Dermatoses

A few specific dermatoses deserve special attention because of certain particular characteristics or due to special public health problems in Colombia; these will be discussed separately.

Cutaneous Leishmaniasis

This parasitic disease is endemic from the Mexico–Texas border throughout Central and South America, including most of Brazil and the northern part of Argentina. It is transmitted by a sand fly of the genus *Lutzomyia*, which feeds from patients that reside, work, or have recreational activities in the vector's habitat.[1]

In recent years, the incidence in Colombia has increased, becoming a public health problem of significance. A remarkable fact is that it has become a problem in suburban areas where the disease had been absent previously.

Parasite Land Vectors

The parasite is a protozoan of the genus *Leishmania*, which belongs to the order Kinetoplastida, family Trypanosomatidae. When in the vertebrate host, they are found as amastigotes or nonflagellated round to oval structures; in the alimentary tract of the sand fly, the parasites are seen as promastigotes or flagellated spindle-shaped organisms. The parasites can be cultured initially in Senekjie's medium and then purified in Schneider's medium. Modern methods for characterization of leishmania species are done with enzyme electrophoresis, restriction endonuclease analysis of kDNA, and molecular karyotyping of nuclear DNA.[4]

At present, according to the newest classification of leishmania,[2] which abolished the trinomial denomination of the parasites, the species affecting the skin and mucosae for the area of Colombia and other Latin American countries, include *L. braziliensis, L. panamensis, L. mexicana, L. venezuelensis, L. guyanensis, L. peruviana, L. amazonensis, L. garnhami, L. pifanoi, L. linsoni*, and the recently described *L. colombiensis.*[5]

Animal reservoirs are mostly forest rodents, sloths, and anteaters. The vectors for American leishmaniasis are phlebotomine sand flies (order Diptera, family Psychodidae) of the genus *Lutzomyia*. The most common reported vectors in Colombia are *Lu. columbiana, Lu. lichyi, Lu. shannoni, Lu. pia*, and *Lu. spinicrassa*.[6]

Life Cycle and Host–Parasite Interactions

The female vector injects the parasites during a blood meal early in the evening. After inoculation, mature promastigotes activate complement, which attract monocytes and macrophages, and become internalized.[7,8] Immature forms are killed by complement-mediated cytotoxicity.[9] Inside the macrophages, the promastigotes lose their flagella and become amastigotes, which replicate by binary fission. After this, the macrophages rupture and release the amastigotes, which are fagocitized by other macrophages to continue the infective cycle and disseminate from the inoculation site.[10]

Studies of initial and recurrent lesions in human leishmaniasis, examining 24 patients on the Pacific coast of Colombia, for distinguishing polymorfirm in strains of *L. brasiliensis* species, demonstrated that 50% of the strains were identical to the initially infecting parasite, supporting endogenous reactivation as the mechanism of recurrence in these patients. The remaining patients showed different strains from the initial one, indicating exogenous reinfection rather than reactivation of the initial parasite.[4]

Clinical features

Two basic cutaneous patterns of most cases of new world leishmaniasis are recognized.

Cutaneous

The two most common species of leishmania producing disease in Colombia, are *L. brasiliensis* and *L. panamensis*. In a recent study, the former was found as the commonest strain (92.5%), followed by *L. panamensis* (7.5%).[11] However, regional or geographic variations may change these figures, as it occurs in the western coastal areas, where *L. panamensis* is the commonest parasite.[12]

The lesions frequently start with macules that originate papules at the sites of inoculation. Within a few weeks, plaques of nodules, single or multiple, develop and may ulcerate, forming shallow craters with raised borders; sometimes, they become infected by bacterial contamination, mostly staphylococci or streptococci. The ulcers are usually asymptomatic, but they may become inflamed and painful. Frequently, satellite lesions, smaller but with a similar configuration around the main ulcers occur. These lesions are said to correspond to multiple vector bites or due to self-induced autoinoculation by scratching. After several months, these lesions heal slowly, leaving depressed scars.

Another clinical presentation, not unfrequently seen in Colombia, is a lymphangitic form resembling sporotrichosis, but with much less tendency to develop inflammatory nodules or ulceration (Fig. 29.2). Sometimes, the lesions consist of large flat plaques with a hyperkeratotic or verrucous surface that makes necessary a differential diagnosis of lupus vulgaris, chromoblastomycosis, or a fixed form of sporotrichosis.

Mucocutaneous (Spundia)

This feature is caused by *L. braziliensis* and may follow the cutaneous stage, usually after healing; however, there is at least one report of *L. guyanensis* causing mucosal disease in Colombia.[12] The parasite reaches the nasal mucosa, probably by hematogenous spread, provoking what has been called "mucocutaneous metastasis." At first, papules, plaques, or merely edema on the tip of the nose are seen. Several months later, ulceration of the cartilage structure may originate nasal destruction and give the patient the appearance of the so-labeled "tapir nose deformity." This parasitic infestation can also involve the pharynx and larynx and, sometimes, the trachea above the carina, provoking dysphonia or dysphagia. This clinical picture does not have a tendency to heal spontaneously, and it must be absorbed at an early stage during the cutaneous phase with appropriate treatment. When mucosal involvement occurs, aggressive treatment is mandatory (Fig. 29.3).

Diffuse cutaneous leishmaniasis is a rare form of cutaneous disease, caused by *L. mexicana*, *L. pifanoi*, and *L. amazonensis*. The affected

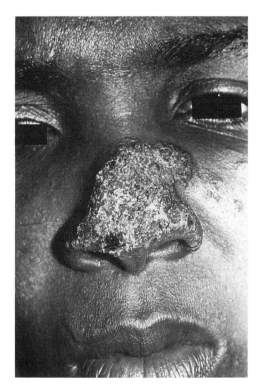

FIGURE 29.3. Cutaneous leishmaniasis. There is verrucous plaque on the dorsum of the nose that must be differentiated from lupus vulgaris, fixed sporotrichosis, and chromoblastomycosis.

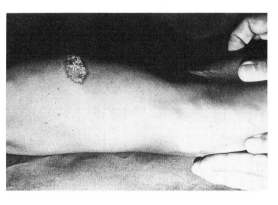

FIGURE 29.2. Lymphangitic leishmaniasis. Several subcutaneous nodules in a linear arrangement and a dry plaque are visualized.

patients develop multiple macules, papules, and nodules, but seldom ulcerate. These indications resemble that of lepromatous leprosy, with abundant parasitized macrophages, poor lymphocytic infiltrate, cutaneous anergy to the Montenegro skin test, and failure to respond to any known chemotherapeutic medications.

Diagnosis

The most useful tools for diagnosis of leishmaniasis are the skin biopsy, a direct smear, and the Montenegro test. The biopsy discloses a granulomatous formation and macrophages with intracellular amastigotes. A direct smear taken by aspiration with a syringe containing saline solution or by simple scrapings from the borders of the ulcer, and then stained with Giemsa are methods that yield a good percentage of positive cases; however, visualization of parasites is different in diverse geographical locations. By immunoperoxidase techniques the number of positive vases can be increased. If a culture medium, such as NNN or Senekjie, is used, a marked improvement in the isolation of promastigotes is obtained, by raising the positive cases to 80%.

The Montenegro skin test, performed with 0.1 ml of a saline suspension of approximately 2×10^6 promastigotes, injected intradermally, causes an induration of 5 mm or more, in positive cases, in 48–72 h. However, in endemic areas, it only has an epidemiological value.

Treatment

The best available therapy for cutaneous leishmaniasis is pentavalent antimonials. Two medications are available: sodium stibogluconate 10 mg/kg/day, 600 mg maximum dose, intramuscularly for 10–14 days, or meglumine antimoniate, 17–28 mg/kg/day for 10–20 days, followed by a 15-day rest period, and a second cycle if needed. However, antimonials can be administered until the lesions heal completely. They are well tolerated, but care should be taken in patients with abnormal EKG findings or during prolonged therapy. In patients with mucocutaneous leishmaniasis, a more aggressive therapy should be performed because a high recurrence rate has been reported after 4 weeks of therapy, even with high doses of antimonials.[13]

A number of diverse medications has also been used with variable success: ketoconazole (400–800 mg for 4–12 weeks), pentamidine (3–4 mg/kg once or twice weekly until healing), and rifampicin (600–1200 mg daily). Other drugs of some value are allopurinol and nifurtimox; cicloguanil pamoate, pirimetamine, and metronidazole are of little or no value. In our hands, none of these medications has been superior to meglumine antimoniate for uncomplicated cases. Amphotericin B, at a maximum dose of 2.5 g, is an excellent second line treatment for patients with cutaneous and mucocutaneous leishmaniasis resistant to antimonials.[3]

Fungal Diseases

Superficial Mycoses

Humidity, heat, and sanitary conditions often interact and produce an increased morbidity for all types of superficial fungal infections. Tinea versicolor, candidiosis, and dermatophytoses are common in Colombia. The most frequent clinical manifestations of dermatophyte infections are T. pedis and T. cruris; onychomycosis is also a very frequent finding, and T. corporis is particularly seen among children. The most important dermatophytes cultured in these clinical presentations are T. mentagrophytes, T. rubrum, and E. floccossum.[14] Therapy is accomplished usually with topical imidazoles and oral griseofulvin, and in case of intolerance, with terbinafine, ketoconazole, or itraconazole.

Subcutaneous and Deep Mycoses

Most of these conditions are prevalent among farmers in rural or isolated communities.

Chromoblastomycosis and Pheohyphomycosis

The former is more frequently caused in Colombia by *Fonsecaea pedrosoi*, and the most commonly affected areas are the lower extremities with chronic verrucous lesions following trauma with vegetable material.

Therapy is accomplished by surgical removal or cryosurgery, when feasible. Systemic medications include amphotericin B, fluorocytosine, and, more recently, itraconazole; this last medication has been employed with noticeable success.[15] It must be differentiated from leishmaniasis, lupus vulgaris or verrucous tuberculosis, and fixed sporotrichosis.

Pheohyphomycosis is much less common than chromoblastomycosis, and it is caused by multiple fungi (i.e., *Exophiala jeanselmei*, black molds, etc.). It is seen either as subcutaneous nodules or affecting the joint areas.

Sporotrichosis

It is of interest that this common mycosis is frequently seen in a fixed form, probably in about half of the cases. The lesions often develop in any area following "a mosquito bite" or trauma with vegetable material. The lymphangitic form does not differ from the classic presentation. The fixed form has the appearance of a chronic pyoderma with crusting, or larger plaques with a verrucous or chronic granulomatous appearance (Fig. 29.4). Crusting and healing may be simultaneous, and a typical micropapillomatous surface is frequently observed in healed areas. The diagnosis is done by culturing *S. schenkii*, but the biopsy helps to rule out other conditions. Fixed sprotrichosis must be differentiated from leishmaniasis, lupus vulgaris, verrucous tuberculosis, and chromoblastomycosis.

Therapy is accomplished with potassium iodide in most cases, but, when contraindicated, oral itraconazole is used with success.[16]

Lobomycosis (*Lobo's Disease, Keloidal Blastomycosis*)

Although a rare disease caused by *Loboa loboi*, this condition is present in Colombia.[17,18] It consists of a granulomatous lesion with a keloidal-like appearance, most commonly affecting the limbs (Fig. 29.5). It runs a chronic course, and it is symptomless, usually developing after traumatic inoculation with vegetable

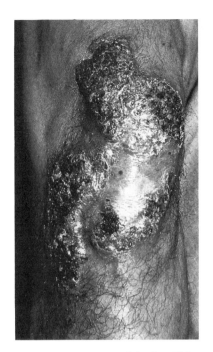

FIGURE 29.4. Fixed sporotrichosis. This patient developed a chronic granuloma disclosing a partially self-healing verrucous surface of several years' duration. Sporothrix schenkii was isolated by culturing.

materials. The diagnosis is made by a biopsy where, besides the chronic granuloma, abundant fungal spores of about 10 μ arranged in groups or chains, frequently six or less, interconnected by narrow tubular bridges are seen.[17,18] The organisms are visualized free in the dermis and within giant cells with routine H & E, but more specifically with silver methanamine and PAS stains (Fig. 29.6). The organism has not been cultured yet. It must be differentiated from keloids, leprosy, dermatofibrosarcoma protuberans, and giant fibrohistiocytomas. Therapy has been unsuccessful with multiple medications, but, in one case, we saw partial resolution with oral itraconazole before the patient was lost to follow-up.

Mycetoma (*Madura Foot*)

The incidence of this condition has somewhat decreased recently in Colombia. It usually presents as single or multiple draining sinuses and granulomatous formations following a

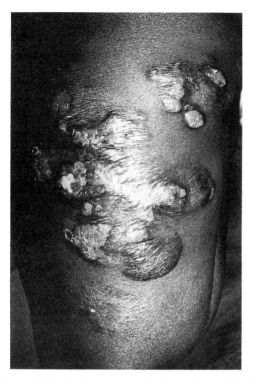

FIGURE 29.5. Lobomycosis. Multiple "keloid-like" asymptomatic lesions on the arm of several years' duration developed after minor trauma with vegetable material.

traumatic inoculation with vegetable material. It may occur in different areas, but it is frequently observed near the joints of the lower limbs and, besides the subcutaneous tissues, it involves the bone structures.

The diagnosis is made by a biopsy of the granuloma where the "grains" disclose either the true fungal structures (eumycetoma) with thick walls and spores surrounded by an infiltrate of polymorphonuclear cells, lymphocytes, and mononuclear cells, or filamentous bacteria (actinomycetomas) with a similar histologic pattern. The "grains" can also be recovered by pressing firmly and obtaining purulent material from the draining sinuses. The most common organism found in Colombia is *Nocardia braziliensis* (actinomycetoma).

The identification of the causative organisms by culture is the ultimate method for classification of mycetoma and for the final decision with regard to therapy. Mycetoma responds with variable success to treatment with trimethoprim-sulfamethoxazole, dapsone, penicillin, streptomycin, amikacin, amphotericin B, and retoconazole[19] or itraconazole. A chronic course can be anticipated in a number of cases.

Paracoccidioidomycosis

This deep mycosis is one of the most common deep fungal diseases with mucocutaneous manifestations, but its frequency has only been estimated in 4 per million inhabitants in endemic countries. It is caused by *Paracoccidioides braziliensis*, a thermally dimorphic fungus that grows in a mycelial form at 26°C (environment) and as a yeast at 37°C (host).

The disease affects primarily men in a

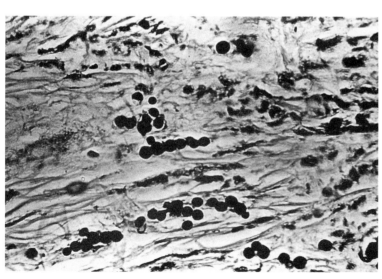

FIGURE 29.6. *Loboa loboi.* Multiple organisms in a biopsy of a patient with lobomycosis are visualized as round or oval spores of about 10 μ, isolated, in groups or in a linear arrangement and interconnected by narrow tubular bridges. (Silver methenamine stain × 400).

proportion of about 14–17:1. The fungus has been found to bear estrogen receptors, which are probably related to female resistance to infection, as mycelial-to-yeast transformation in the early phase of the disease is necessary for the organism to start the invasion sequence in the host. At this stage, female estrogens can inhibit this important step and block its initial colonization.[20]

In the cell wall of the *P. braziliensis* yeast, a polysaccharide, Alpha-1,3 glucan has been found, which has been postulated as a shield against the host's defense mechanisms; phagocytes may lack Alpha-glucanase, being unable to destroy the yeast forms of the fungus, which then multiply and spread.[21,22]

Clinical Aspects

The most frequent manifestation is the development of an erosive granuloma affecting the oral cavity, lips, pharynx, and larynx. The lesions can be highly destructive and dysphonia or odinophagia are not infrequent. Less frequently, cutaneous granulomas, with plaque formation disclosing a raised border and surrounded by satellite papules, are seen. The lungs are believed to be the major portal of entry of the disease and are frequently affected, but the radiologic findings are more prominent than the clinical symptoms. Other organs may be affected, but the adrenals follow to the lungs in frequency.

Diagnosis

The simplest method is the visualization of the multiple budding yeasts ("pilot's wheel") by direct examination, taken from mucosal lesions by superficial scraping (Fig. 29.7). However, the biopsy and fungal stains are of great value. Cultures of fluids, pus, biopsy material, and sputum, at 37°C, on chocolate or blood agar, disclose the yeasts in 7–10 days; at 26°C on Sabouraud glucose agar, this fungus grows in 20–30 days. A simple and reliable method for diagnosis and treatment evaluation is the detection of antibodies by immunodiffusion.[23] This mycosis should be differentiated from other pulmonary diseases, such as tuberculosis, histoplasmosis, coccidioidomycosis, and so on.

Treatment

For a long time, sulfonamides were used as the treatment of choice, the most common one being sulfadiazine 0.5–1.0 g, every 4–6 h; this medication has been replaced by trimethoprim-sulfamethoxazole 80/400 mg, twice daily. A long therapy course and prolonged therapy after healing are recommended. Low cost is the main advantage with these drugs.[24] Amphotericin B was also used for moderate to severe resistant cases, or in case of intolerance to sulfonamides. More recently, ketoconazole 200 mg daily for 6–12 months[25] and itraconazole 100 mg daily for 4–10 months[26] have become the drugs of

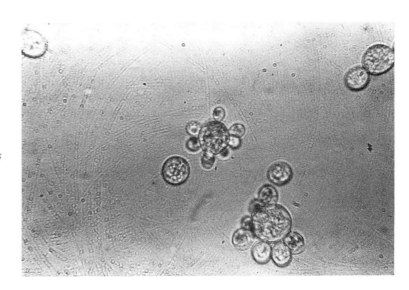

FIGURE 29.7. *Paracoccidioides braziliensis.* A direct smear taken from the granulomatous surface of a patient with mucosal involvement discloses the typical diagnostic multiple budding yeasts ("pilot's wheel").

choice. The percentage of relapse has decreased from 20–30% with sulfonamides to less than 7–10% with the newer azoles.

Actinic Prurigo

This photoermatosis, also known as hereditary light eruption, has been reported and studied in Colombia. It consists of chronic eczematoid changes, papules, crusts, nodules, and erythema, limited to sunlight-exposed areas associated with marked pruritus and multiple self-induced excoriations (Fig. 29.8). It is a condition affecting primarily subjects of Indian extraction and begins early in childhood, persisting throughout life. Although it has been seen usually in geographic areas around 2000–3000 m above sea level, a recent report indicates that it is also present at sea level in the northern regions of Colombia.[27] The findings of two HLA alleles, B40 and CW3[28] in Indian communities, which are frequent in American Indians, and later on CW4, means that at least part of the susceptibility for the development of actinic prurigo depends on the HLA system.[29]

The disease is incapacitating and becomes an occupational dermatosis, as most of the affected individuals are exposed daily to sunlight during their work activities.

Actinic prurigo was initially treated with success with thalidomide, but recurrences soon occur after discontinuing therapy.[30] More recently, therapy with tetracycline 1.5 g (as a superoxide scavenger) or vitamin E 400 mg daily (as an antioxidant) has been used with promising results.[31] In addition, a combination of a UVA sunscreen (avobenzone, Parsol 1789) and a UVB sunscreen (padimate O) seems very effective in decreasing the photosensitivity in these patients.[32]

Vitiligo and Other Types of Leukoderma

Vitiligo and other depigmented conditions in Colombia have a similar prevalence to that of other countries, but the lack of pigmentation originated in these dermatoses cause much concern to patients who suffer them, mainly in dark-skinned individuals.

When vitiligo, particularly the segmental forms and other stable leukodermas, such as piebaldism, posthydroquinone leukoderma, and postburn leukoderma, do not respond to diverse medical therapies because melanocytes have been completely destroyed or are absent, but if the disease is stable a good option to restore the normal pigmentation is by melanocyte transplantation. Two of these methods were developed in Colombia and used successfully for repigmentation of untractable leukoderma unresponsive to medical forms of therapy. These methods are minigrafting (1.2-mm grafts transplanted from normally pigmented skin to achromic skin)[33–35] and epidermal grafting (suction grafts obtained with negative pressures of 200–300 mm Hg).[36,27] In vitro cultured epidermal sheets bearing melanocytes are presently under investigation for extensive depigmented defects and the reports are encouraging.[38,39]

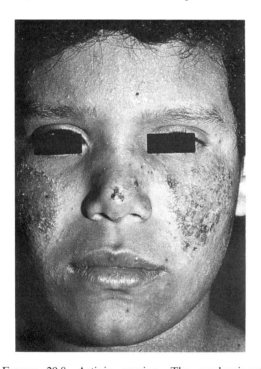

FIGURE 29.8. Actinic prurigo. The predominant features include plaquelike chronic eczematoid changes with crusting, multiple papules, and excoriations, due to frequent scratching in sun-exposed areas.

Leprosy

As a tropical country with many of the conditions that favor communicable diseases, Colombia does not escape the specter of leprosy, with a prevalence of about 0.09%.

The most significant peculiarity in regard to this condition is that 70% of the cases belong to the lepromatous pole, and the remaining 30% to the tuberculoid and other types of leprosy. This particular situation indicates that there are a fair number of patients with multibacillary disease that may contribute to the spread of this ailment. Nevertheless, an active sanitary campaign is permanently run by governmental agencies and, as new cases are discovered, they are treated at an early stage in an attempt to decrease the rate of morbidity.

Histoid (Fig. 29.9) and diffuse leprosy of Lucio are unfrequent, but reactional leprosy, mainly of type II or erythema nodosum leprosum reaction, is not uncommon, and it is treated with thalidomide, when available.

The treatment is furnished entirely free by the Ministry of Health, and the therapeutic rules of World Health Organization are followed for the diverse types of leprosy. The basic medications used for this condition are dapsone, rifampicin, and clofazimine. It is hoped that in the next years, with more active campaigns and by raising the standards of living, thus improving the sanitary conditions, nutrition, and other environmental factors, the morbidity rates will decrease gradually. New drugs and eventually the development of a vaccine will certainly have a great impact on eradicating this disease.

References

1. Walton BC: Leishmaniasis: A world-wide problem. *Int J Dermatol* 1989;**28**:305–307.
2. Lainson R, Shaw JJ: Evolution, classification and geographic distribution. In: Peters W, Killick-Kendrick R, eds. The Leishmaniasis in Biology and Medicine, Vol. 1, London: Academic Press, 1987: 1–120.
3. Wyler DJ, Marsden PD: Leishmaniasis. In: Warren KS, Mahmoud AAF, eds. Tropical and Geographical Medicine. New York: McGraw-Hill Book Co., 1984: 270–280.
4. Saravia NG, Weigle K, Segura I, et al: Recurrent lesions in human Leishmania braziliensis infection. Reactivation or reinfection? *Lancet* 1990; **336**:398–402.
5. Kreutzer RD, Corredor A, Grimaldi G, et al. Characterization of Leishmania colombiensis sp. N (Kinetoplastida: Trypanosomatidae), a new parasite infecting humans, animals, and phlebotomine sand flies in Colombia and Panama. *Am J Trop Med Hyg* 1991;**44**:662–675.
6. Warburg A, Montoya-Lerma J, Jaramillo C, et al: Leishmaniasis vector potential of Lutzomyia spp. in Colombian coffee plantations. *Med. Vet Entomol* 1991;**5**:9–16.
7. Mosser DM, Wedgewood JF, Edelson PJ: Leishmania amastigotes: Resistance to complement-mediated lysis is not due to failure to fix C3. *Am Assoc Immunol* 1985;**134**:4128–4131.
8. Sacks D, Hieny S, Sher A: Identification of cell surface carbohydrate and antigenic changes between non-infective and infective developmental stages of L. major promastigotes. *Am Assoc Immunol* 1985;**135**:564–569.
9. Hoover DL, Berger M, Hammer CH: Complement-mediated serum cytotoxicity for L. major amastigotes. *Am Assoc Immunol* 1985;**135**:570–573.

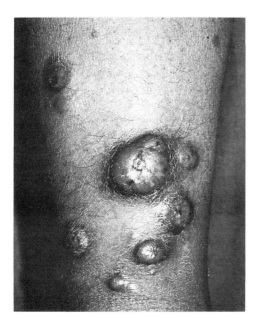

FIGURE 29.9. Histoid leprosy. An uncommon leprosy manifestation also seen in patients with dapsone resistance. Characteristic lesions have a tumoral rather than an infiltrative appearance, resembling large histiocytomas.

10. Hill JO: Pathophysiology of experimental leishmaniasis. Pattern of development of metastatic disease in the susceptible host. *Infect Immunol* 1986;**52**:364–369.

11. Montoya J, Jaramillo C, Palma G, et al. Report of an epidemic outbreak of tegumentary leishmaniasis in a coffee-growing area of Colombia. *Mem Inst Oswaldo Cruz, Rio de Janeiro* 1990;**85**: 119–121.

12. Santrich C, Segura I, Arias AL, et al. Mucosal disease caused by Leishmania braziliensis guyanensis. *Am J Trop Med Hyg* 1990;**42**:51–55.

13. Franke ED, Wignall S, Cruz ME, et al: Efficacy and toxicity of sodium stibogluconate for mucosal leishmaniasis. *Ann Int Med* 1990;**113**: 934–940.

14. Alvarez MI, González-De Polanía LA: Diagnóstico de las Dermatofitosis por el Laboratorio. Examen Directo o Cultivo? *Colombia Med* 1991;**22**:61–63.

15. Restrepo A, González A, Gómez I, et al: Antifungal drugs. *Ann NY Acad Sci* 1988;**544**: 504.

16. Restrepo A, Robledo J, Gómez I, et al: Itraconazole therapy in lymphangitic and cutaneous sporotrichosis. *Arch Dermatol* 1986;**122**: 413–417.

18. Rodriguez-Toro Gerzain: Lobomycosis. *Int J Dermatol* 1993;**32**:324–332.

19. Palestine RT, Rogers RS, III: Diagnosis and treatment of mycetoma. *J Am Acad Dermatol* 1982;**6**:107–111.

20. Restrepo A, Salazar ME, Cano LE, et al: Estrogens inhibit mycelium-to-yeast transformation in the fungus Paraccocidioides braziliensis: implications for resistance of females to parcoccidioidomycosis. *Infect Immun* 1984; **46**:346–353.

21. San Blas G: Cell wall of fungal human pathogens: its possible role to host–parasite relationships. A review. *Mycopathologia* 1982;**79**:159–184.

22. San Blas G, San Blas F: Molecular aspects of fungal dimorphism. *CRC Crit Rev Microbiol* 1985;**11**:101–127.

23. Cano LE, Restrepo A: Predictive value of serologic tests in the diagnosis and follow-up of patients with paracoccidioidomycosis. *Rev Inst Med Trop Sao Paulo* 1987;**29**:276–283.

24. Negroni P: Prolonged therapy of paracoccidioidomycosis: Approaches, complications and risks. In Proceedings of the 1st Pan American Symposium on Paracoccidioidomycosis, Medellin, Colombia, 1972. Science Publications No. 254. Pan American Health Organization. 1972: 147–155.

25. Restrepo A, Gomez I, Cano LE, et al: Treatment of paracoccidioidomycosis with ketoconazole. A 3-year experience. *Am J Med* 1983;**78**:48.

26. Naranjo MS, Trujillo M, Munera MI, et al: Treatment of paracoccidioidomycosis with itraconazole. *J Med Vet Mycol* 1990;**28**: 67–76.

27. Duran MM, Bernal J, Ordóñez CP: Actinic prurigo at sea level in Colombia. *Int J Dermatol* 1989;**28**:228–229.

28. Bernal JE, Duran MM, de Brigard D: Human lymphocyte antigen in actinic prurigo. *J Am Acad Dermatol* 1988;**18**:310–312.

29. Bernal JE, Duran MM, Ordóñez CP, et al: Actinic prurigo among the Chimila Indians in Columbia: HLA studies. *J Am Acad Dermatol* 1990;**22**: 1049–1051.

30. Londoño P. Thalidomide in the treatment of actinic prurigo. *Int J Dermatol* 1973;**12**:326–328.

31. Duran MM, Ordóñez CP, Prieto JC, et al: Management of actinic prurigo. *J Am Acad Dermatol* 1993 (submitted for publication).

32. Fusaro RM, Johnson JA: Topical photoprotection for hereditary polymorphic light eruption of American Indians. *J Am Acad Dermatol* 1991;**24**: 744–746.

33. Falabella R: Repigmentation of stable leukoderma by minigrafts of normally pigmented, autologous skin. *J Dermatol Surg Oncol* 1978;**4**: 916–919.

34. Falabella R: Treatment of localized vitiligo by autologous minigrafting. *Arch Dermatol* 1988; **124**:1649–1655.

35. Falabella R: Grafting and transplantation of melanocytes for repigmenting vitiligo and other types of stable leukoderma. *Int J Dermatol* 1989;**28**:363–369.

36. Falabella R: Epidermal grafting: An original technique and its application in achromic and granulating areas. *Arch Dermatol* 1971;**104**:592–600.

37. Falabella R: Repigmentation of leukoderma by autologous epidermal grafting. *J Dermatol Surg Oncol* 1984;**10**:136–144.

38. Falabella R, Escobar C, Borrero I: In-vitro cultured epidermis bearing melanocytes for repigmenting vitiligo. *J Am Acad Dermatol* 1989;**21**:257–264.

39. Falabella R, Escobar C, Borrero I: Treatment of refractory and stable vitiligo by cultured epidermal autografts bearing melanocytes. *J Am Acad Dermatol* 1992;**26**:230–236.

30

Mexico

Luciano Domínguez-Soto

Mexico is located between Central America and the United States and belongs to the North American continent. It was conquered in 1521 by Hernán Cortes and named New Spain.

In this country, the Spanish population mixed with the native Indians, which resulted in the race that currently lives in the Mexican territory. Different types of skin can be seen according to these racial mixtures, ranging from dark brown to light brown, and includes various skin tones that give the different appearances of dermatologic conditions. There is also a smaller number of Caucasion people, and on the Pacific coast, black or negroid populations are found, but these are relatively small as compared to the black population of the United States, Brazil, Venezuela, or Peru.

It is important to consider that dermatologic conditions in Mexico are influenced by racial, ecologic, geographic, and socioeconomic factors.

The expanse of the country is wide and irregular, with sierras, plains, and tablelands. The weather is variable (warm, cold, or mild) depending on the location of the territory within the Tropic of Cancer, which determines two areas: a lower intertropical area and an upper extratropical area. There is a large number of microclimates that, together with occupational aspects, plays an important role in the dermatologic conditions in the country.

Dermatoses

The main cutaneous manifestations found in Mexico may be considered as cosmopolitan, such as immunodermatoses, tumors, atopic dermatitis, and psoriasis; however, other relevant conditions that could be considered regional and are influenced by environmental factors are also present, including leishmaniasis, onchocerciasis, and pinta, found in the southern part of the country where the weather is tropical with high humidity.

Coccidioidomycosis is found in the northern region of Mexico where the weather is dry and hot due to the desert and semidesert areas.

Pellagra, tuberculosis, and leprosy are closely related to poverty, malnutrition, and overcrowded conditions. In the large cities, occupational dermatoses resulting from industrial activities are observed as in other parts of the world. The mongolian spot is seen in practically all the Spanish–Indian (mestizo) population.

We have chosen two special dermatoses that exist on the American continent; these are actinic prurigo and ashy dermatosis. Both are sometimes misunderstood in other latitudes and they are mistaken and misclassified by most authors in other countries.

Actinic Prurigo

Synonyms

Polymorphous light eruption (prurigo type), hereditary polymorphous light eruption (in native Americans), guatemalensis cutaneous syndrome, solar prurigo.

197

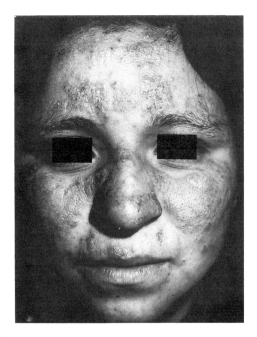

FIGURE 30.1. Actinic prurigo.

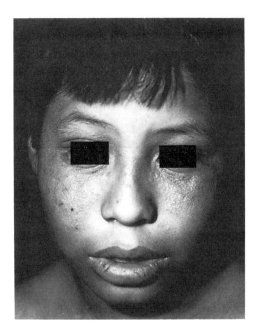

FIGURE 30.2. Actinic prurigo.

Clinical Descriptions

Actinic prurigo is a dermatosis that appears in sun-exposed areas and is characterized by polymorphous lesions (papules, erythematous plaques, lichenification, scabs, and excoriations) (see Figs. 30.1 and 30.2; also color insert). The lips and conjunctivas are affected in a large number of cases. It predominates in females and, according to our experience, the ratio is 5:1. The onset is at an early age and follows a chronic course, which is always quite itchy with exacerbation in summer months and is present in light-brown-skinned individuals of low socioeconomic status who live in high-altitude zones (over 1000 m above sea level).[1-13] These patients probably have specific histocompatibility antigens.[14,15]

The histopathology shows unspecific characteristics even though a lymphocytic infiltrate and polymorphonuclear cells distributed in clusters or "follicles" were found in 80% of our cases.[7,8]

With phototesting procedures, it is possible to reproduce the clinical lesions with UVA and UVB in all patients.[10,16]

Proposed clinical markers that are definitive for the diagnosis of actinic prurigo are presented in Table 30.1.

TABLE 30.1. Clinical markers for the diagnosis of actinic prurigo

Major	Minor
1. Sun-exposed areas affected	1. Polymorphous lesions (mainly lichenification)
2. Race (skin color type III–IV)	2. Early onset
3. Itching	3. Female predominance
4. Chronic course, exacerbation in summer months	4. Family history of actinic prurigo
5. Lips and conjunctivas affected	5. Non atopic personal or familiar background
6. Phototesting (reproduction of lesions with UVA and UVB)	6. Living in towns above 1000 m altitude
7. Excellent response to thalidomide	7. Clinical correlation with the histopathological findings

Note: To diagnose actinic prurigo, it is necessary to have five or seven of the major clinical markers and three or more of the minor clinical markers.

Significant Differential Diagnosis

Actinic prurigo is frequently mistaken for photosensitized atopic dermatitis, photocontact dermatitis, drug photosensitivity dermatitis, and seldom with disseminated discoid lupus erythematosus.

Photosensitized atopic dermatitis is the greatest problem because it affects children, and in many cases, the lesions are so extensive that they involve not only flexural folds but also the sun-exposed areas. Some atopic markers or a certain family history, which is infrequent in actinic prurigo cases, can be detected as a result of a careful search. The photosensitized atopic dermatitis patients have longer remission periods and they show a better response to topical and/or systemic steroids and oral antihistaminics.

Photocontact dermatitis may appear chronically among Latin-American individuals as a result of the prolonged use of numerous prescription and over-the-counter drugs that cause conditions that could clinically simulate the morphologic characteristics of actinic prurigo. The patient responded very well to topical steroids and, obviously, drugs that caused the reaction are discontinued.

Something similar happens with drug photosensitivity dermatitis where the prolonged intake of prescription or over-the-counter drugs, which is especially common in Latin American countries, can result in lesions that sometimes simulate actinic prurigo. The adequate investigation of the possible substances that are responsible for this and their consequent discontinuation, together with the use of topical and/or systemic steroids and oral antihistaminics, as well as the application of sunscreens and general sun protection measures, may solve this problem.

Disseminated discoid lupus erythematosus may less often resemble actinic prurigo lesions, but in this case, this histopathology is decisive in support or ruling out clinical assumptions.

Treatment

This disorder is particularly resistant to all treatments, such as sunscreens, which are not tolerated in the acute stage; chloroquines and antihistaminics have not been useful in our experience. Topical and/or systemic steroids and antibiotics are used when the disease becomes more serious or when there are complications.

Thalidomide, which was initially used by Londoño for this disease,[17-20] is excellent and the good response obtained in virtually all patients has made it a diagnostic test.

In our experience, the initial dose used was 100–200 mg, which can be lowered depending on the clinical improvement, and 50 mg is the maintenance dose for several months. Concerning side effects, we have seen few (sleepiness and increased appetite) without serious effects such as neuritis.

Ashy Dermatosis

Synonyms

Erythema dyschromicum perstans, Ramírez' disease.

Clinical Description

Ashy dermatosis is a pigmentary disorder that appears mainly in the trunk or arms, not involving the hairy skin, palms, soles, and mucous membranes, but can affect other sites. It consists of ashy, grayish blue macules, which are not precisely limited—from 0.5 to several centimeters in size.[21] (Figs. 30.3 and 30.4). A characteristic ring-shaped and erythematous border may be seen at the initial stages, which disappears after several weeks or months.[22] The course is chronic and asymptomatic.

Epidemiology

Ashy dermatosis is prevalent in women and it usually appears during the second or third decades of life; it is more common among brown-skinned individuals and occasionally occurs in Caucasians. It is possible that hybrid races in Latin America react and produce this type of pigmentation, whereas the white, yellow, or black races cannot.

This disease is found worldwide. Cases have been described in several countries with very

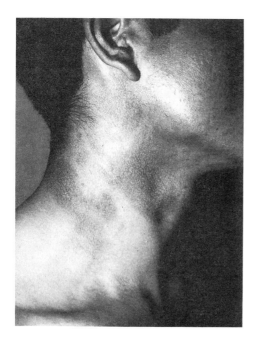

FIGURE 30.3. Ashy dermatosis.

different racial, geographic, and socioeconomic characteristics. Some questionable cases have been studied along a well-defined zone that is limited in the north by Finland[23] and in the south by Ecuador, but most of the patients have been found in Mesoamerica.

Athough the etiology of this dermatosis remains unknown, occupational, pharmacological, contact, and genetic factors have been mentioned.[24] Cellular hypersensitivity seems to play an important role in its pathogenesis as a result of the interaction between lymphocytes and melanocytes, which causes vacuolar degeneration of the dermoepidermal junction and pigment incontinentia. Some authors[25] believe that this is a variety of lichen planus because of the similarity of the immune and pathologic data. This situation has resulted in confusion between these two diseases.[26,27] We don't agree with this hypothesis. The immunofluorescence reports are few and not conclusive.[28] In some of our cases, direct immunofluorescence was negative.

Diagnosis and Differential Diagnosis

The misdiagnosed dermatologic conditions are occupational dermatoses with hyperpigmentation, especially argyria and caloric dermatitis; drug-related dermatoses such as fixed drug reaction and the pigmentary reactions to carbamazepine. In the histology, they only present melanin drop, with pinta in the early stage; in fact, the first cases of ashy dermatosis observed by Convit in Venezuela were diagnosed as pinta. This skin dyschromia is endemic in certain areas with defined ecologic

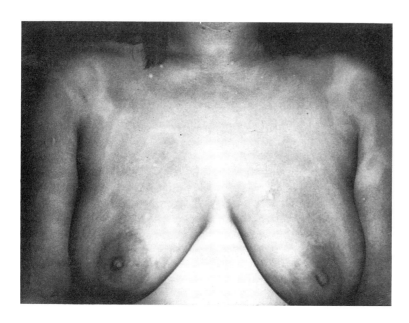

FIGURE 30.4. Ashy dermatosis.

characteristics, but it is about to disappear because of its response to penicillin. It has also been confused with Gougerot and Carteaud's reticulated and confluent papillomatosis,[29,30] Addison's disease, melasma, macular amyloidosis, and ochronosis.

The greatest confusion and controversy is with pigmented lichen planus.[31–33] This dermatosis presents a histopathologic picture with a lichenoid pattern and this is where confusion originates[34,35] because pigmented lichen planus is very similar to erythema dyschromicum. Although the lesions are pigmented, they are macules, papules, or light brown plaques.

Management and Treatment

There is no effective treatment for ashy dermatosis due to the lack of knowledge on its etiopathogenicity. Multiple drugs have been used, such as topical and systemic steroids, oral antihistaminics, keratolytic agents, and others.

Good results have been obtained recently with clofazimine.[36,37] According to our experience, some improvement was observed in early cases but none was totally cured.

References

1. Londoño F, Mundi F, Girald F, et al: Familial actinic prurigo. *Dermatol Latin Am* 1968;**3**: 61–71.
2. Everett MA, Crockett W, Lamb JH, et al: Light sensitive eruption in American Indians. *Arch Dermatol* 1961;**83**:243–248.
3. López-González G: Prúrigo solar. *Arch Argent Dermatol* 1961;**11**:301–318.
4. Jonquieres ED, De-Garrido RCB: Prúrigo actínico familiar. *Med Cutan Latin Amer* 1973;**5**: 319–326.
5. Birt AR, Davis RA: Photodermatitis in North American Indians. Familial actinic prurigo. *Int J Dermatol* 1975;**10**:107–114.
6. Hojyo-Tomoka MT, Domínguez-Soto L: Clinical and epidemiological characteristics of polymorphous light eruption in Mexico. *Castellania* 1975;**3**:21–23.
7. Hojyo-Tomoka MT, Domínguez-Soto L, Vargas-Ocampo F: Actinic prurigo: Clinical–pathological correlation. *Int J Dermatol* 1978;**17**:706–710.
8. Corrales-Padilla H, Domínguez-Soto L, Hojyo-Tomoka MT, et al: Polymorphous light eruption. Some interesting aspect. Dermatology. Proceedings of the XV International Congress of Dermatology, Mexico. *Excerpta Medica* 1979; 365–375.
9. Birt AR, Hogy GR: The actinic cheilitis of hereditary polymorphic light eruption. *Arch Dermatol* 1979;**115**:699–702.
10. Vega-Memije ME, Ortega-Estrada S, Hojyo-Tomoka MT, et al: Queilitis. Correlación clínico–patológica. *Dermatología Rev Mex* 1991; **35**:212–217.
11. Epstein JH: Polymorphous light eruption. *J Am Acad Dermatol* 1980;**3**:329–343.
12. Pizzi N, Parra CA, Brugnoli O, Spitalieri C: Conjunctivitis exubernate pigmentada en prúrigo solar. *Rev Argen Dermatol* 1982;**63**:249–252.
13. Fletcher DC, Romanchuk KG, Lane PR: Conjunctivitis and pterigium associated with American Indian type of polymorphous light eruption. *Can J Ophthalmol* 1988;**23**:30–33.
14. Sheridan DP, Lane PR, Irvine J, et al: HLA typing in actinic prurigo. *J Am Acad Dermatol* 1990;**22**:1019–1023.
15. Bernal JE, Durán MM, Ordoñez CP, Duran C: Actinic prurigo among the Chimila Indians in Colombia: HLA studies. 1990;**22**:1049–1051.
16. Hojyo MT: Reproduction of clinical lesions of actinic prurigo with UVA and UVB. Proceedings of the XVII World Congress of Dermatology. Berlin: Springer-Verlag, 1987: 885–888.
17. Londoño F: Prúrigo actínico. A propósito de su tratamiento con Talidomida. In: Sintesis Dosmil CA, ed. Memorias del VII Congreso Ibero Latino Americano de Dermatología. Caracas: Venezuela, 1971: 475–483.
18. Londoño F: Thalidomide in the treatment of actinic prurigo. *Int J Dermatol* 1973;**12**:326–328.
19. Flores O: Prúrigo solar de altiplaniciie. Resultados preliminares de tratamiento con talidomida en 25 casos. *Dermatol Rev Mex* 1975;**19**:26–39.
20. Saúl A, Flores O, Novales J: Polymorphous light eruption, treatment with thalidomide. *Australas J Dermatol* 1976;**17**:17.
21. Ramírez CO: Estado actual de la dermatosis cenicenta. *Med Cutan Latin Am* 1984;**12**:11–18.
22. Convit J, Kerdel-Vegas F: Erythema dyschromicum perstans: a hitherto undescribed skin disease. *J Invest Dermatol* 1961;**36**:457–462.
23. Holst R, Mobacken H: Erythema dyschromicum perstans (Ashy dermatosis) report of 2 cases from Scandinavia. *Acta Derma Venereol (Stockh)* 1974; **54**:69–72.

24. Navarro Jiménez BR, Sánchez Navarro LM: Dermatosis cenicienta. Estudio prospectivo de 23 pacientes. *Med Cutan Latin Am* 1988;**16**: 407–412.

25. Bhutani LK, Bedi TR: Lichen planus pigmentosus. *Dermatologica* 1974;**149**:43–50.

26. Naidorf KF, Cohen SR: Erythema dyschromicum perstans and lichen planus. *Arch Dermatol* 1982;**118**:683–685.

27. Berger RS, Hayes TJ: Erythema dyschromicum perstans and lichen planus. Are they related? *J Am Acad Dermatol* 1989;**21**:438–442.

28. Miyagawa S, Komatsu M, Okuchi T: Erythema dyschromicum perstans. Immunopathologic studies. *J Am Acad Dermatol* 1989;**20**:882–886.

29. Gougerot MH: Lichens atypiques ou invisibles pigmentogenes revelie par des pigmentations. *Bull Soc Fr Dermatol Syphil* 1935;**42**:792–794.

30. Gougerot MH: Lichens atypiques invisibles pigmentogenes. *Bull Soc Fr Dermatol Syphil* 1935;**42**:894–898.

31. Byrne DA, Berger RS: Erythema dyschromicum perstans. A report of two cases in fair-skinned patients. *Acta Derma Venereol (Stockh)* 1974;**54**: 65–68.

32. Leonforte L, Pelaez DB: Eritema discrómico persistente versus liquen plano. *Med Cutan Latin Am* 1987;**15**:89–92.

33. Pozo TR, Pintado HB: Liquen plano pigmentoso. Aportación de un caso y revisión de la literatura. *Actas Dermo-sif* 1988;**79**:681–686.

34. Pinkus H: Lichenoid tissue reactions: a speculative review of the clinical spectrum of epidermal basal cell damage with special reference to erythema dyschromicum perstans. *Arch Dermatol* 1973;**107**:840–846.

35. Tschen JA, Tshen EA: Erythema dyschromicum perstans. *J Am Acad Dermatol* 1980;**2**:295–302.

36. Piquero-Martin J, Pérez AR: Clinical trial with clofazimin on treating erythema dyschromicum perstans. Evaluation of cell mediated immunity. *Int J Dermatol* 1989;**28**:198–200.

37. Woodley DT: Clofazimine and its uses in dermatology. *J Assoc Mil Dermatol* 1982;**8**(2): 41–46.

31

Venezuela

Mauricio Goihman-Yahr

Few big cities are homogeneous. Nevertheless, the heterogeneity of big Latin American cities is so great that a study of dermatology in a city such as Caracas, Venezuela, provides a cosmic scope to the findings of such study. Other Latin American cities may show features similar to those of Caracas. In all, history is the clue to the present.

Historical Survey

Early History

Spanish conquistadores founded Caracas in 1567; its name was inspired by the Caracas Indian tribe. Spaniards were not amateurs in city planning and building. Caracas sits in a narrow valley in the Venezuelan coastal mountain range, about 3000 ft above sea level. Weather was (and still is) mild. There is never a need for heating, and hot weather is not excessive. The sea is very near "as the crow flies" but is separated from Caracas by the mountains. There is abundant rain particularly from May to October. There are several creeks that converge to the Guaire river, a small tributary of the river Tuy.

The slope of the land allows for drainage. The land is fertile and plantations blossomed around the city.

Initial city plans had a good design. With growing political importance, the city soon had a cathedral, governmental buildings, military forts, and a university.

Spanish administration provided medical care for destitute individuals, burial grounds, hospitals, a board of medical examiners, pharmacies, and a medical school (since 1777). Public health measures, such as antismallpox vaccination, appeared as early as 1804. The city had no malaria, and yellow fever was a rarity.

Population growth was progressive. At the beginning of the 19th century, Caracas had more than 30,000 inhabitants.[2,5,8] Social classes were stratified. Full-blood negroes were enslaved, but individuals of mixed ethnic origin (i.e., "Pardos") were mainly free and in charge of most crafts and plastic arts. Native whites (creoles) were land owners, members of the clergy, lawyers, physicians, and handled municipal affairs. Spaniards (*peninsulares*) were in charge of high political offices and senior military posts. The 19th century was chaotic. Caracas was severely damaged by the 1812 earthquake.[5] The fabric of government and of social strata was markedly altered by the long and bloody war of independence (1811–1821)[5] and afterward by civil wars, including a prolonged Federal War (1859–1863).[5] Nevertheless, by the end of the century, Caracas had been rebuilt. There were new public buildings erected in the 1870s and 1880s. A great new city hospital, the Vargas, opened in 1891. Caracas had running water, electricity, telephones, and telegraph. The overall plan of the city was still that of its Spanish origin. Some European migration had taken place (mainly Spanish, German, Italian, and some French), but most inhabitants came from families that had dwelt in the city for generations.

The population at the turn of the century was about 90,000[2,15] (about 4% of the country's population).

Modern History

The 20th century brought air and mechanized road transportation, radio and television, oil, and increasing resources. The old oligarchy was stretched and fragmented. The aftermath of World War II brought a flood of immigrants from Europe; mainly from Italy, Spain, and Portugal, but also from Greece, Germany, Russia, Romania, and Poland. Chinese and citizens from Arab countries also came.

Increased oil production and enhanced participation of Venezuelan government in oil revenues created additional economic opportunities. These attracted people from all over Venezuela to the cities. Countrysides and small towns were emptied and cities (particularly Caracas) grew and grew.

Starting in 1936, advances in public health (adequate sewage disposal, clean water, child vaccination, DDT, and antituberculous therapy) plus lack of birth control spawned a marked increase in population. By 1979, the net growth was about 3% per year.[2,15] In the seventies and eighties, a new migratory wave reached Venezuela, originating from impoverished and convulsed Latin America. Argentina, Cuba, and Chile provided individuals fleeing from dictatorship or social unrest. Poverty was the main reason for migration from Ecuador, Colombia, Peru, and from Trinidad, Haiti, and the Dominican Republic.

Current Situation

The current tableau may be summarized thusly: Metropolitan Caracas has about 4 million people.[2,15] Neighboring towns push this figure to more than 5 million. This is about 25% of the country's population.

Caracas is tightly packed. The weather is still mild but hotter than before. Office buildings need air conditioning. All public services are overburdened, and creeks and rivers are now carriers of liquid waste.

Clean water comes from an elaborate and far-flung system of intercommunicating reservoirs. These are extremely vulnerable and easily damaged. Water rationing and lack of supply is common during the year because of relative drought or more commonly because of maintenance and repair.

About 35% of the population lacks true running water, either because of lack of pipes or the impossibility of water to reach high altitudes. Drainage is also in jeopardy. Pipes for clean water or for sewage tend to burst frequently.

Tropical rains may flood streets, and traffic may be paralyzed for hours. In addition, traffic is very heavy. Going from one place to another may take 5 min or 3 h depending on the time of the day. The subway was started in the late seventies and finished portions of it are very helpful and well kept.

Population is extremely heterogeneous in terms of education, income, and ethnicity. Its distribution is very haphazard. City planning existed in theory but has collapsed.

The old center of the city and newer developments called *urbanizaciones* (mostly located where old plantations used to be) show some degree of rational planning; but as there is no planned lodging available for the multitude of poor individuals, they live as squatters in huts called *ranchos*. Several of these are in near proximity or in the midst of urbanizaciones or of downtown. Most poor individuals come from rural areas of Venezuela or elsewhere. In the midst of Caracas, they have created compressed huddled "pueblos" with an admixture of some modern amenities (e.g., TV sets). Efforts were made in the late fifties to stem the tide. Huge inexpensive apartment buildings were built, and some hills were reforested. Some housing developments for low–middle class families were built by the government in the late sixties and early seventies, and a few are being finished even today. Regretfully, this effort was not sufficient and has practically come to a halt. What is being done now is to provide the ranchos (early barrios) with certain modern facilities such as water by means of pipes, fountains, or trucks electricity, concrete stairs to climb the hills, and nuclei of medical care called *módulos*. These are staffed by fledgling physicians who have to spend 1 year in this endeavor in return for a practically free medical education. Although it is difficult to disparage measures that soften life's hardships for the poor, what has been done in the "barrios marginales" will never turn them into truly livable neighborhoods. It is difficult to envisage how módulos could provide adequate medical care. These measures may, nonetheless, prevent or delay blatant social unrest. As in many big cities, personal safety is waning in Caracas and crime is waxing.

Lack of Social Unheaval

There are redeeming features that explain why matters are not worse and why widespread social unrest is the exception and not the rule:

(a) There is freedom of speech and of opinion.
(b) The weather is mild; no one dies from cold in an unheated room. No one suffocates in the extreme heat of summer. There is no need to purchase varied sets of clothing according to season. Relatively light meals suffice throughout the year.
(c) Public transportation is not optimal, but it is cheap and it does function. Jeeps will carry people close to their dwellings, even high in the hills. No one is isolated and a great deal of time is spent in the streets where cheap food, produce, and clothing are available from vendors.
(d) There is remarkably little race hatred or even race consciousness. Speech and accent are more distinctive features than skin color and there is little bitterness, except lately, and that is against foreigners from neighboring countries (mainly Colombia). Colombians and Venezuelans are similar in many ways and only competition for work begets tension.
(e) Families may not be well structured according to orthodox criteria; a mother, elder brother, or some relative becomes head of the household.
(f) The government has subsidized foods and medicines in the past and kept gasoline

prices low. There are retirement and other pensions, but there is no widespread distribution of welfare cheques to individuals. Thus, no one can really live without working at something or doing something.

Overview of the Health System

Venezuelan governments have shown interest and spent much money on medical care and public health. In 1936, the Ministry of Public Health and Welfare was created.[13] The Venezuelan Institute for Social Security was formed in 1946 and[9] funded by compulsory payments from employers and employees. Monies are administered by a government agency.

The Institute provides ambulatory and hospital-based care to members and their closest relatives. Pensions and sick and maternity leaves of absence are also included. Not all workers participate; rural and household workers as well as certain other categories do not belong.

In addition to the above, there is a university hospital in Caracas and the city administers other hospitals (including huge children's and obstetrics hospitals) as well as ambulatory health facilities. There are also free hospitals owned by the Church and other private institutions. Private (paying) clinics and hospitals also exist, and are on the rise.

In theory, the Ministry of Health is the ruling body, and there have been plans to create a truly National Health Service but there is no completely effective central coordinating authority. Some individuals may have simultaneous and overlapping coverage, whereas many (as will be discussed later) have none.

Despite genuine governmental interest in health and the high proportion of the budget allotted to it, there were always deficiencies in the system. Hospitals were not run according to modern methods. There was never adequate maintenance of equipment and no well-organized system of visiting health workers. Except for vaccination programs, units of child care, and the obvious control of water, sewage, foods, and medications, the health system of the city was and is oriented toward treatment rather than prevention. Critics were active in the sixties, but it is apparent that the situation then was not so bad.

The seventies and eighties brought a dramatic increase in population and a cancerlike growth of unsanitary dwellings in the hills. The financial crisis of 1983 created a new situation. Hospitals and other health providers do not work well not only because of poor administration but because now they do not have enough resources. The state does not have sufficient money to continue subsidizing the cost of medicines and many of these are now at international prices. Regretfully, Venezuelan monthly minimum wage is now about US$ 100. Low salaries also affect physicians, nurses, laboratory technicians, and all kinds of paramedical personnel. Strikes have become common. New equipment is difficult to buy and spare parts and skilled repair technicians are scarce.

Low–middle and mid–middle class individuals who were previously able to afford private medical care must turn now to public facilities that are worse off than ever. Paradoxically, the very poor are not coming to clinics. One reason is that they cannot afford the costs of medications. Consultations in public hospitals used to be free. Now hospitals charge a fee for several services. Fees are low enough not to solve the financial problems of hospitals but high enough to be a burden for the poor. A differential tariff would be appropriate, but public hospitals do not usually provide the type of service that the rich would care to use.

Dermatology in Medicine

There are more than 100 dermatologists in metropolitan Caracas.[11] Dermatology was a specialty restricted in numbers, practiced by men, and many had trained abroad. Dermatologists is now very much sought after; most dermatologists are young women who have trained in Venezuela.

With current salaries, it is difficult to have only one activity or only a single source of employment. Most dermatologists will spend some hours in a salaried appointment at a Social Security dependency or at a city health-providing institution. University positions are an alternative for a few, but *ad-honorem* or "clinical appointments" do not exist as such. Private practice in one or more locations complements the income of most (but not all) dermatologists.

Some dermatologists receive patients from private or governmental companies for a prearranged reduced fee. There is no system by which a patient may preserve free choice and yet have his fees paid or reimbursed by public funds.

Caracas monopolizes public dermatological care in the country. There are two full-fledged departments of dermatology, with access to a preestablished number of hospital beds and with training and research programs. Both belong, at least in part, to the Central University of Venezuela. A third program trains residents and is supervised by university authorities but does not carry out research projects and does not have a fixed complement of hospital beds. Departments of dermatology are a rarity in the interior of the country; dermatology clinics exist everywhere but are under the aegis of departments of medicine.

In a public outpatient clinic in Caracas, a dermatologist will see the population of a given geographic segment of the city, including working individuals, their relatives, and a great number of persons from marginal areas. Some have been long-time city dwellers. Others are newly arrived from rural areas from Venezuela or elsewhere. Special clinics exist in pediatric or obstetric hospitals. A dermatologist may attend one of these clinics and then participate in one of the clinics of the university hospitals. Finally, a few hours are spent in a private office where the system is fee for service, but where tradition rules that poorer patients may still be seen for a lower fee or even no fee at all. Richer individuals may send servants or people that perform certain jobs for them.

Diseases Observed

What is the pathology seen? The key point is that races, occupations, social standing, and ways of living are more mixed than in more stratified societies. In the barrios most frequent ailments are acne, contact dermatitis, scabies, and pediculosis, superficial mycoses, and pyodermas; in individuals of more than 40 years of age, varicose veins and stasis ulcers are most frequent. Contact dermatitis and dermatitis medicamentosa are more common in poorer individuals and more so in the past when topical sulfonamides and penicillin were widely used. Interestingly, actinic keratoses, chronic actinic damage, and skin cancers are fairly common in individuals from rural areas in the Andes mountains. Andinos may be fair and blue eyed and they receive considerable ultraviolet light working outdoors in the mountains.

Besides "standard" pathology, people from rural areas have brought additional diseases to Caracas (see Fig. 31.1). Leishmaniasis, paracoccidioidomycosis, and sporotrichosis occur near Caracas in townlets that were previously isolated but are now linked to the city by highways. Old plantations were turned into residential, resort, or industrial areas, and some (particularly near the coast) are microfoci of leishmaniasis. This disease is on the rise.[3,10,12] I have seen youngsters who have spent a weekend camping near the city return with leishmaniasis.

Leprosy is another such condition. Caracas now has about 1400 known cases.[4] Patients are either Venezuelans coming from the Andean states or the plains, or else Colombians with the condition. Risk of transmission is not great. There are only about 36 cases of leprosy actually acquired in Caracas.[4] The Vargas Hospital has a leprosy clinic staffed by residents and senior physicians.

Sexually transmitted diseases (STDs) have increased in Caracas, as they have elsewhere, and with similar features. Chancroid, lymphogranuloma venereum, and granuloma inguinale are relatively rare (about 200 cases of chancroid in metropolitan Caracas during 1990),[4] although they were relatively common decades ago. Gonorrhea, nongonococcal urethritis, herpes, and condylomata are very common. Syphilis is also on the increase. Dermatologists working in obstetric hospitals are once again seeing congenital syphilis. AIDS is also present. It started, as elsewhere, among male homosexuals. These were initially rich and/or

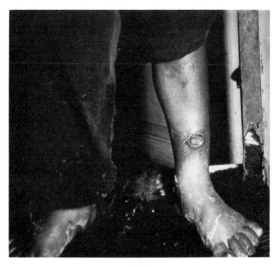

(a)

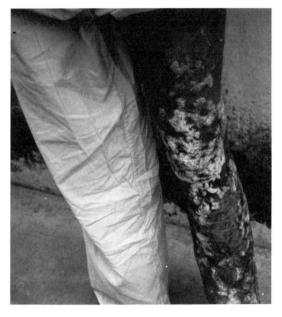

(b)

FIGURE 31.1. Two cases of "rural" diseases customarily seen in the Vargas or other Caracas hospitals. (a) Leishmaniasis, (b) chromomycosis. Lower extremities are commonly affected.

educated individuals who traveled a great deal and brought the disease from New York, San Francisco, or Paris. There have been cases in hemophiliacs, and lately AIDS is appearing among drug users. Venereal diseases were once under fair control. Prostitution is not illegal, there is no penalty for cohabitating with prostitutes, and little, if any, stigma attached to this. The Division of Venereal Diseases (now Department of Sexually Transmitted Diseases) of the Ministry of Health has always been directed by a dermatologist. Many of the venereal disease (VD) clinics were in the hands of expert dermatologists who would also care for VD patients in their offices.

The situation has deteriorated since the late fifties. The upper echelons of the Department of STD are still occupied by competent dermatologists but control is not as good. There are too many cases. Prostitution is no longer confined to "red light districts" but is widespread. Male and female streetwalkers roam the avenues at night.

The change in sexual mores is such that control of prostitution does not mean control of sexually transmitted diseases. In addition, poor salaries, low prestige, and the fear of AIDS has taken dermatologists out of venereology, although residents in training still attend VD clinics and receive adequate basic training.

Overview of Research

Venezuela does not stand at the forefront of research activities in the world. It does not have the private industrial basis that would use research findings and would finance further activity and development.

Biomedical research is basically funded by the government, either through the National Research Council or the universities. Drug trials are sponsored by pharmaceutical houses, but usually on the third phase.

Remarkably, dermatologists have been pioneers in Venezuelan research. The first independent chair of dermatology was created in Caracas around 1908.[1] Future dermatologists trained in Europe and (later) in the United States and brought back interest and knowledge in research techniques. They were able to make original contributions to universal knowledge in the fields of leprology, mycology, treponemal diseases, histopathology, and lately in histochemistry, biochemistry, and immunology.[6,7]

Several dermatologists or individuals con-

nected with dermatology have sat on the Executive Board of the National Research Council and have helped to plan the country's overall research strategy. The largest and perhaps most productive research group in the medical schools of Caracas is primarily connected with dermatology and was founded and is directed by a dermatologist. The successful strategy was to study diseases that were peculiar or common to Venezuelan environment, employing modern research tools and concepts. In this way, there was a logistic advantage over developed countries, the results wee germane to the country's situation, and their value could be understood by politicians and granting agencies. Thus, Venezuelan dermatology could contribute to international medical knowledge.

The recent economic crisis and overall disorganization of the society have hampered development and training at the precise time when new technology is making the "new knowledge" of the sixties and seventies obsolete. Venezuelans were able to purchase scintillation counters and ultracentrifuges and to train individuals capable of planning research projects and of using this equipment. They are now short of computerized equipment, cell sorters, and biotechnology. It is difficult to attract young dermatologists to research careers.

Conclusions

The gist of dermatology in Caracas is that it encompasses at the same time preindustrial and most modern aspects of the specialty. It is not simply a question of ministering to the rich and the poor. The Caracas rancho dweller is different from the slum dweller of U.S. cities. A dermatologist will in the same day or even hour embrace centuries in the pathology that he sees and in the psyche of those seen by him. The old, the new, the growing, and the decaying are intermingled. Life in Caracas is like a tropical jungle. The jungles have an immense variety of life and of decay; of trees that reach the sky and branches that rot. This is no less beautiful but is vastly different from the majestic growths of the Pacific Northwest.

In Caracas, dermatology has been been

neither a late comer in the development of medicine nor a leader in advances pioneered by other branches of medicine, but rather a torch lighting the way. From this complex milieu, important advances could have developed in the knowledge of skin and its functions. The economic crisis, which has turned into a crisis of society itself, has seemingly hampered progress. Whether this is just a passing phase or not will be seen in the next two decades.

Acknowledgments. Research in the author's laboratory is financed in part by grants from CONICIT (Venezuela) and the Congress of the Republic of Venezuela through Fundación Fagocitos. Jaime Piquero-Martín, M.D., Antonio José Rondón-Lugo, M.D., and most particularly Leonardo García, M.D., provided pertinent information. Evenz Arismendi E. typed the manuscript.

References

1. Alarcón CJ: La Enseñanza de la dermatología en las escuelas de medicina de Venezuela (Teaching of dermatology in Venezuelan schools of medicine). In: Goihman-Yahr M, Di Prisco J, eds, La Dermatiología en la Medicina, IIIrd Bolivarian Congress of Dermatology, Maracaibo, Venezuela, 1975: 11–18.
2. Beroes PM: Caracas. In: Pérez-Vila M, Director of Editorial Group, Caracas: Editorial Ex-Libris, Diccionario de Historia de Venezuela (Dictionary of the History of Venezuela), 1988: 562–567.
3. García L: Personal communication.
4. García L, Zúñiga M: Situación de la lepra en la región capital (Status of leprosy in Caracas' Metropolitan area). In preparation.
5. Gil-Fortoul J: Historia Constitucional de Venezuela (A Constitutional History of Venezuela) 3rd ed. Caracas: Editorial Las Novedades, 1942.
6. Goihman-Yahr M: La investigación en dermatología (Research in Dermatology). In: Goihman-Yahr M, Di Prisco J, eds, La Dermatología en la Medicina. Publ. of the IIIrd Bolivarian Congress of Dermatology. Maracaibo, Venezuela, 1975: 57–61.
7. Goihman–Yahr M: The international origin of knowledge. Coincidence and reality. *Int J Dermatol* 1990;**29**:21–23.
8. Humboldt A von: Viaje a las regiones equinocciales del nuevo continente (Voyage to Tropical Regions of the New Continent) Alvarado L, Röhl E, transl. Caracas: Monte Avila Publishers, 1985.
9. Pérez OA: Seguro Social Obligatorio (Compulsory Social Security) In: Pérez-Vila M, Director of Editorial Group, Diccionario de Historia de Venezuela. Caracas: Editorial Ex-Libris, 1988: 564–565.
10. Piquero-Martín J, Amini-Köves S: Primeras causas de consulta de las enfermedades de la piel en Caracas (hospitalario y privado) (Most common consultations in dermatology in Caracas, both in private and hospital practice). *Dermatologia Venezolana* 1986;**24**:21–24.
11. Piquero-Martín J:·Personal communication.
12. Rondón-Lugo, AJ: Personal Communication.
13. Silva-Alvarez A: "Salud" (Health) and "Balmis, FJ," In: Pérez-Vila M, Director of Editorial Group, Caracas: Editorial Ex Libris, Diccionario de Historia de Venezuela, 1988;**28**:510–518.
14. Ministry of Health. Department of Sexually Transmitted Diseases. Figures for 1988–1990.
15. Ministry of Environment and Renewable Natural Resources. Direction of National Cartography. Atlas of Venezuela, 2nd ed. Caracas: Litografia Tecnocolor, 1979.

32

Europe

Germany

Günter Stüttgen

All characteristics of the skin have been shown to be dependent on sex, age, constitution, race, and environment in the broad sense.[1] This statement made by Hermann Pinkus (1905–1985) is aimed at anatomic conditions but can be extended to the reactivity of skin. In various European regions, these factors are discretely reflected in the respective dermatoses; between the continents, the differences are more significant.[18] These are shown especially with respect to genetically caused forms of skin pigmentation and influences of exogenous factors such as climate and sun.

Traditional environmental factors play a role such as in India where the chewing of betel nuts and simultaneous smoking are important factors in the high frequency of cancer of oral mucosa. In the genetically different populations of Europe, exposure to sun and smoking habits are important in terms of cheilocarcinoma/labial cancer.

In 1975, Cabré demonstrated light-dependent skin carcinoma dependency in Andalusian farmers (Cadiz) to me. I could not report a similar frequency in a corresponding group of patients in Nepal (1980–81), despite the altitude of approximately 4000 m and the intense solar radiation. My objective will be to discuss dermatology only to the extent that dermatoses can be observed in the German linguistic areas as opposed to neighboring countries. Such characteristics can present themselves due to exposure to substances of the environment such as occupational hazards or from hobbies, including traditional habits in some regions.

Botanical characteristics[6] are important in the correlation between woods and vectors for infections via contact with insects (borrelioses). Plant allergens show their importance in variants throughout the country. The varying exposure to environmental substances in a limited European region is indicated in the list of allergens, which shows a marked differentiation between the European countries and also emphasizes the substance distribution in quantitatively (see Tables 32.1 and 32.2).

In the field of therapy programming, the European nations differ considerably, a fact that has developed from the traditional philosophies of the respective medical schools. Today, a different therapy in internal medicine is more markedly pronounced than in dermatology, even more so as alternative groups have not won favor within European dermatology as extreme variations to a specific medical conception. In Europe, this also becomes evident in the cases of physiotherapy, homeopathy, and in the relationship to "traditional medicine."

Significant History

The term regional dermatology under the heading "Germany" includes dermatology within today's state boundaries of the Federal Republic of Germany. Together with the termination of the power and political ambitions of the German emperor and the criminal aggression of the Nazi period,[8] today's current

TABLE 32.1. Common contact allergens (type IV) (1987) compared between Graz (Austria) and Munich (Germany).

Men	Graz (%)	Munich (%)	Women	Graz (%)	Munich (%)
Peru-Balsam	15.9	5.7	Nickel Sulfate	37.4	13.7
Diaminodiphenylmethane	15.0	—	Peru-Balsam	17.4	6.8
Neomycin sulfate	12.3	3.0	Cobalt chloride	10.0	5.9
Potassiumdichromate	8.8	5.1	Neomycin sulfate	7.7	3.4
Nickel sulfate	7.1	2.6	Diaminodiphenylmethane	7.1	—
Cobalt chloride	7.1	3.0	Colophony (rosin)	6.5	2.9
Benzocaine	6.2	3.3	Eucerine	5.9	2.9
Parabene	6.2	1.5	Formaldehyde	5.9	3.8
Paraphenylendiamine	6.2	4.3	Wool wax alcohols	5.3	4.7
Colophony	6.2	2.5	Paraphenylendiamine	5.0	3.9

TABLE 32.2. Common contact allergens (1980) in various countries. (According to the International Contract Dermatitis Research Group 1980.)

Denmark	Switzerland	Spain	United States
Nickel	Turpentine	Nickel	Nickel
Chrome	Nickel	Chrome	Chrome
Peru-Balsam	Chrome	Cobalt	Local anesthetics
Wood tar	Mercurials	TMTD	Peru-Balsam
Carbo mix	p-phenylendiamine	p-phenylendiamine	p-phenylendiamine
Wool wax alcohols	Peru-Balsam	Mercurials	Äthylendiamine
Neomycin	Cobalt	Local anesthetics	Neomycin
Cobalt	Parabene	Neomycin	Formaldehyde

borders of the Federal Republic of Germany became consolidated after the unification process between East and West Germany. When comparing this political term "Germany" with the tradition of today's German Dermatologic Society (GDS), which celebrated its 100th birthday in 1989, the dermatology of Austria and German-speaking Switzerland is incorporated in this society. Under the president of the GDS, Oscar Gans (1888–1983), the additional definition of the GDS, namely a society of German-speaking dermatologists, was an invitation to such dermatologists speaking the German language outside the political boundaries (1953).

Austria and the German-speaking part of Switzerland are very conscious of their rank with respect to the term German dermatology and its development. The *Deutsche Dermatologische Gesellschaft* was established in Prague in 1889, along with the foundation of the *Achiv für Dermatologie und Syphilis* (Archives for Dermatology and Syphilis) by Auspitz (1835–1880) in Vienna, in and Pick (1834–1910) in Prague 1869. Undoubtedly, Austria/Vienna and the German Karls-University of those days in Prague played an important role in the presentation of dermatology not only in the German-speaking areas. Today's scientific dermatology is based on the establishment of scientific principle by von Hebra (1816–1880) and his successors. The influence of German-speaking dermatology in Switzerland is connected with the names of Bruno Bloch (1887–1933 Zürich), Julius Jadassohn (Breslau/Bern, 1863–1936) and Guido Miescher (1887–1961). The comprehensive history of names and places in Germany on the history of German dermatology was given by G. W. Korting (see Table 32.3).

I will restrict the term German dermatology to the German-speaking area, thus accentuating

TABLE 32.3. Frequency of some dermatoses in Germany (BRD), average data.

Dermatomycoses
Onychomycoses: 10% of the population
Psoriasis: 1–2% of the population
Atopic diseases: 10% of the population
  (allergic rhinitis, allergic asthma, neurodermitis atopica constitutionalis)
Acne vulgaris: 80% of younger people; 36% men, 16% women
Eczemas of allergic and toxic pathogenesis: 20% of all professional diseases, 5% of the outpatients
Urticarias
Skin rashes: 3% of the patients
Basel cell carcinomas/other carcinomas in relation 3:1: 5% of the patients older than 60 years
Melanomas: 10/100000: 10% of all malignant skin tumors with possibilities of metastases.
Erythematodes with skin eruptions 10/100000
Sarcoidoses: 13/100000
Lyell syndrome: (Drug-induced TEN) 0.7/1000000
Drug reactions at least 5% of the patients in the clinic and outpatients
Lichen planus: 0.28% of the outpatients
Granuloma anulare: 0.16%
Pityriasis rosea: 0.7%
Zoster: 0.5%
Varicose ulcer/varices: 10/1000

Therapy: In principle, no differentiation from the other European countries.

Basel cell and other carcinomas of the skin: surgical dermatology.
Melanomas: the excision at the earliest by dermatologists.

the linguistic mutuality rather than the political differences. The forced emigration of Jewish dermatologists from Nazi Germany led to an exodus mainly to England and the United States. Owing to the initiative of Oscar Gans and Alfred Marchionini (1889–1965) and his friends outside Germany, the door to Anglo-American dermatology was opened to the young dermatologic postwar generation, a process that had a basic effect on today's dermatology in the Germany-speaking area.[21] Due to today's exchange of information that knows no political boundaries, this historic introduction now belongs to the past; however, it shows the roots that are still important for regional characteristics of dermatology in Germany today.

Discussion of the Problem

Environmental Dermatology

The term environment does not only pertain to the animate and inanimate parts of a given substantial situation but also includes influences by upbringing/education, nutrition/diet, and living habits. Finally, therapy with its side effects is also incorporated in this observation, regardless of whether the therapeutic principles are rooted in traditional medicine or popular belief.

With respect to the climate, the German-speaking area differs little from the neighboring countries. The same factors for the development of dermatoses are present as in England and France, for example. This is especially valid for exposure to the sun. Here different genetic dispositions are in the foregound when evaluating the damage pattern by exposure to solar radiation. As in other countries of the world, the frequency of basal cell cancer and carcinomas is mainly due to the intensity of the exposure to sun for whatever reason.

Approximately 20% of the German population are to be classified into type I and type II according to Fitzpatrick (Boston), and these are the key to the frequency of epithelial malignant growths that have an occurrence of approximately 10% in the age group of about 60 years. Approximately 10 million Germans choose such countries for their vacation in which exposure to sun is a dominating element, and according to our research, every person of the age of 50 has suffered at least 20 sunburns in his life. Thus, the frequency of cutaneous-helial tumors in Germany is mostly a function of insolation in combination with genetic disposition (Fig. 32.1). The intensive use of light filters for exposure to sun, due to the information by mass media and dermatologic enlightenment, will show only in 10–20 years even if the massive exposure to sun could be balanced by the use of sunscreen agents for preventing skin cancer/carcinoma cutaneum. The German melanoma register does not show a direct statistical correlation between sun exposure and melanomas but people with red hair have a incidence which is 4.7 higher than people with black hair.

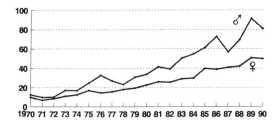

FIGURE 32.1. Incidence-rates (per 100,000 inhabitants and year) of epithelial malignant tumors of the skin without melanomas (age-adjusted for the European standard population) according to the cancer register of the Saarland which is representative for the German population (C. Garbe).

Blond hair people have only a small increase of 1.5 (C. Garbe). In Berlin, age-adjusted incidence rates are with 9.8 for men and 7.8 for women during 1985–1986 were found clearly higher than in the more rural Saarland area at 6.1 cases per 100,000 inhabitants and year. The incidence in the Turkish population of Berlin (110,000) was more than 5 times lower. Men developed melanomas on the upper part of the trunk 31% vs. 16.6% whereas women showed most frequently the tumor on the lower extremities. 42.1% vs. 17.2% in men. The similar data have been presented in the region of Trento (Italy).

Germany is a country abounding in woods. Furthermore, there is a tendency for the population to frequent these regions for short vacations. Beyond all doubt, a great number of ticks can be found in German forests, especially in the region of the Taunus and toward the Pfälzer Forest and on the way to the Bohemian Forest. Borrelioses with their clinical dermatologic appearances as erythema migrans, acrodermatitis atrophicans Herxheimer, and benign lymphomas are valid proof of this.

Furthermore, Germany is decidedly an industrial country focusing on chemistry, steel, and iron. Allergic contact dermatitis to metals are present in all countries which have become extremely industrialized. This can be recognized in the German area by the fact that nickel sulfate is the most frequent allergen in the hit list of positive patch tests. The sensitization, apparently by early contact of women with

metal "jewelry" during youth, favors a later development of metal sensitization.[17]

The recompense provided by law of occupational diseases in dermatology with proof of the allergens and evidence of the degree of the disease has greatly supported the recognition of exogenous factors in the development of dermatoses. Regionally, the contacts that are in connection with occupational exposure can be gathered from this (such as the synthetic rubber industry in Hanover).

Air pollution together with the intensification of industrialization and traffic has become the number one topic of the nation. The extent of air pollution in its actual sense, the deposit of soot and the percentage of sulfur dioxide, has not been successfully connected to characteristic dermatoses. As a current subject of interest, the development of allergic diseases of the mucous membranes, such as allergic rhinitis and asthma, are in the center of discussion.[17] The increased sensitivity of the mucous membranes due to sulfur dioxide and further industrial gases is recognized as paving the way for allergic reactions by increasing the aggressivity of allergens of plants origin as pollen together with a given genetic disposition.[11] Thus, the pattern of the proportional distribution of dermatoses in Germany remains similar to that of other European countries.

Body care products and their intensive use are a much discussed sector in the field of skin tolerance and intolerance to perfumes, preservatives, and bases of cosmetics. A correlation between cosmetics and allergic toxic dermatoses cannot be recognized in a statistical sense.

Approximately 3–8% of the total allergic reactions that develop in Germany are attributed to contact with cosmetics. As in other countries, anecdotal individual cases are published with priority and even repeatedly, thus giving the impression that a certain frequency is developing. Nevertheless, the surprising recommendation of oleum laurinum, known to be an allergen in dermatology, as a cosmetic was the cause for a dramatic increase of allergic contact dermatitis in the Berlin area from 1970 to 1975 (see Fig. 32.2). Following an educational campaign to the population and to the manufacturers, this ratio decreased substantially to

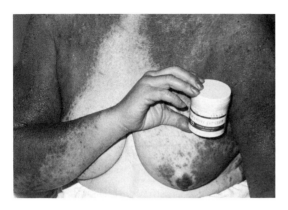

Figure 32.2. Patient 45 years old with allergic contact dermatitis to laurel oil 2% in an ointment base, 6 weeks after the application for cosmetic reasons.

psychogenic factors in the new habitat. As an example, psoriasis can be noted, which developed after resettling in Germany, together with many anecdotal individual cases. A similar story can be told for dermatitis herpetiformis. Neurodermatitis and atopic dermatitis, with their known tendency to depend on psychosocial and climatogenous circumstances, are conditions also seen in this modern voluntary exodus to the industrial center, Germany (see Table 32.3).

Development of Therapy

the level before the endemic increase. Vegetable materials in various cosmetics are the reason for an intolerance today, especially as Germany promotes self-made cosmetic preparations.

Genetic Features for the Development of Dermatoses

If we consider Germany from a genetic point of view, the borders are characterized by a constant coming and going of various population elements.

When looking at old textbooks and atlases, it is remarkable that especially the dermatologic school in Breslau could present immune diseases in its surroundings, such as pemphigus vulgaris, but also mycosis fungoides in a remarkable variety. This experience can also occur today in cooperation with dermatologists in Poland (Stefania Jablonska). Due to the transistory or long-term immigration of Turkish families who had accepted the invitation to participate in the rebuilding of the productive capacity of German industry, interesting aspects have resulted that are, however, not yet substantiated by solid statistical data. After all, Behçet's disease is not an exception in Berlin anymore, especially as more than 200,000 Turks live in this area.

Other interesting aspects show that dormant dispositions became evident by resettling and by

Treatment of skin diseases in the German-speaking area preceded the development of field dermatology by many centuries and was derived from folk medicine and especially from monastic documents [Hildegard von Bingen (1089–1170) et al.]. Skin diseases were considered to be in the field of general medicine and were thus not differentiated as such. Therapeutically, there was remarkable uniformity such as sulfur baths and herbal concoctions. These types of treatments appeared in the Middle Ages when combating the national epidemic, syphilis; here the emphasis was on mercurial preparations and tropical woods. In this regard, the sulfur springs of Äachen were of special importance around the turn of the century, mainly for the remedy of damages caused by antisyphilitic therapies, namely, mercury and arsenic and the assumed emission thereof.

Only since Hebra (1810–1880) and Kaposi (1837–1902) do we speak of skin therapy that is based on pathologic anatomy and physiology. Twenty-five years later the ideas of P.G. Unna (1859–1929) were generally accepted. Unna requested a scientific basis for internal and external therapies of dermatoses. The derivation of local therapies based on the already chemically comprehensible basic phenomena in histology and the concept of reductive and oxidative therapeutic agents was the beginning of a biochemical approach.

This scientific approach could be derived mainly from the behavior of the pathologically altered skin toward staining methods in the histology. The biochemical approach was promoted in therapy as well, due to the close contact between venereologists and chemotherapists around the turn of the century [Paul Ehrlich (1854–1915) and Karl Herxheimer (1861–1942)], later between Domagk (sulfonamides) and German dermatologists and venereologists, and finally the acceptance of a professorship for dermatology by Kimmig (1909–1976), primarily a chemist. The trend to favor molecular biology in dermatology as it is presented in Cologne by Th. Krieg (connective tissue) and H. Merk (drug research), in Kiel by E. Chrisophers and J. M. Schröder (psoriasis), in Münster by Th. Luger and T. Schwarz (cytokines), and in Berlin by B. Czarnetzki (mast cells) and C. Orfanos (hair and tumor research) includes immunology, as well as physiology and pharmacology of the skin, which is combined with the integration of appropriate scientific co-workers.[2,15] The physical non-invasive examination of the skin runs parallel to the success in biochemistry. Recognition of the heat pattern of the skin using thermography[22] and subtle analyses of microcirculation by angiodynography and measurement of tumor proliferation by ultrasound[1] are examples of the direct evaluation of clinical parameters in dermatology in accordance with bioengineering of the skin.

The development of subdisciplines in dermatology is connected with the progress in science and therapy but also with the charisma of scientists (Table 32.4).

Characteristic Subdisciplines of Dermatology

Around the turn of the century, *surgical dermatology* developed mainly in the German linguistic area. The personality was a deciding factor for the success of these therapeutic concepts, this can be demonstrated especially with the example of Max Joseph (1860–1932) in Berlin, who was a pioneer for aesthetic surgery at this time. Surgical dermatologic therapy was accepted and considered in health insurance settlements.

TABLE 32.4. Subspecialties in German dermatology according to the specialty regulations of the German government (1992).

General Dermatology and sexually transmitted diseases
Allergies
Proctology
Male diseases
Operative Dermatology
Phototherapy

The concept of aesthetic medicine includes *dermatological cosmetology*, which is integrated in the clinic and in practice. The aesthetic and clinical aspects of topical vitamin A-acid treatment began in Germany in (1959) in collaboration with Hoffman-la Rocho in Basel (see Fig. 32.3).

X-rays were soon integrated into dermatology. The idea of superficial X-ray therapy with special consideration of the dermal layers reached by radiation energy and their absorptive capacities, thus decreasing the risk of tissue destruction to a large extent, was advanced by the collaboration of dermatologists with corresponding radiation equipment, such as the chairman of dermatology and chairman of the department of X-ray therapy H. Th. Schreus (1892–1970). X-rays as a therapeutic tool in dermatology have lost their former importance today because of progress in laser-therapy and the therapeutic use of gene-technological drugs such as interferon and cytocines, treatment with the development in chemotherapy of malignancies of the skin.

The particular attention to X-ray therapy in the United States can be traced to H. Goldschmidt (1923) and his training in Marchionini's clinic in Munich before his emigration to America.

Phototherapy with UV-radiation (UVB, UVA 1, UVA 2, PUVA) shows promise in the treatment of suitable dermatoses such as high doses of UVA 1 in atopic dermatitis.[5,13] Finally, the treatment of hypertension with infrared-radiation by shifting the blood in the reservoirs of the skin was demonstrated at the Charité in Berlin.[15] Obviously, dermatology provides additional information to general medicine, as was demonstrated some decades ago by H. Ippen

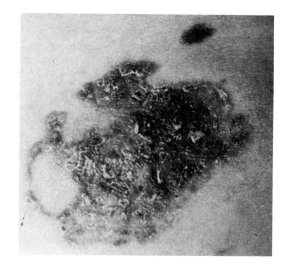

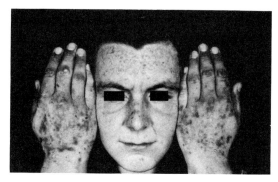

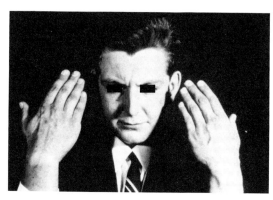

FIGURE 32.4. A. Patient, 18 years old, with porphyria cutanea tarda. B. The same patient at 20 years old, after 8 liter blood bleeding (phleboctomy) (courtesy of Professor H. Ippen, Göttingen).

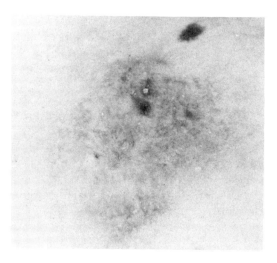

FIGURE 32.3. Superficial basalioma. Therapy with topical application with vitamin A acid ointment 0.1%, 2 times daily for 3 months. A. Before treatment. B. Three months after discontinuation of the local treatment.

who inaugurated phlebolomy in cases of porphyria cutanea tarda.[10] (see Fig. 32.4).

In this connection, the subdiscipline *phlebology* must be mentioned; it originated from the sclerosing of varicose veins by P. Linser (1871–1953) in Tübingen. Phlebology was submitted as an area of responsibility to dermatology by Oscar Gans in 1957. *Dermatologic angiology* is a special field in the German-speaking area that led to the formation of appropriate departments at universities in Essen, Tübingen, and Aachen. In the German-speaking area, the treatment of diseases of the legs, especially ulcers has always been a domain of dermatologists and has belonged to the scope of duties of dermatology for more than 50 years. Today, phlebology and peripheral angiology show the trend to be integrated in non-dermatological disciplines. Proctology and the treatment of hemorrhoids also belong to dermatology in Germany.

Therapy of *allergic skin and mucous membrane* diseases shows a very tight compound system between immunologists, allergologists, and pulmonologists and has, thus, opened possibilities for appropriately trained dermatologists to become active in the ever-increasing field of recognition and treatment of allergic diseases, which exceeds contact allergies. The additional designation allergology is characteristic of this, and approximately 10% of the dermatologists avail themselves to it.

Clima-therapy of atopic diseases in suitable dermatologic clinics at the sea-side in Germany (North Sea) or in the higher mountains (Davos) is indicated if conventional dermato-therapy in combination with the rehabilitation process shows therapeutic advantages that one can be deduced from an environment with fewer allergens, more sun radiation, and psychotherapeutic effects.

TABLE 32.6. Services billed by Dermatologists in Order of Occurence

No.		%
1	Allergies	34.2
2	Consultation, physical examination	26.7
3	Operative dermatology	4.7
4	Therapy involving dressing changes	4.2
5	Phototherapy	3.0
6	Microbiology-histology	1.7
	Total:	75.0

Sexually Transmitted Diseases (STDs)

The term venereology is now replaced in the European Community by the term sexually transmitted diseases. The tradition of treatment is not affected by changing the designation. Dermatology in Germany is concerned with the diagnoses and treatment of STDs.

Concerning the treatment of syphilis, so-called short-term therapy with a 3-day large-dose, pulsed intravenous therapy (28 mill units penicillin) has become an alternative to the conventional 2-week penicillin treatment with low dosage penicillin.[23] The short-term therapy was developed in 1974 in Berlin and taken over in the former German Democratic Republic. This therapy can be an alternative in distinct cases of syphilis, but has not replaced the conventional treatment today. The therapy of gonorrhea is complicated in Germany by an increasing resistance against conventional antimicrobial treatments, especially in the big seaports.

Some *data of the professional organization of the German dermatologists* presented by R. Fritz and J. A. von Preyss as a poster on the last World Congress of Dermatology in New York (1992) complete this short survey and make it evident that dermatologists play an important role in medicine in Germany. (See Tables 32.5 and 32.6).

TABLE 32.5.

Number of practicing physicians (male and female) in Germany:	244,238
Number of practicing dermatologists (male and female) in Germany:	3,452
Dermatologists practicing only in a hospital setting:	671
Dermatologists practicing only in an out-patient office setting:	2,577
Number of hospitals with dermatological wards: (only West Germany)	102
Of those—number of University Hospitals:	36
Total number of hospital beds on dermatological wards:	5,242

Financing of Medical Care in Germany
90% through sickness funds* and welfare (minimal)
10% privately including private health insurances

* Sickness funds are not-for-profit compulsory health care insurances financed by employer and employees equally according to gross income of employee.

References

1. Altmeyer P: Dermatologischer Ultraschall-gegenwärtiger Stand und Perspektiven. *Z Hautkr* 1989;**64**:727–728.
2. Braun-Falco O, Geiler G, Jablońska St, eds.: Die Haut als Abwehrorgan. Stuttgart: Wissenschaftliche Verlagsgesellschaft mbH, 1991.
3. Garbe C, Thieß S, Nürnberger F, Ehlers G, Albrecht G, Lindlar F, Bertz J: Incidence and Mortality of Malignant Melanoma in Berlin (West) from 1980 to 1986. *Acta Derm Venereol (Stockh)* 1990;**71**:506–511.
4. Gailhofer G, Ludvan M: Zur Änderung des Allergenspektrums bei Kontaktekzemen in den Jahren 1975–1984. *Dermatosen* 1987;**35**:13–16.
5. Grewe M, Gyufko K, Block R, Parlow F, Schöpf E, Krutman J: Transcript levels of the T-cell derived cytokines interferon α and interleukin-4

in lesional atopic skin in patients undergoing High-Dose-UVA1 therapy. XX. Jahrestagung der Arbeitsgemeinschaft Dermatologische Forschung November 1992.

6. Hausen B: Allergiepflanzen Pflanzenallergene. Landsberg/München: Ecomed Verlagsgesellschaft, 1988.

7. Hebra FV: Handbuch der speziellen Pathologie. 2. Auflage in Virchow, R. Erlangen: Ferdinand Enke, 1872.

8. Hollander A: Jüdische Dermatologen vor und während des Naziregimes, Auswanderung und Wiederaufbau. In: Nürnberger F, ed. Die Berliner Dermatologische Gesellschaft (1886–1986), Die Hautklinik im RVK (1906–1986). Berlin: Grosse Verlag, 1987.

9. Hornstein P, Nürnberg, eds: Externe Therapie von Hautkrankheiten Pharmazeutische und medizinische Praxis. Stuttgart: Georg Thieme Verlag, 1985.

10. Ippen H: Long-term prognosis of cutaneous Porphyrias. In: Kukita A, Seiji M, eds. Proceedings of the XVIth International Congress of Dermatology, May 1982 Tokyo, University of Tokyo Press, 1983: 271–274.

11. Kainka-Stänicke E, Behrendt H, Friedrichs KH, Tomingas R: Mögliche Einfluße von Luftverunreinigung, Klima und Urbanität auf allergische Rhinitis. Autorenreferat 2. Allergologischer Workshop der Deutschen Gesellschaft für Allergie-u. Immunitätsforschung, 9. März 1990 in Mainz. Allergologie 1990: Jg. 2, Heft 2: 67.

12. Korting GW: Some aspects of the genesis and development of German dermatology. In: Herzberg JJ, Korting GW, eds., On the History of German Dermatology. Berlin: Grosse Verlag, 1987: 117–130.

13. Krutmann J, Grewe M, Christoph H, Block R, Schöpf E: Ultraviolet immunomodulation: high-dose UVA1 therapy for atopic dermatitis. In: Burgdorf WHC, Katz SI, eds., Dermatology Progress & Perspectives. The Proceedings of the 18th World Congress of Dermatology, New York, June 1992. New York, Casterton, London: The Parthenon Publishing Group: 1993: 562–565.

14. Meffert H, Hecht HChr, Günther H, Scherf HP, Schumann E, von Ardenne M, Sönnichsen N: Biophysikalische Ergebnisse des klinischen Tests der IRA-Therm-Hyperthermietechnik der 2. Generation. *Thermo Med* 1990;**6**:71–78.

15. Orfanos CE: Die Integration der DDG in die Naturwissenschaften. In: Stüttgen G, ed., Standort und Ausblick der deutschsprachigen Dermatologie. Zum 100 jährigen Bestehen der Deutschen Dermatologischen Gesellschaft. Berlin: Grosse Verlag, 1989: 56–69.

16. Pinkus H: Die makroskopische Anatomie der Haut. In: Jadassohn von J, ed., Handb. d. Haut- u. Geschlechtskrankheiten. Berlin: Springer-Verlag, 1964.

17. Ring J: Angewandte Allergol. Vieweg: MMV Medizen Verlag, 1988.

18. Spitzer R: Geographische Verteilung der Hautkrankheiten. In: Handb. d. Haut- u. Geschlechtskrankheiten. Berlin: Springer-Verlag, 1964: 1–40.

19. Scherf HP, Meffert H, Bäumler H, Dittmann K, Siewert H, Strangfeld D, Winterfeld HJ, Hecht HChr, Schumann E, Sönnichsen N: Wirkung einer einmaligen milden Infrarot-A-Hyperthermie auf Körpertemperatur, Herzfrequenz, Blutdruck und Blutviscosität bei Gesunden und Patienten mit arterieller Hypertonie der Stadien I und II. *Dermatol Mon. schr* 1989;**175**:733–740.

20. Stüttgen G: Historical perspectives of tretinoin. *J Am Acad Dermatol* 1986;**15**:735–740.

21. Stüttgen G: A short history of German dermatology. *J Am Acad Dermatol* 1987; 1061–1064.

22. Stüttgen G, Flesch U: Dermatological Thermography, eds.: Engel JM, Ring J. Weinheim: VCH Verlagsgesellschaft mbH, 1985.

23. Wecke J, Bartunek J, Stüttgen G: Treponema Pallidum in Early Syphilitic Lesions in Humans during High-Dosage Penicillin Therapy. An Electron Microscopical Study. *Arch Derm Res* 1976;**257**:1–15.

33

Greece

John D. Stratigos, A. Katsambas, and D. Rigopoulos

Historical Data

The University of Athens, Greece's first university, was established in 1837, only 7 years after the end of the War of Independence against the Ottoman Empire, a harsh battle that lasted 9 years. In 1837, the medical school was founded, with Greek professors coming from European universities. Dermatology and venereology were initially taught to a limited degree by professors of hygiene and, afterward by surgeons.

Immediately after the turn of the 20th century, a rudimentary interest in dermatovenereology emerged, namely, the course began to be taught by relatively specialized medical doctors, and a primitive hospital of venereal diseases (not dermatologic ones) was founded to treat prostitutes, primarily. It was the only one of its kind in Greece and operated under appalling conditions.

These elementary measures, taken within the framework of the antivenereal disease struggle, were absolutely necessary, as the rampant spread of venereal diseases everywhere was terrifying. During the first two decades, two events of decisive significance took place. Moreover, the state took several necessary measures that had strong and beneficial effects on the elimination of venereal diseases.

They were the following:

1910 The new hospital for the management of venereal and skin diseases, with perfect specifications for its time, was built and donated by Ifigenia A. Sygros in memory of her husband Andreas Sygros [named:

A. Sygros Hospital for Skin and Venereal Diseases–University Clinic].

1920 G. Photinos was appointed professor of dermatology and venereology at the university and director of this hospital. He was a man with a dynamic and creative personality and fruitful postgraduate studies in Paris, Berlin, London, and Vienna.

Despite the unfavorable conditions arising from the successive liberation wars and World War I, during the second decade (1910–1922), Photinos, in collaboration with the state, succeeded in:

- Organizing a pioneer hospital, according to international standards
- Implementing regular and responsible teaching for medical students
- Establishing specialties and training of doctors in the hospital
- Founding the renowned Moulagen Museum, realizing the need for combining "visual recognition" and "visual memory" in the teaching of students
- Founding and running the Hellenic Dermatological and Venereological Society
- Making a decisive contribution to the legislative reform on the management and elimination of venereal diseases
- He also succeeded in:

  1917   Establishing a similar albeit smaller hospital in Thessaloniki [60 beds]

1915–1920   Founding special antive-
            nereal disease centers:
            three such centers for sea-
            men and six medical la-
            boratories for venereal
            diseases
1929   Establishing an anti-Han-
            sen's disease center
1932   Founding the Faculty of
            Venereal and Skin Dis-
            eases at the University of
            Thessaloniki and incor-
            porating it in the afore-
            said hospital.

A few years later, dermatology was neglected. Generally speaking, there had been an apparent stagnation in the academic development of dermatology since 1935. World War II and the occupation put an end to all progressive activities and scientific endeavors for long after the end of the war. Inertia in dermatovenereology continued despite the sporadic appearance of noteworthy scientists during this period.

The new era started during the seventies and, in the eighties, a new dynamic effort in dermatology had already been consolidated. The outpatient clinics of A. Sygros Hospital University Clinic carried the burden of work. Table 33.1 shows the progressive increase in the number of patient visits from 1931 to 1990. In 1992, there were 600 dermatologists throughout the country (total population of Greece is approximately 10 million).

In addition to the older university hospitals (A. Sygros Hospital in Athens and another in Thessaloniki), four well-organized dermatological departments are already operating in four new universities.

A good collaboration is already under way between the dermatological centers of Greece with respective centers abroad in the field of medical education as well as in the field of research work.

Finally, we would like to point out that, in general terms, the scientific activities in the field of dermatology–venereology is far more developed than in 1910, 1950, or part of 1970.[1]

Diseases of Major Significance and Major Effect During the First Half of the 20th Century

Syphilis

Syphilis, and gonorrhea to a lesser degree, were the most significant disease at the beginning of the century. The effects of the disease were important, not only because of the effective treatment but also mainly because of the lack of prevention.

Syphilis is an extremely severe disease with multiple medical, social, and economic consequences. Apart from that, people lived for decades with the notion that it was an incurable disease with terrible hereditary distribution.

At the beginning of the century, the annual number of deaths of adults and newborns due to syphilis was approximately 20,000. Due to health measures taken during 1915–1920, the epidemic of the disease was significantly limited during the thirties and forties and was decreased to a minimum during the fifties with the use of penicillin.[2]

A. Sygros Hospital–University Clinic (Control Centre of STDs) provided the following data which are indicative for the course of the disease in time:

Frequency of syphilis among the examined

1910	49.2%
1911	47.7%
1912	51.2%
1983	0.83%
1984	0.81%
1990	0.69%

In conclusion, despite the minor fluctuations of epidemiological parameters, syphilis in Greece has been dramatically limited from the point of

TABLE 33.1. A Sygros Hospital comparison in the rate of increase in patient visits.

Period (duration)		Number of visits
1931–1936	(5 years)	49.383
1971–1980	(10 years)	596.158
1981–1985	(5 years)	429.277
1986–1990	(5 years)	405.137

view of frequency toward the end of the 20th century, although it had been a real plague during the first decade of the century.

Leprosy

Leprosy was frequent in Greece during the 19th and at the beginning of the 20th century. Apart from the fact that the disease was endemic in certain parts of the country, it appears that, up to a certain degree, it was a disease imported from the countries of the Middle East due to transit trade.

In Greece, the disease appeared at the beginning of the 4th century B.C., when the troops of Alexander the Great returned from India. It was then called "leontiases" or "satiriasis," afterwards "elephantiasis," and finally "leprosis" by Hippocrates (460–377 B.C.).

It is obvious that, at the beginning of the 20th century, it was a medical and social problem. The total number of lepers amounted to 1000.

In 1902, at the island of Crete, where the disease was endemic, the number of lepers amounted to 600.[3] The list of dates when antileprosy stations and hospitals were established and abolished reflects the course of epidemiological parameters of the disease during the 20th century and is presented in Table 33.2.

The above mentioned Anti-Leprosy Station of Athens operates only partially, as an institute where old patients with leprosy stay or where new cases are admitted.

TABLE 33.2. Antileprosy stations in Greece.

Center station	Year of establishment	Year of abolishment
Leper hospital of Crete, island of Spinalonga	1903	1957
Leper hospital of the island of Chios	1973	1960
Leper hospital of the island of Samos	1895	1970
Leper hospital of Iviron Monastery Agio Oros	Established at Byzantium era but has ceased to operate for years	
Antileprosy station of Athens	1929	—
Antileprosy station of Thessaloniki	1920s	

In Greece, the disease is controlled. The very few new cases which may arise annually—no more than 10—are registered and are stateprotected.[3]

Diseases of Major Significance of Endemic Nature

These diseases are divided in two groups. The first group includes skin diseases that preexisted in the country but their study was neglected during the first half of the century, although they were stressed during the recent decades and their identity and significance was established.

These diseases include the following:

(a) Cutaneous leishmaniasis
(b) Classical Kaposi's sarcoma
(c) Meleda disease

Cutaneous leishmaniasis is an endemic skin disease that can be found in certain parts of Greece under several synonyms. From 1950 on, interest was focused on issues of clinical manifestations, morphology, and initially histological classification. Finally, during the recent decades, wide epidemiological, clinical, and therapeutic reevaluation of the matter was initiated in collaboration with similar international centers.[4]

Classical Kaposi's sarcoma (Mediterranean type—KS) is quite common in Greece and has a characteristic (peculiar) geographical distribution. There is high concentration of KS patients in the peninsula of Peloponnisus, southern Greece.

The disease was present for a long time in Greece; however, there are no data that prove that its presence was identified and its neoplasmic nature had been evaluated. Very few moulages in the museum of 1666 moulages and very few simple descriptions have been found. This was due either to the fact that endemic areas could not easily communicate by way of transport means with A. Sygros Hospital or to the fact that it was considered as a localized disease of slow development, namely, of little significance. Thus, from 1936, when the first data were registered, to 1975 only 40 cases were announced. Since 1976, a significant follow-up of these patients began and the total number has exceeded 250 cases. It is now understood that it is a systematic angiopathy with distribution to other organs and particularly to the intestines, such as the gastroenteric duct, the liver, the bones, and so on. Moreover, the simultaneous presence of other diseases of a neoplasmatic nature is being examined, such as lymphomas and paraproteinaemias. This study was stressed after the appearance of AIDS-Kaposi. The etiopathogenesis of KS is still unknown.

Classical KS, although not a new disease in Greece, has recently been identified and constitutes a classical sample of endemic disease.[6]

Mal de Meleda is a rare inherited disease. The disease affects mainly members of isolated population groups and influences socially and economically the affected individuals.

Until now, the disease was rare in Greece, as in the rest of the world, and its incidence was estimated to be four new cases in every 1 million people. The few reported cases were on the island of Naxos and Evia.[7,8]

Due to the massive migration of the Greek-origin population from north Ipirus, now part of Albania since 1940, toward Greece, the incidence of this palmoplantar keratosis has increased due to new cases that were found among these immigrants.

The existence in Albania of population groups that seem to be isolated due to nationalistic or religious reasons explains the presence of these cases because these isolated genetic groups are reproduced by marriage between relatives.

The gene prevalence of Mal de Meleda is not obligatorily higher in these isolated groups of people but, due to "endogamy," which is mainly observed among them, the genes of the disease, which are recessively inherited, now have more opportunities to coexist as homozygotes and so there is a higher chance for the clinical appearance of the disease.

The second group includes two types of dermatomycosis due to the impressive change in epidemiological parameters during the 20th century.

Dermatomycoses had extremely high distribution during the first half of the 20th century and up to 1960. The problem of hair growth seemed unsurpassable at the beginning of the 1950s. It was estimated that 400,000 children suffered from tinea capitis, out of a total population of 9 million. This was mainly due to the agricultural nature of the population, improper diet, and lack of hygiene; to a certain degree, it was the result of the wars that had just ended. During the 1980s cases of tinea capitis were rare, whereas cases of tinea corporis are more frequent.

On the contrary, during the second half of the century, there was a significant increase in the distribution of candidiasis. Perhaps this is due to the fact that greater attention was paid to simple zymomycoses of the past or to the increases of diabetes mellitus and to diseases of intense immunosuppression or, finally, to the increased use of antimicrobial and immunosuppressive medications.

New Diseases of Major Significance

The new diseases are:

1. Acquired immunodeficiency syndrome— AIDS
2. Lyme borreliosis

Acquired immunodeficiency syndrome is a new disease for all countries. In Greece, the first case was diagnosed in 1983 (A. Sygros Hospital University Clinic). By September 1992, the total number of patients reached to 145.

This disease is classified, to a certain degree in the field of dermatovenereology for two reasons. The first reason is that it is sexually transmitted and the fact that, consequently, its epidemiological behavior is connected to and harmonized with the behavior of sexually transmitted diseases (STDs). The other reason is that there is an extremely large variety of skin manifestations accompanying its presence, mainly manifestations of Kaposi's sarcoma.[9]

The epidemiological behavior and natural course of Lyme borreliosis does not differ from those already described internationally. The first case was reported in Greece in 1991.

However, there is a comment and a question. Approximately 20 years ago and continuously after that time, scleroderma and morphen were treated by high doses of penicillin for 4 weeks in conjunction with very low doses of cortisone.[10] The results were rather good. Was it or was it not Borreliosis?

Psoriasis and Skin Lymphomata

Psoriasis was much less in the forties, during World War II and one or two decades later (1938: 2.5%; 1941: 1.15%; 1953: 2.89%; 1960: 3.40%)[11]. It cannot be maintained that this was due only to the fact that skin diseases were then treated with indifference, whereas today attention is paid due to improvement of cultural and economic levels. Hypoprotein diet was then discussed, which was compulsory for that time and which is compatible with the special hypoprotein Grutz diet.

Just as with the undoubtedly higher frequency of skin lymphomata, it is possible that this increased distribution is due to better diagnosis conditions or to an inexplicable real increase.

References

1. Stratigos J: Dermatology and venereology in Greece. Yesterday and today. *Int J Dermatol* 1988;**27**:723–729.
2. Photinos G: The anti-venereal disease struggle in Greece. Dean's speech of March 14, 1938. Archives of "A. Sygros" Hospital, 1938.
3. Kontochristopoulos G: Immunochemical study in leprosy. Thesis. University of Athens, 1992.
4. Stratigos J, Tosca A, Nicolis G, Papavassiliou S: Epidemiology of cutaneous leishmaniasis in Greece. *Int J Dermatol* 1980;**19**:86–88.
5. Kaloterakis A: Kaposi's sarcoma in Greece. Epidemiology, clinical laboratory investigation and treatment. Thesis. University of Athens, 1984.
6. Rappersberg K, Tschachler E, Zonzits E, et al: Endemic Kaposi's sarcoma in human. *J Invest Dermatol* 1990;**95**:371–381.
7. Zaganiaris A, Demertzis D, Venios E: Meleda disease. Archives of "A. Sygros" Hospital, 1937: 405.
8. Fotinos P, Kanitakis C: 3 cases of mal de Meleda. Archives of "A. Sygros" Hospital, 1955:529.
9. Stratigos J: 2nd Greek Congress in AIDS disease, Athens, 1991.
10. Seretis I, Pateraki E, Stratigos A, Kilafis G: Lyme disease (stage II). The first diagnosed case in Greece. *Hellenic Dermato-Venereol Rev* 1990;**1**: 39–43.
11. Stratigos J: Study on metabolic disorders of psoriasis. Thesis. University of Athens, 1962.

34

Malta

Joseph L. Pace

The Maltese Islands lie in the center of the Mediterranean Sea some 60 miles from Sicily and 180 miles from North Africa. The population is around 360,000, almost uniformly of southern European extraction. The climate is mild with most people leading an "outdoor" life as much as possible between June and September. The major industry is tourism, and the population increases dramatically in the summer months, straining severely the islands' infrastructure. Winter tourism is also popular. Malta has established itself as a center for teaching English, and large numbers of students of all ages attend the numerous language schools. In addition, large numbers of Maltese regularly return home on long visits from their adopted countries of Australia, Canada, and the United States.

Other than tourism, Malta has a fishing industry, some agriculture, and a large deep-water harbor.

Medical Facilities

Malta has a long proud tradition of first-class medicine. The medical school is over 300 years old, and Maltese physicians occupy positions of eminence all over the world. Malta's current medical system comprises a mix of state and private medicine with easy access to both facilities. Private fees are low, well within reach of the average income. All medicines are available and these are supplied free of charge to low-income earners and those suffering from certain chronic diseases such as diabetes and, very recently, from psoriasis.

Dermatology

Until relatively recently, dermatology was a "cinderella" with one dermatologist looking after the island's needs. Today, however, the small university department of dermatology is a highly sought after post for residents with the number of requests for trainee posts far outnumbering what can be offered. Two consultants, three residents, and two interns manage to see over 15,000 patients annually. As in European countries, a dermatologist's responsibilities encompass also venereology (and AIDS with all its problems), and leprology.

Clinical Dermatology

In Malta, one meets the conditions encountered in any dermatological department in Western Europe with certain differences related to:

1. Climate and life-style
2. Population movements resulting from tourism, returning emigrants, and, lately, immigrant workers.

In addition, the relatively low average income in spite of an acceptable standard of living has to be kept in mind when prescribing more expensive medication.

The following are of interest:

1. Cutaneous leishmaniasis
2. Leprosy
3. HIV-associated disease
4. Acne
5. Skin cancer
6. Drug eruptions—sun and nonsun-related
7. Herpes zoster
8. Trepohematoses

Cutaneous Leishmaniasis

The Mediterranean region is endemic for the leishmaniases, but cutaneous infection was not recorded in the Maltese Islands until very recently, although visceral infection has been around since time immemorial. In 1980 the first case of cutaneous leishmaniasis (CL) was reported from the small village of Qala on the island of Gozo, a 15-minute ferry ride from Malta. Since that time, about 65 cases have occurred with the very great majority originating from Gozo. Cutaneous leishmaniasis is infinitely more prevalent on Gozo, but the opposite is true of visceral leishmaniasis (VL). Furthermore, the causative organism seems to be *L. donovani infantum* rather than *L. tropica*. According to a recent study,[1] it is likely that the animal host is the dog rather than rodents, which have not been found to be infected locally. To the contrary, at least 70% of the dogs tested positive (ELISA). The reason for the occurrence of a new focus of CL on Gozo is, as yet, unexplained. An awareness campaign for local doctors, dog owners, and others is under way and it is hoped to make testing of dogs compulsory in the immediate future. The lesions respond well to cryotherapy, but systemic treatment with rifampicin/INH[2] has been needed on some occasions. Ketoconazole was not effective in the single patient for whom it was prescribed (see Fig. 34.1).

Leprosy

Leprosy has been endemic in the Mediterranean littoral for centuries and persists as small endemic foci that are difficult to eradicate. Malta has proved to be no exception.

A decrease in new cases occurred in the pre-dapsone era and paralleled improved socioeconomic conditions. A further decrease

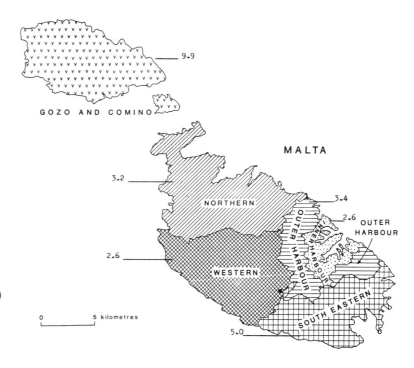

FIGURE 34.1. Reported average incidence (per 10^{-5}) of leishmaniasis for Malta and Gozo (1984–1989) by region.

followed the introduction of dapsone mono-therapy in 1948. In 1972, the Leprosy Eradication Programme was initiated with the support of the Sovereign Military Order of Malta and the German Leprosy Relief Association. The program was under the direction of the Borstel Research Institute of the Federal Republic of Germany. In the first ever large-scale application of multidrug therapy (MDT) in leprosy, 201 patients were treated with a combination of four antileprosy drugs. The results were excellent, and although regular clinical and bacteriological follow-up are still carried out, no relapse has been reported to date.[3] According to Noordeen,[4] "MDT has been the most important development in the field of leprosy control," and the WHO recommendation on MDT represents "a landmark in the history of leprosy."

New cases have become a rarity and the problem has largely disappeared from public attention. Only three new cases have been reported in the past 3 years. Newly reported cases over the past 15 years have been middle aged or elderly with lepromatous or borderline lepromatous leprosy. No new case with tuberculoid leprosy has occurred since 1975. Epidemiologically, this is in keeping with a reduction in disease transmission. The main problem is now to deal with residual disabilities requiring continued care. The leprosy clinic is now part of the dermatology service to further reduce any stigma, and medical education at both undergraduate and postgraduate levels is directed at maintaining awareness of the disease to enable early recognition of any new cases that might occur. To this end, medical students are encouraged to spend a period of time in countries where the disease is still highly prevalent.

HIV Infection

Because of the "STD" connotation, the dermatology department has been given the responsibility of "managing" the HIV problem for the past years. Initially at least, cases were confined to the hemophiliacs, 100% being affected[38] from a single batch of imported blood from the United States in 1983. To date, many have died,

but much experience has been gained in the overall management of these complicated problems. We recognize that our main problem is the possibly imported HIV infection both from the tourists coming to Malta in ever-increasing numbers and also from Maltese returning home from countries with life-styles far different to what is found here. With Malta being an all-year holiday resort, sexual adventures are far from difficult and particular care has been taken in this respect to direct HIV information programs to young people and tourism workers, groups perceived to be at particular risk. Far more serious is the possibility of HIV being disseminated among intravenous drug users (IVDUs) because drugs are a problem locally and Malta is surrounded by countries with considerable drug problems, particularly Italy where IVDUs surpass sexual transmission of HIV. Sterile needles and syringes are freely available, but the fight against organized crime with all its resources must be stepped up if a widespread HIV problem is to be avoided. (See Figs 34.2 and 34.3). Visceral leishmaniasis has occurred as a concomitant infection in AIDS patients, in line with the experience reported from Spain and other Mediterranean countries.

Acne

Acne is an important cosmetic problem in Maltese adolescents, and numerous patients with late-onset acne are also seen. If topical therapy proves unsuccessful, patients need (and demand) systemic treatment.

In the 1970s, tetracycline was the first-line drug with clindamycin a second-line treatment for "tetracycline-resistant cases;" however, clindamycin was abandoned following warnings of associated pseudomembranous colitis.[5] Erythromycin and co-trimoxazole proved little better than tetracycline with considerable side effects (nausea with erythromycin and dermatitis with co-trimoxazole). We were unhappy to use long-term hormonal therapy especially with the high estrogen content of the cyproterone "combination" available at that time.

Because all other medication was proving

FIGURE 34.2. Projected AIDS
cases. WHO model applied
to Malta—cumulative
incidence.

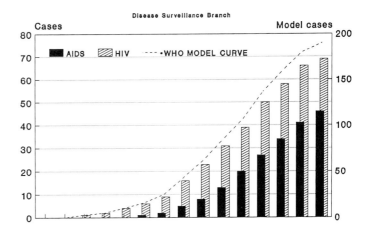

unsatisfactory, clindamycin was reintroduced initially only for patients with severe acne who had not improved with 1 gm tetracycline daily for 6 months. Great care was exercised in view of the dire warnings appearing in the literature.[6] Patients were repeatedly warned about possible bowel problems, and we went to the extreme of giving anyone going on holiday while on clindamycin a supply of vancomycin for emergency use. Patients were delighted with the improvement in their acne . . . and nobody used vancomycin. Gradually, confidence in clindamycin increased, although the literature did not make for comfortable reading and it is doubtful whether this treatment would get through a 1991 medical ethics committee.

The advent of minocycline suggested that perhaps we would now stop playing as gastroenterologists, because surely no more clindamycin would need to be prescribed. Unfortunately, although minocycline is probably almost as effective as clindamycin in severe acne, the numerous side effects that have occurred in our patients have made us rule out this drug except when clindamycin is contraindicated. Young females especially have suffered from headaches and dizziness severe enough to warrant discontinuation of therapy.[7] Benign intracranial hypertension[8] and severe pigmentation both on the skin and also internally[9] have been reported.

Clindamycin has therefore been retained as

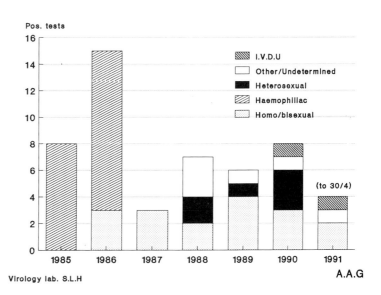

FIGURE 34.3. Known HIV
seropositive patients.

the oral antibiotic of choice in acne. Initially used in severe cases only, experience with thousands of patients has resulted in its being used (albeit in smaller doses of 75 mg daily) as an alternative to tetracycline. The advent of Isoretinonin has enabled us to define more clearly the place of clindamycin in acne management. Because of the teratogenic potential and the extremely high cost (around $1000 for a 16-week course of treatment—equivalent to 6 weeks' wages for a shop assistant), Accutane is a last resort therapy and clindamycin is routinely employed in doses of 150–225 mg daily before Accutane is prescribed. Many of these patients manage to do without Accutane.

Finally, a recent study[10] confirmed both the efficacy and safety of clindamycin when used in small doses in a healthy age group. This point has been made previously[11] but needs re-emphasis: side effects described in patients with multisystem diseases and on numerous types of medication do not necessarily apply when a different (lower) dosage is used in an otherwise healthy population.

Skin Cancer

Malta has not been spared the current worldwide increase in skin cancers. From preliminary survey results, it appears that the Maltese are getting nonmelanoma skin cancers more frequently than their counterparts in Northern Italy, France, or Germany. The darker skins of the Maltese are, therefore, only protective up to a point and a "sun care campaign" is more than warranted, given the outdoor life-style so beloved of the Maltese. In addition, it appears, (but the figures are too small to be sure) that melanomas are on the increase. The dermatology department has managed to persuade the authorities that sun blocks of SPF 15 or higher are to be rated as medicinals rather than as cosmetics with the price expected to drop by almost 70%. This has given a tremendous boost to our campaign with the public realizing that the medical profession is actually doing something very positive on their behalf. The widespread use of Retin

A among women has also boosted the sensible use of sun blocks.

Drug Eruptions

These occur as frequently as elsewhere and are related to prescribing habits and the sunny climate. Fixed eruptions have become infrequent since Malta followed other countries in banning the pyrazolone group of analgesic/antispasmodic agents. These were the commonest causative agents in a study carried out in Saudi Arabia.[12] In addition, first reports of vasculitis following loxacin[13] and mefloquin[14] have emanated from Malta. Photosensitive eruptions are, as elsewhere, common with thiazides, NSAIDs, sulfa drugs, and tetracyclines. Of particular interest is the occurrence of explosive pemphigus erythematosus in a patient inadvertently treated with liquid nitrogen for a facial lesion while on captopril,[15] and of previously undescribed pigmented lesions on exposed areas in a patient on etretinate for ichthyosis.

Herpes Zoster

Although Maltese physicians were among the first to remark on the apparent value of acyclovir in severe varicella-zoster infections (Symposium on Acyclovir, Malta, 1984), the prohibitive cost of the drug in the recommended dose makes it a nonstarter for all but the very wealthy. Fortunately, the medication is available free of charge for hospitalized patients. For the rest, because concomitant treatment with probenecid is known to increase serum levels of acyclovir,[16] we have quite empirically been using half the recommended dose of acyclovir (i.e. 400 mg five times daily) together with 1 g of probenecid daily, and to date have been impressed with the apparent lower morbidity in these patients compared with the pre-acyclovir era. Scientific studies are needed to establish whether this regime can be improved on and whether it is scientifically acceptable. Meanwhile, patients are getting better at half the cost.

Treponematoses

With Malta's position between Europe and Africa as the crossroads of the Mediterranean, the possibility of a nonvenereal treponemal infection as a cause of a reaction specific test for syphilis must be kept in mind in patients of Arab or African origin. A misdiagnosis of a sexually transmitted disease might be socially catastrophic in this situation.[17] Furthermore, a single injection of long-acting penicillin might prevent serious involvement of bone or skin later.

References

1. Tsankor, NK: Kamarasher, JA: Rofampin in dermatology. *Int J Dermatol* 1993;**32**:401–406.
2. Pace JL: Rifampicin in cutaneous leishmaniasis. *Arch Dermatol* 1982;**118**:880.
3. Freerksen E, Depasquale G: In: Freerksen E, ed. The Malta Project—A Leprosy Eradication Programme. German Leprosy Relief Association, 1987.
4. Noordeen SK: Recent status of leprosy in the world, and WHO's approach to the problem. International Seminar on Leprosy, Istanbul, September 1991.
5. Cohen LE, McNeill CJ, Wells RF: Clindamycin associated colitis. *JAMA* 1973;**223**:1379–1380.
6. Gurwith MJ, Rabin HR, Love K: Diarrhea associated with clindamycin and ampicillin. *J Infect Dis* 1977;**135** (suppl):104–110.
7. Claussen CF, Schneider D, Claussen E: Equilibriometric measurements of central vestibular dysregulation following administration minocycline. *Artzneimittelforschung* 1987;**37**:950–953.
8. Lubvetski C: Hypertension intracranienne bengin et minocycline. *Rev Neurol (Paris)* 1988;**144**:218.
9. Wolfe, ID, Reichmister J, Minocycline hyperpigmentation skin: tooth, nail and bone involvement. Curtis 1984;**33**:457–458.
10. Sammut A: Systemtic treatment of acne with special reference to clindamycin. Thesis. University of Malta, 1990:43–69.
11. Ad Hoc Committee on the Use of Antibiotics in Dermatology: Systemic antibiotics for treatment of acne vulgaris—efficacy and safety. *Arch Dermatol* 1975;**111**:1630–1636.
12. Pace JL: Fixed drug eruptions in Saudi Arabia. *Saudi Med J* 1984;**5**:315–318.
13. Pace JL, Gatt P: Fatal vasculitis with ofloxacin. *BMJ* 1989;**299**:658.
14. Scerri L, Pace JL: Mefloquin associated cutaneous vasculitis. *Int J Dermatol* 1993; **32**: 517–518.
15. Pace JL, Calnan C, Soler D: In: Panconesi E, ed. Captopril induced pemphigus erythematosus in Dermatology in Europe. Oxford: Blackwell Scientific Publications, 1991:946–948.
16. Zovirax: in 1994 Physicians Desk Reference. Montvale, NJ. Medical Economics Data Production 1994:765–772.
17. Pace JL, Csonka GW: Endemic non-venereal syphilis in Arabia. *Br J Venereol Dis* 1984;**60**: 293–297.

35

Poland

Stefania Jablonska

Dermatology in Poland is very similar to that of other European countries but has some peculiarities of middle Europe. In the past, there was an endemic area of rhinoscleroma, specifically in Galicia. Presently, there are sporadic cases of sarcomatosis, Kaposi sarcoma of the Mediterranean type, and acrodermatisis atrophicans, sometimes with sclerodermatous indurations.

History

Dermatology became a separate specialty in 1863 with the creation of the first chair for dermatology in Cracow, the former capital of Poland and one of the most important cities of Galicia.[1,2] Hospitals for skin and venereal diseases existed since the end of the 15th century, the time of the epidemics of syphilis in Poland. This epidemic started in Cracow. In the old annals, there is a description of the first case brought to this country by a pious woman who went on a pilgrimage to Rome and came back with the allegedly new disease which started to devastate the country, especially the upper classes of the society, and, therefore, regarded as a courtly disease.

It is of interest that in Cracow, in the famous Gothic altar of Vit Stoss in St. Mary Church, built before the discovery of America, the crucified robbers were found to have saddle noses typical of congenital syphilis.[3,4] The Cracow researchers F. Walter and K. Lejman claimed that this favored the existence of syphilis in Europe before the return of Columbus. In Cracow, the venereal diseases were treated in the St. Roch Hospital opened in 1528, and in Warsaw in St. Lazarus Hospital created in 1591. Since 1756, St. Lazarus Hospital was used exclusively for the management of venereal diseases, mainly in the treatment of prostitutes.[2]

The Warsaw University Department of Dermatology, created in 1866, became, in 1869, a part of the Russian University at Warsaw which had been boycotted by the Polish population. Since that time, St. Lazarus Hospital gained much authority as a counterpart of the Russian University dermatology department. It should be stressed that in the period 1898–1916 the head of the Warsaw Department was an eminent Russian dermatologist, Nikolski.

The Department of Dermatology of the Warsaw University was created after World War I in 1920 by Fr. Knysztatowioz and Marian Gnybowski.

The other important center of Polish dermatology was Lwów (Lemberg), a Polish city surrounded by Ukranian villages. The Medical Faculty was created in 1784 after the city became a part of the Austrio-Hungarian monarchy, but the dermatology chair was organized first in 1898. Due to the close connections with the eminent School of Dermatology in Vienna, Lwów developed into the leading center of the Polish medical sciences. Both of these schools, Vienna and Lwów, contributed greatly to the study on rhinoscleroma.

Rhinoscleroma

Rhinoscleroma, an endemic disease in the 19th century in Galicia, is almost extinct. As a new entity it was first recognized in 1870 by Hebra (Vienna), who believed it to be a special form of neoplasia in the spectrum of sarcoma. The exact clinical description was given by Kaposi (1870) who stressed the presence of abundant round cell infiltrates and connective tissue proliferation, nonconsistent with malignancy. The detailed pathologic study by Mikulicz (1876) disclosed, besides inflammatory infiltrates surrounding the blood vessels, large vesicular, multinucleated cells, which were referred to as Mikulicz cells. He also stressed the significance of fibrosis believed to be a hallmark of the disease. Some years later, Frisch (1882) detected in the Mikulicz cells the presence of specific microorganisms similar to Friedlanders bacilli. Also characteristic of the disease are round Roussel's hyaline bodies, more abundant in older lesions besides pronounced fibrosis. Roussel bodies appear to be a product of degeneration.[5,6]

Rhinoscleroma was endemic in Galicia, but several cases were reported also from the eastern Polish cities outside Galicia—Lublin, Chelm, and Grodno. The clinical features were very characteristic: wooden hard submucosal sclerosis of the nosopharynx and nasal skin in otherwise healthy young people, without any visceral involvement. There was no special risk of infection from the surroundings, favoring genetic background and individual predisposition to the disease.

The greatest series of rhinoscleroma cases was collected by Zalewski of the Laryngology Department of Lwów University—457 cases seen in the period of 10 years. The disease was rare even in this endemic area, only about 1.5% of all hospitalized cases in Lwów were rhinoscleroma.[6] The course of the disease was variable but usually slowly progressive or stationary. The sclerotizing process was, in general, progressive, involving the nasal mucosa and the skin, reducing the nasal and the mouth orifices. In the past, there was no effective treatment. Surgery was the only mode of therapy that produced relief. After antibiotics (penicillin, streptomycin) were introduced, rhinoscleroma disappeared. We have now a few abortive cases that in the past had no sufficient therapy with antibiotics, or were not treated at all. In spite of the disappearance of rhinoscleroma, it is still possible that Frisch bacilli, in the future, will gain resistance to the antibiotics used presently in therapy. Thus, a revival of this unexplained endemic disease is a possibility, although a remote one.

Kaposi's Sarcoma

Another peculiarity of Polish dermatology is an eastern European variant of Kaposi's sarcoma. This disease also has an endemic character, occurring almost exclusively in Eastern Europe but is of the same type as in the Mediterranean area, especially in Sicily.[7] Affected almost exclusively are old people, vascular infiltrates and tumors are limited to the distal parts of the extremities, visceral involvement is rare, and general health usually unaffected.[7,8] Although the pathologic picture is very similar or identical to Kaposi's sarcoma associated with HIV infection, the course is entirely different.

The tumors are well demarcated, usually large and flat, sometimes coalescent, whereas the hemorrhagic lesions of sarcoma Kaposi associated with HIV are mostly small and disseminated. However in some traumatized areas, especially in the mouth, tumors can be proliferative and indistinguishable from the Kaposi not related to HIV. (See Fig. 35.1).

Another cutaneous variety of Kaposi's sarcoma is the African variant, with large tumors all over the body and, not infrequently, visceral involvement. In contrast to the East European variety, the course is severe and the outcome very often unfavorable. Very rare in Poland are cases of Kaposi sarcoma having characteristics of this disease in Africa, with more extensive cutaneous involvement, large ulcerating tumors, enlarged lymph glands, and occasionally visceral changes. The course of these cases is severe, often with a fatal outcome.

We have seen three cases of European Kaposi's sarcoma coexistent with lymphatic

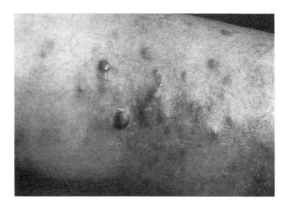

FIGURE 35.1. Kaposi's sarcoma on the leg. Numerous small violaceus tumors, with no tendency to ulceration and deeper penetration.

leukemia that might be due to infection with another HTLV (human T lymphotropic virus). In these cases, the prognosis depends on the generalization of the process.

Acrodermatitis Atrophicans

Another rare disease occurring in Poland and in other middle and northern European countries is acrodermatitis chronica atrophicans found to be associated with borreliosis.[9] In center Poland, as elsewhere, borreliosis is associated mainly with lymphodenosis cutis benigna and erythema chronicum migrans. The latter is still not an infrequent disease, especially in some forested areas of Poland.

Acrodermatitis chronica atrophicans was a common disease in prewar Poland, and until the 1950s when, owing to the widespread use of antibiotics, it disappeared almost entirely. Sporadic cases are seen in the last years in all regions of the country.[10] Characteristic of the disease are flat violaceous infiltrates on the distal parts of the extremities, spreading proximally in the lower limbs not beyond the groins and buttocks (Figs. 35.2 and 35.3), and in the upper extremities not beyond the elbows. The infiltrates are gradually replaced by atrophic wrinkled, cigarette-paper-like skin with veins shining through the atrophies. In later stages, at the elbows may develop fibrous nodules or fibrotic bands extending along the ulna from

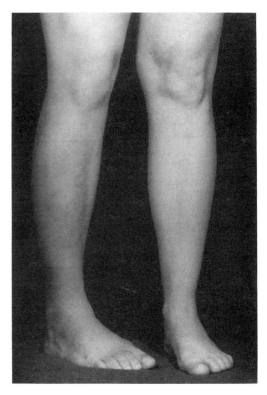

FIGURE 35.2. Acrodermatitis chronica atrophicans. Reddish-violaceus, not well-demarcated, plaque extending from the dorsum of the foot beyond the knee. The skin of the leg is thinned and the whole leg shows atrophy.

the elbow to the wrist (so-called ulnar streaks). On the lower extremities, within the atrophies may develop indurations closely resembling morphea (Figs. 35.4 and 35.5), regarded by some authors as the coexistence of morphea and acrodermatitis atrophicans, and by others as pseudoscleroderma.[10] Gottron[11,12] collected 54 cases of this type and believed them to be a coexistence of acrodermatitis and morphea. We have observed 26 cases, all in the lower extremities. Indurations developed within the foci of atrophies, usually symmetrically on both limbs, or only on one leg.

The violaceous surroundings of the sclerodermatous lesions were suggestive of the extensive lilac ring of morphea. We also had cases of the coexistence of morphea en plaques on the trunk or elsewhere, and acrodermatitis atrophicans on the legs, with characteristic histological features in both.

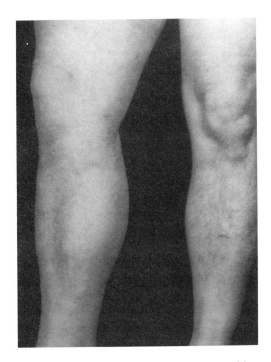

FIGURE 35.3. Acrodermatitis chronica atrophicans. Violaceous, slightly unfiltered lesions involving the leg and a part of the thigh, well demarcated on the thigh. Beginning whitish discoloration on the leg.

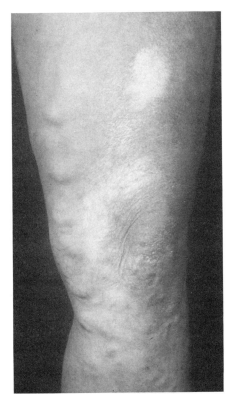

FIGURE 35.4. Acrodermatitis chronica atrophicans sclerodermiformis. Sclerodermalike indurations within violaceus atrophic lesion on the lower extremity, with protruding tortuous veins.

Penicillin therapy is as effective for sclerodermatous indurations within the atrophies of acrodermatitis atrophicans as for other forms of borreliosis.

We have observed a patient living in the forested area of northern Poland who developed simultaneously lesions of erythema migrans on the forearm, acrodermatitis atrophicans on the legs, and morphea with pronounced inflammatory reaction on the back. All lesions had characteristic histological pattern. After intensive penicillin therapy, there was a complete regression of inflammatory plaques within several weeks, and of indurations of morphea type within several months. The high titers of anti-*Borrelia burgdorferi* antibodies dropped, after regression of the lesions, to the normal level. The causal relationship of morphea with borreliosis is of special interest but the reports from various parts of the world are controversial. Some authors, mainly Austrian—based on serology and presence of spirochetes in the tissue—believe *B. burgdorferi* to be

a causative agent in localized scleroderma in general.[13,14] Swedish and Danish authors did not find any increased number of positive serology in scleroderma patients as compared to the controls in the same areas.[15,17] These discrepancies might be due to the geographical distribution of *B. burgdorferi*, and possibly also to various borrelia strains in different parts of the world. Another contributing factor might be nonstandardized ELISA and immunofluorescence tests for borrelia, and the different strains of *B. burgdorferi* used as an antigen.

In Poland, we have strong support for the association of some morphea cases with *B. burgdorferi*. Due to a wide use of antibiotics, cutaneous borreliosis—previously an endemic disease—became rarer. Specifically, sclerodermiform acrodermatitis atrophicans is seen only sporadically, but in recent years more often than in the 1960s and 1970s, and this might be due to

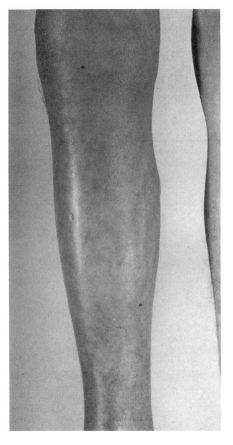

FIGURE 35.5. Sclerodermalike indurations on the leg developed in acrodermatitis chronica atrophicans. This lesion is indistinguishable from linear scleroderma.

a slowly developing resistance to antibiotics. It could be presumed that in the United States there are also cases of acrodermatitis atrophicans that remain unrecognized.

The Effect of Hunger on Skin Diseases—the Experience of the Nazi Occupation of Poland and the War Period (1939–1945)

We have some medical observations on the skin diseases in people put into concentration camps and ghettos, living in extremely poor conditions,

on hunger diets. Unexpectedly, in the starving people psoriasis regressed spontaneously, and even erythrodermic changes cleared completely. The role of nutrition was best evidenced in people who were moved from the camps to slave labor in private German farms, where the food was abundant but the nervous tension usually persisted. In those conditions, psoriasis tended to relapse. It is conceivable that in emaciated persons the diminished production of proteins is not sufficient to sustain psoriatic lesions. This aspect of psoriasis is not well known and merits investigation.

References

1. Jablonska S: In: Burg G, ed. Dermatologie in Polen und Osteuropa in Dermatologie. München Wien, Urban-Schwarzenberger, 1988: 117–138.
2. Stapiński A: Fight Against Syphilis and Gonorrhoea in Poland. Warsaw: Polish Medical Publishers, 1979.
3. Walter F: Vit Stoos, Sculpture of Skin Diseases. Cracow, Art Society, 1933.
4. Lejman K: Dermatologie und Kunst. *Hautarzt* 1964;**15**:89–91.
5. Jakowski M, Matlakowski W: O twardzieli nosa (Rhinoslceroma Hebrae). *Gazeta Lekarska* 1987; **7**:994–998.
6. Pieniążek S: Das Rhinosklerom. In: Heymann P, ed. Handbuch der Laryngologie und Rhinologie, Vol. 3. Die Nase. Wien: A. Hölder/publ./ 1990:965–984.
7. Kalamkarian AA: Kliniczeskije aspekty sarcoma Kaposi. *Westn Wenerol* 1978;**1**:3–8.
8. Zabel J, Karaś Z: Sarcom Kaposi. *Przegl Dermatol* 1984;**71**:141–144.
9. Asbrink E, Hovmark A, Hederstedt B: The spirochetal etiology of acrodermatitis chronica atrophicans Herxheimer. *Acta Dermato-Venereol (Stockh)* 1984;**64**:506–512.
10. Jablonska S: Acrodermatitis atrophicans and its sclerodermiform variety: related to scleroderma. In: Jablonska S, ed. Warsaw: Scleroderma and Pseudoscleroderma. Polish Medical Publishers, 1975:58–593.
11. Gottron HA: Glichzeitiges Vorhandensein von Acrodermatitis chronica atrophicans and circumscripter Sklerodermie. *Zbl Haut Gschlkr* 1938; **57**:7.

12. Gottron HA: Gleichzeitiges Vorhandensein von Acrodermatitis und circumscripter Sklerodermie. *Zbl Haut Geschlkr* 1943;**70**:594.

13. Aberer E, Stanek G: Histological evidence for spirochetal origin of morphea and lichen sclerosus et strophicans. *Am J Dermatopathol* 1987;**9**:374–379.

14. Aberer E, Klade H, Stanek G, Gebhard W: Borrelia burgdorferi and different types of morphea. *Dermatologica* 1991;**182**:145–154.

15. Hoesly JM, Mertz LE, Winkelmann RK: Located scleroderma (morphea) and antibody to Borrelia burgdorferi. *J Am Acad Dermatol* 1987;**17**:455–459.

16. Asbrink E, Hovmark A: Cutaneous manifestations in Ixodes-borne Borrelia spirochetosis. *Int J Dermatol* 1987;**26**:215–223.

17. Halkier-Sørensen L, Kragballe K, Hansen K: Antibodies to the Borrelia burgdorferi flagellum in patients with scleroderma, granuloma annulare and porphyria cutanea tarda. *Acta Dermato-Venereol. (Stockh)* 1989;**69**:116–119.

Africa

Malawi

Gunnar Lomholt

Malawi—formerly Nyasaland—is a part of southeast Africa. It is a longitudinal inland country with no harbor, situated west of Lake Malawi. The central part is a highland 1100 m above sea level. The northern part is a sparsely populated mountain area. The southern part is a lowland around the Shire Valley with a warm, humid climate. The population was 8.8 million in 1990, mainly belonging to two tribes.

For several years Malawi has had a university, but only since 1991 has a medical school been attached. Seventeen medical students, who have had 2 years premedical training in the United Kingdom, started clinical training in the country.[1] Hitherto, medical training has only been given at Lilongwe School of Health Sciences. The students from this school have formed the core of medical services to the population as clinical officers with 4 years, and medical assistants with 3 years, of training.

Malawi has two central hospitals situated in Blantyre and Lilongwe. In addition, it has 21 district hospitals and a number of mission hospitals. A total of 253 Health Centers each with one medical assistant and one nurse, serve the population. There are only 120 medical doctors, mostly young expatriates, and only 30 Malawians trained abroad who are mainly involved in administration. Figures from 1989 reported one physician per 80,000 people—some hospitals are without a medical doctor. Nurses are trained at Kamuzu College of Nursing in Lilongwe. The training includes midwifery.

Malawai, as do most countries in Africa south of the Sahara, belongs to the 31 least developed countries (LDCs).[2] In 1989–90 the budget for the Ministry of Health (MOH) was 23 million dollars (U.S.) or 5.2% of the central governments total recurrent expenditures. Free medical care including prescriptions is provided by MOH.

The clinical picture is dominated by the poor socioeconomic situation. Malaria and tuberculosis are the most common diseases, together with diarrhea and malnutrition in small children. A high mortality rate for small children and maternal death in connection with delivery are important health problems. The life expectancy was 44.6 years for the years 1982–87. Recently, there has been a seriously high prevalence of HIV infection and patients with AIDS.

Dermatology

Dermatology is a new specialty in the country. A leprosy campaign was started in Blantyre by LEPRA (the British Leprosy Relief Association) in 1965, and covered the southern part of the country. In 1973, MOH took over the responsibility of leprosy for this region and LEPRA transferred its activities to the central and northern regions.

Dermatology as a specialty was first introduced in 1977 by Gooskens at the Central Hospital in Blantyre. When he left the country 3 years later, the clinic was continued with only one clinical officer trained by him. By establishing the skin clinic at Kamuzu Central Hospital in connection with Lilongwe School of Health Sciences in 1984, dermatological care was offered to the central and to part of the northern region. This clinic is still functioning with the support of the Danish Red Cross. One Scandinavian dermatologist is head of the clinic. The project has gradually expanded to cover four district hospitals and has taken over leprosy control as well.

The clinic is responsible for teaching dermatology, venereology, and leprology to medical students and student nurses. Leprosy assistants trained by LEPRA have gradually received special training in dermatology and are now involved in dermatological care as well.

The skin clinic in Lilongwe has been received by the population. The number of new patients attending the clinic in 1990 was 26,000 and, in addition, 11,000 were seen in the four district clinics.[3] The skin clinic in Blantyre has at present no permanent clinical officer and is without a dermatologist. It is uncertain if the country in the future will have even one dermatologist.

Common Skin Diseases

Because the skin clinic in Lilongwe is an open clinic without a referral system, it presumably mirrors the situation in the population. Because of the low socioeconomic situation mentioned, infestations with scabies and bacterial skin infections dominate the clinical picture. Scabies accounts for not less than 37% of the patients attending the clinic, and 28% are suffering from skin infections.[4] Most patients are small children.

A source of medicines for this group of patients is the main problem. Even when only the most simple remedies are required, the government has great difficulties in supplying benzyl benzoate for scabies and penicillin, pastes and ointments with sulfur for pyodermas. The Central Medical Store is often out of stock of these essential drugs. It is even more difficult to obtain medicine for the districts. They are often left with only gentian violet. This is one of the greatest problems for the future of dermatology in Malawi—and other developing countries.

Even when the paramedical staff is reasonably well-trained, dermatological care suffers, from lack of available therapy.

The skin clinic has worked out a simple list of drugs needed to cover the most prevalent conditions[3] Gooskens and Chalila have published a small textbook for treatment of dermatological conditions for paramedics working in Malawi.[5]

Except for scabies and pyodermas, it is not possible to give real figures about the prevalence of other skin conditions. The only clinic attracts many patients with unusual and often severe skin diseases. Figures would, however, not mirror the situation in the country even when the relative frequencies were given. The following is only an estimate based on the conditions seen. The diagnoses are in most cases made on the clinical features only because of lack of laboratory facilities. Even biopsies are of little value because the specimens have to be sent abroad for evaluation and the answer delayed for at least 6 weeks.

Miliaria and *papular urticaria*, together with *Tunga penetrans*, are some of the main reasons for secondary skin infections. *Pediculoses corporis* is quite common, but *pediculosis capitis* is nearly unknown. This contrasts to the situation in Uganda where head lice infestation is very common. The extensive use of vaseline on the scalp is presumably the reason for this difference.

Dermatophytoses in different forms are a great problem. A survey from Uganda covering 3 schools with 2,000 pupils showed a prevalence of 4–8%, and in 1 school even 40%.[4] Tinea of the skin is treated with a modified Witfield's ointment (benzoic acid compound ointment), but for the many cases of tinea capitis—mainly due to *Microsporum canis* and *Trichophyton violaceum*—griseofulvin is essential but usually out of stock (Fig. 36.1).

Eczemas are high on the list, commonly affecting the lower aspects of the legs in the form of the nummular or acneiform type (sycosis cruris) caused by the extensive use of vaseline. Heavily infected dermatitis in children is, however, the most impressive (Fig. 36.2).

Among the eczemas, it is worth mentioning a not uncommon special condition not previously

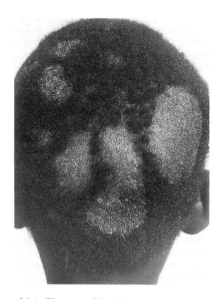

FIGURE 36.1. Tinea capitis, Microsporum canis.

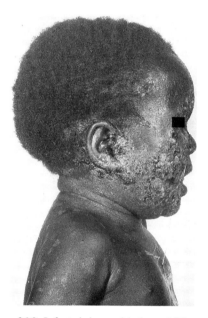

FIGURE 36.2. Infected dermatitis in a child.

country is less industrialized, but one cannot exclude that dark skin might have a higher tolerance to allergens. Atopic dermatitis is seen every day, usually with secondary infections.

Seborrheic dermatitis (Fig. 36.3) is extremely common, often with extensive follicular keratoses even in small children. Many of these patients have later been found to have AIDS. The frequent intertriginous dermatitis in the folds of the anogenital and inframammarian regions and in the deep folds of the neck in small children is usually treated with gentian violet or with potassium-permanganate baths.

It is important to realize that *psoriasis* is common in East Africa[7] and also in southern Africa while being very common on the western coast of the continent. Dithranol is well tolerated but usually not available. The extensive forms can be beneficially treated with methotrexate.

Lichen planus seems to be more common than in Europe and North America, usually as widespread disseminated eruptions which respond well to a short course of oral corticosteroids. The local hypertrophic form is more unusual, although one might see the tropical hyperpigmented type on the face. Oral lesions are extremely rare but cheilitis does occur.

Pityriasis rosea is one of the conditions seen very often. In contrast to the usual experience, this condition in this part of Africa presents equally in the papular and macular type. It is

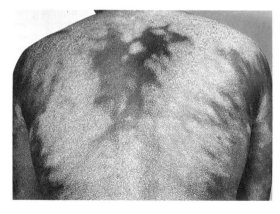

FIGURE 36.3. Extensive seborhheic dermatitis with follicular keratoses.

described, *neurodermatitis lienaris traumatica* (*Nyirenda*).[6] It is customary that the local people when affected by a skin condition try to eliminate it by rubbing it with a stone. When the lesion is on the hand or foot, it presents as linear neurodermitic lichenification along the tendons leaving the skin between unscathed.

Allergic dermatitis is much less common than in the Western World; perhaps because the impressive that the lesions often affect the face. Even an experienced physician might not reliably differentiate this disease from secondary syphilis. Serological testing for syphilis should be part of the routine.

Hyperpigmentation in the form of melanoderma is usually seen in connection with nearly every long-standing condition and eruptions caused by internal medication including fixed drug eruptions.

Hypopigmentation is less common but is usual in *tinea versicolor*, a condition nearly universal in humid climates. It is usually no indication for treatment but the patient often confuses this hypopigmentation with leprosy. *Vitiligo* is a more disturbing disease in dark skin than in fair skin as it presents itself much more impressively and might cause erythematous irritation in the strong sun. It presumably never causes cancer of the skin.[8] In contrast, *albinos* and patients with *xeroderma pigmentosum* always develop malignancies in the form of basal cell or squamous-cell carcinomas and melanomas resulting in an early death usually before the age of 20–25 years. *Actinic cheilitis* on the lower lip is a common feature.

Acne vulgaris is presumably not less common than elsewhere. Usually only cases with acne conglobate will present for treatment.

Malnutrition and *malabsorption* are common problems among small children. They present with a dry scaling skin and commonly with red hair with the most advanced cases known as *kwashiorkor*. This last condition has a mortality rate of 25% among children admitted. *Pellagra* (Fig. 36.4) is seen in still increasing numbers. It is a common disease among people with a stable diet of maize and bananas. One might say that these people have a predisposition for latent pellagra. Among the 900,000 refuges from Mosambique in 1990 living in camps in Malawi, the prevalence was as high as 6.5%.[9] The response to nicotinic acid is very dramatic.

Impressive But Less Common Skin Diseases

Onchocerciasis is usually seen along the Shire River but is very uncommon in the northern part of the country. *Larva migrans* is best treated with freezing with ethyl chloride because of a lack of thiabendazole. *Loa loa* is not found in East Africa. A high number of patients suffered from *chronic urticaria*. The first case was reported from Uganda. Later, it was found not to be very uncommon. *Guinea worm* is occasionally seen.

The deep mycoses in the form of *Madura foot*, *chromoblastomycosis*, *African histoplasmosis*, and *subcutaneous phycomycosis* are occasionally diagnosed and present a great therapeutic problem. The same is true for the classical nodular type of *Kaposi's sarcoma* and *Burkitt's lymphoma*.

The term *tropical ulcer* is confusing; most ulcers are registered as pyoderma. *Buruli ulcer*, well known in Uganda, is not diagnosed. *Venous ulcers* of the legs are uncommon. The same is found among Eskimos in Greenland, which is quite astonishing because in both areas women give birth to many children and the conditions

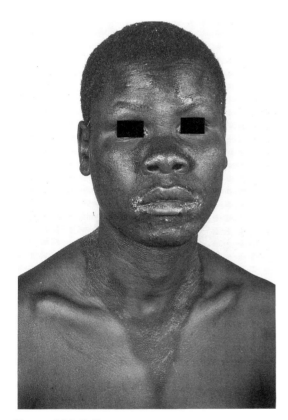

FIGURE 36.4. Pellagra.

in connection with delivery are highly unacceptable.

Melanoma is not more common than in other parts of the world, but when seen is found in the soles. *Basal cell cancer* is extremely uncommon in the Malawis except in albinos and patients with xeroderma pigmentosus. *Squamous cell cancer* is not unusual.

With the high prevalence of tuberculosis it is impressive to find very few cases of *lupus vulgaris* and *erythema nodosum*. The first case of *sarcoidosis* was diagnosed in Uganda in 1970. *Lupus erythematosus* is, however, not unusual, and in many cases extensive. The systemic form is also seen. *Dermatomyositis* is one of the more common collagenosis in Africa.

Bullous diseases seem to be more prevalent than usual. Many cases of *juvenile pemphigoid* and *dermatitis herpetiformis* among children are seen (Fig. 36.5). The same accounts for *erythema multiforme* in the form of *Stevens-Johnson's disease*. Of the other bullous diseases, *pemphigus erythematosus* and *pemphigus foliaceus* are

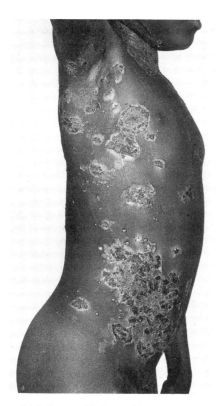

FIGURE 36.5. Dermatitis herpetiformis in a child.

regularly seen and seem to be relatively frequent in East and South Africa. *Toxic epidermal necrolysis* and *staphylococcal scalded skin syndrome* are also conditions with which one should be familiar.

Leprosy

In 1968, the estimated number of patients suffering from leprosy in Uganda was as high as 140,000 with only about 40,000 known. The number of patients in Malawi in treatment was 18,862 in 1980. Since the implementation of the multidrug treatment (WHO), the number has fallen dramatically. In 1990, only 1,773 were in treatment. Of these patients, 18.2% were suffering from the multibacillary type. Children accounted for 7.7% of the total number and the disability rate was as high as 23.8%. The Karonga Prevalence Study covering a population of 140,000 in the most northern part of Malawi was launched in 1986. This is a vaccination program using Convit's vaccine. It will take 10–15 years to evaluate if this vaccine is effective.[10]

Sexually Transmitted Diseases

Sexually transmitted diseases (STDs) are known to have a high prevalence in Africa. From the Skin Clinic at Makerere University, Uganda, an extraordinary high prevalence was reported.[11] In 1972, 19,000 cases with gonorrhea, 2,000 with early contagious syphilis, 40 with early congenitas syphilis, 1,000 with chancroid, and 40–50 with lymphogranuloma venereum were diagnosed. Of the men with syphilis, 75% were diagnosed in the primary stage and 75% of the women in the secondary stage. A frequency of not less than 7% of biological false positive tests (BFP) was demonstrated,[12] and even more astonishing was that among darkfield positive secondary syphilitic patients 12% were seronegative using the VDRL test. During the years 1969–73 only 10 cases of gummata in the skin were found. General paresis (GP) was diagnosed in 1–3% of new patients admitted at the large mental hospital.[13] The first case of tabes dorsalis in East Africa was diagnosed in the skin clinic. In the Department of Medicine, cardiovascular syphilis amounted to 4–6%.[14] There is a disturbingly high number of congenital syphilis, which commonly presents as pseudoparalysis caused by osseous changes.[14] Late congenital syphilis was, however, never found. This might be because these children succumbed to the disease or that the extensive use of antibiotics has finally cured them.

The prevalence of STDs in Malawi is not known. A pilot study[15] among a group of unselected outpatients has, however, shown a prevalence of 4.4%. "Ulcer diseases" (syphilis, chancroid, and lymphogranuloma venereum) represented 67% of the patients involved. Among patients with gonorrhea, 53% had penicillinase-producing *Neisseria gonorrhoeae* (PPNG). Sexually transmitted diseases remain a huge problem for the population and the administration. There is, however, no special clinic and the patients are still diagnosed and treated by paramedicals in general outpatient clinics. The established skin clinic in Lilongwe has neither space nor staff to take responsibility for further evaluation, especially if the high frequency of genital sores and strains of PPNG is alarming.

Infection with HIV

Infection with HIV is a great epidemiological problem in all sub-Saharan countries. The prevalence in Malawi is not known—lack of screening kits is one of the difficulties. Surveys in antenatal clinics and among blood donors seem to show it to be about 18%. The steep increase in young adults suffering from severe *herpes zoster* with 840 cases diagnosed in 1990[3] compared with 133 in 1986 and only 10 in the skin clinic in Uganda in 1972 raises the suspicion of additional HIV infection.

The number of patients who developed AIDS is high and increasing. A reduction of the African population might be feared in the years to come.

References

1. The Economist Intelligence Unit. Government Report No. 4, 1990.
2. *WHO Chron.* Anonymous. The last developed countries: a substantial new programme of action for the 1980's. 1981;**35**:223–226.
3. Vik IL: Annual Report from the Skin Clinic in Lilongwe, 1990.
4. Lomholt G: Conditions for dermatological treatment in a developing country. *Int J Dermatol* 1990;**29**:511–514.
5. Gooskens V, Chalila L: Common skin diseases in Malawi and their treatment, Private printing 2nd ed. 1991.
6. Lomholt G: Dermatology in Malawi. *Int J Dermatol* 1988;**27**:501–503.
7. Lomholt G: Psoriasis in Uganda: a comparative study with other parts of Africa. In: Farber EM, Cox AJ, eds. Psoriasis: Proceedings of the International Symposium. Stanford University Press, 1971:41–48.
8. Marshall J: Skin Diseases in Africa. Cape Town. Maskew Miller, 1964.
9. Center for Disease Control: Outbreak of pellagra among Mozambican refugees, Malawi 1990. *Arch Dermatol* 1991;**127**:791–792.
10. Gjalt B: Personal communication, 1991.
11. Lomholt G: Venereal problems in a developing country. *Trop Doctor* 1976;**6**:7–10.
12. Masawe AEJ, Lomholt G, Aho K, Lassus A: Unusual behavior of serological tests for syphilis. *Br J Vener Dis* 1972;**48**:345–348.
13. Masawe AEJ, German AG: Neurosyphilitic psycosis in psychiatric practise in Uganda. *J Afr Sci* 1972;**3**:195–197.
14. Lomholt G: Bone involvement in early congenital syphilis. *Arch Dermatol* 1977;**113**:1300–1301.
15. Kristensen JK: The prevalence of symptomatic sexually transmitted diseases and human immunodeficiency virus infections in outpatients in Lilongwe, Malawi. *Genitourin Med* 1990;**66**:244–246.

37

Nigeria

Yetunde Mercy Olumide

Nigeria is one of the largest countries in Africa. It lies wholly within the tropics along the Gulf of Guinea, on the western coast of Africa. There are two well-marked seasons—the dry season lasting from November to March, and the rainy season from April to October. Temperatures at the coast seldom rise above 32°C, but humidity can be as high as 95%. The climate is drier further north where extremes of temperature are common, sometimes ranging from 36°C to 42°C. Nigeria covers a total geographical area of 923,768 square kilometers. The population of the country is about 100 million. This population is made up of multiethnic groups with highly diversified cultural practices. The country is a federation of 30 states. Peasant farming is largely practiced in the rural areas; the major cities are highly industrialized. The federal, state, and local governments carry out, in a co-ordinated manner, a three-tier system of health care, namely; primary health care, secondary health care, and tertiary health care.

The Problem

About 30% of patients seeking medical help suffer from skin afflictions, and of this, about 65–70% are communicable diseases.[1-5] Other identified problems are the dearth of personnel to manage these dermatoses at all levels of health care delivery, the often conflicting therapies from the herbalists, inadequate laboratory services, prohibitively expensive health care services in the absence of medical insurance,

and the atavistic fears and opprobrium from certain dermatoses.

Incidence of Skin Diseases

Skin diseases constitute the commonest indication for seeking medical advice in our environment because of highly conducive ecoclimatic, cultural, and other socioeconomic factors, and partly because a skin disease can be seen even when asymptomatic. The fear of contagion (often erroneously ascribed to skin diseases) and the attendant ostracism encourage people to seek medical advice however, socioeconomic determinants largely influence the high rate of infective dermatoses. Some of these factors are listed in Table 37.1.

Personnel

There is a dearth of dermatologists in Nigeria with 20 dermatologists to over 100 million people. Obviously, only a minute fraction of cases with skin disease can have access to dermatologists who are largely in tertiary institutions. It has been observed that very often dermatologists are presented with the complication of initial mismanagement. There is a general misconception by general practitioners that no prior diagnosis need be made as far as skin diseases are concerned and that no harm is done if a system of "trial and error" is adopted in the management of these patients. The repercussions of this misconception is that the patient becomes physically, emotionally, and financially impoverished. This pitiable state of affairs has been enhanced because of the dearth of teachers in dermatology in most training institutions for medical personnel in the country. It has also been observed that the majority of industrial-site clinics are managed exclusively by nurses. The

TABLE 37.1. Factors that promote increase in infective dermatoses.

Inadequate Water Supply
  Scarcity of water to wash body and clothes
  Personal hygiene becomes poor or impossible
Poverty
  Cannot eat well
  Cannot buy soap for bathing and washing clothes
  Cannot buy water (when needed)
  Cannot live in a decent and clean home
  Cannot buy drugs (when needed)
Polygamy and Uncontrolled Birth Rate
  Leads to more poverty as it overstretches the meager money available
  Leads to overcrowded living conditions
  Every effort at improving health care delivery is rendered ineffective
Inadequate Supply of Drugs—Prohibitive Cost of Drugs
  Affected individual not treated or inadequately treated, disease persists, spreads further, and resistant strains develop
Sky-Rocketing Inflation
  Prohibitive costs of basic items like soap and detergents
Unstable Political Climate and Frequent Changes in Government
  Associated changes in health policies and direction of emphasis and priorities
Absence of Consistent or Corroborative Health Policies Between Federal and State Government
  Some states have free health services; some do not. Communicable diseases do not respect state boundaries.
  Even the free health service had its own disadvantage: People seem to find it cheaper to consume drugs that they do not pay for than to avoid disease
National Economic Recession
  Less money available to promote health policies
Loss of Income by Farmers
  Majority of rural dwellers are peasant farmers
  Farm crops perish due to inadequate storage facilities and inadequate transport facilities to convey the crops to the cities
  This results in more poverty to the farmer and more inflation to the general public and the vicious cycle continues
Ignorance
  Traditional beliefs about the causes of diseases die hard. Even if health education is vigorously and resolutely pursued, the target audience must have the desire to practice the ideal

name of a consulting physician may be floated, just for the records. As a result, quite a sizable percentage of patients referred are from these nurses, who have simply abandoned hospital nursing care, for which they are trained, to more financially rewarding industrial clinics, where they play the role of doctors.

The Herbalist

One also has to contend with the herbalist and other traditional healers. Herbalists abound in all marketplaces. The ubiquitous presence of the herbalists facilitates casual consultation. Therefore, the majority of patients would have had prior treatment with herbal concoctions, and only consult with a physician when the lesion fails to heal or gets worse. Even the few patients who consult with a physician at the inception of the disease get impatient when response is not initially dramatic or fast. Friends and relations readily advise to seek alternative remedies. When such a patient returns for follow-up visits, one finds it difficult to assess response to prescribed drugs, because a superimposed contact dermatitis from the herbal concoctions may have developed.

Furthermore, all drugs are marketed as over-the-counter drugs in Nigeria. So, when taking a medical history, one needs to specifically inquire about consumption of both prescribed and unprescribed drugs. Patients are usually shy or afraid (for fear of resentment) to release the fact that they have consulted the herbalist. Therefore, a history of herbal consumption has to be literally "dragged out" of the patient.

All referred patients are seen promptly on the day they present their referral letters, without any previous appointment. If they are sent away and asked to return at an appointed day, they invariably start to self-medicate and they return with complications. Therefore, only follow-up cases are seen on appointment.

Cost of Health Services

There is no health insurance in Nigeria. Provision of health services has become prohibitively expensive, particularly since the structural adjustment policy which led to the fiftyfold devaluation of the Nigerian currency (the naira). Most of the drugs and hospital equipment are imported by multinational companies. With the devaluation of the naira, these companies simply multiplied the cost of the drugs fiftyfold. As a result of this, some of the simple dermatological preparations like benzyl benzoate lotion or selenium sulphide could cost about 50% of the minimum wage of a worker.

Not even tertiary institutions can boast of adequate laboratory diagnostic facilities. One histopathology department serves all the departments in the hospital, and some private hospitals also send their specimens to this same department for processing and interpretation. Consequently, biopsy results are received after several weeks or months, often after the patient has been treated and discharged. Furthermore, the same blade is used for sectioning all tissues—liver, kidney, skin, and so on. Naturally, this affects the quality of the skin section and eventually the interpretation.

Even where the facilities exist, some "routine" and largely confirmatory laboratory tests are deliberately not done because of the high cost of such investigations. In the Lagos University teaching hospital, patients pay for all laboratory tests and all drugs. The cost of a simple investigation like culture and resistogram for pyoderma or mycology culture may be equivalent to a patient's income for the month. A physician then has to decide on priority—spending money to investigate or spending money to purchase the required curative drugs?

The occupation of a hospital bed is very expensive. Therefore, hospitalization of patients is reduced to the barest minimum. Only about 0.5% of patients seen are hospitalized when they are deemed too ill to be managed on an outpatient basis. At times, when a patient is very ill and still cannot pay the heavy deposit necessary for admission, he/she is treated on a couch in the Accident and Emergency (A & E) unit for some hours to several days and sent home for outpatient follow-up.

Integrated Clinics

There is an integrated approach to the care of patients with skin disease, leprosy, and sexually transmitted diseases (STDs).

Apart from economic considerations, it has been observed that patients with Hansen's disease (HD) or sexually transmitted diseases (STDs) are not happy patronizing clinics so labeled.

Recommendations

Because the majority of dermatoses are under the influence of socioeconomic determinants that are essentially alterable, it becomes obvious that the provision of health is inextricably linked with integrated rural development, controlled birth rate, health insurance, the local development of the petrochemical industry for local drug manufacture, research for integrating modern and traditional medicine, a well-articulated basic dermatological training for all cadres of health care delivery personnel, and a sustained health education program for the people in order to improve their personal hygiene and positively influence their attitudes and beliefs. The need for stable democratic governments that can formulate and sustain well-directed and coordinated national health policies cannot be overemphasized.

Various Dermatoses

Because it is not possible to discuss all the dermatoses or even the relevant ones in detail, only the salient variations in presentation will be discussed. They will be discussed under the various headings highlighted in Table 37.2.

Fungal Infections

Fungal infections constitute 15–25% of dermatoses in Nigeria.[1-3] This high prevalence is largely due to the prevailing environmental heat and humidity, and partly to poor hygienic conditions.

TABLE 37.2. Some diseases influenced by eco-climatic, socioeconomic, or genetic factors.

Hot and Humid Environment
   Tinea corporis
   Tinea versicolor
   Flexural candidiasis
   Miliaria and periportis
Other Ecological Factors
   Papular urticaria   Larva migrans
   Onchodermatitis   Myiasis
   Loiasis   *Mycobacterium ulcerans*
   Elephantiasis   Histoplasmosis
   Blister beetle dermatitis
Overcrowded Living Conditions
   Scabies
   Leprosy
   Zoonosis from animal parasites
   Impetigo contagiosa
Inadequate Potable Water
   Guinea worm
   Infective dermatoses
Malnutrition and Inappropriate Nutrition
   Kwashiorkor
   Phrynoderma
   Pellagra
Wearing Apparel
   Shoe dermatitis
   Nickel dermatitis
   Clothing dermatitis
   Marginal alopecia
Cosmetic Habits
   Ochronosis, striae, acne, and folliculitis
   Oil acne (dermatitis cruris pustulosa et atrophicans)
Complications of Therapy
   Dermatitis, drug eruptions
   Exacerbations of existing dermatoses
Miscellaneous Dermatoses
   Folliculitis keloidalis nuchae
   Seborrheic dermatitis
   Dermatosis papulosa nigra
   Pseudofolliculitis barbae
   Sarcoidosis

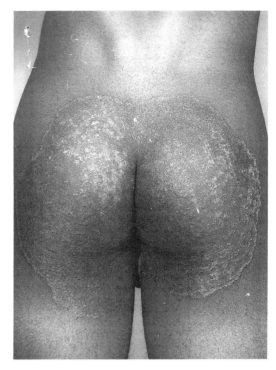

FIGURE 37.1. Tinea cruris spreading to the buttocks.

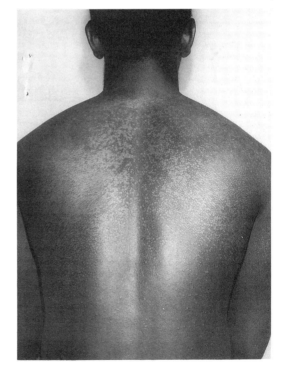

FIGURE 37.2. Disseminated tinea versicolor.

The prevailing heat and humidity also promote the spread of the lesion. The cheap pants that are available are often made of thick polyester (crimplene) or nylon fabrics that further promote sweating and maceration. Tinea cruris often presents as very extensive lesions spreading directly to the buttocks and belt line as shown in Fig. 37.1. Tinea versicolor also tends to be disseminated (Fig. 37.2), involving both seborrheic and nonseborrheic areas.

Miliaria (Heat Rash)

Miliaria is also a common disturbing problem. It presents most often in babies because they are often overdressed with thick woolen or polyester fabrics due to a popular misconception that babies must be kept very warm. Older children try to relieve themselves of the heat by playing about only in pants. The vigorous exercise often engaged in by children promotes severe sweating, which fails to evaporate due to the prevailing humidity. Periporitis (Fig. 37.3), particular to the forehead, which sweats most, is a common complication.

The pruritus provoked by a hot and humid environment is a major exacerbating factor in atopic dermatitis.

Papular Urticaria (Strophulus infantum)

Papular urticaria is frequently caused by the bites of sandflies and mosquitoes.

Children after infancy and before puberty are classically affected. The persistent papules are found mainly in exposed areas of the body—legs and forearms (Fig. 37.4). The papules last for several days and old sites flare up with new bites, so that lesions are profuse. The lesions are extremely itchy. The excoriated papules often become weepy and crusted from impetiginization. There is often regional lymphadenopathy.

Although papular urticaria is notoriously a disease of childhood, it is not uncommon to find papular urticaria in adults, particularly young women, as a personal idiosyncrasy when the skin continues to behave like that of a child, with distinct, persistent papules, rather than evanescent wheals, when bitten by insects. At times, papular urticaria develops for the first time among teenagers and young adults, who were born and had lived in temperate countries, and so have not had the opportunity to get sensitized due to inadequate exposure to arthropod bites.

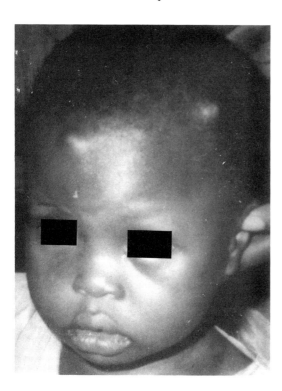

FIGURE 37.3. Periporitis.

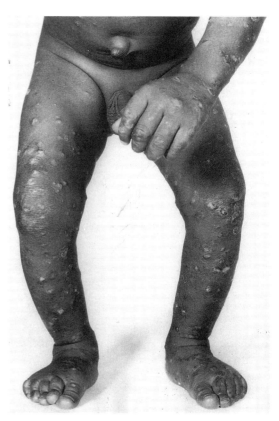

FIGURE 37.4. Papular urticaria.

Children who are carried about strapped on the backs of their mothers also develop papular urticaria on the face.

Differential Diagnosis

The significant diseases to be excluded are scabies, onchodermatitis, and papulo-necrotic tuberculids. Scabetic lesions are found on both exposed and covered parts of the body, and the hands are fairly regularly affected. A fairly constant history that other members of the family are scratching is often obtained in scabies. Onchodermatitis largely affects adults; covered and uncovered parts of the body are affected, and eczematization and lichenification of the lesion often develops. Papulo-necrotic tuberculids are found predominantly in adults. Extensor surfaces of the elbows and knees are favored sites, accompanying lymphadenopathy is significant, and there may be an accompanying history of cough and wasting.

Onchocerciasis (African River Blindness)

Onchocerciasis is a disease caused by the filarial worm, *Onchocerca volvulus*. The vector of the disease is the tiny black fly, *Simulium damnosum*. Studies conducted in Nigeria showed an overall prevalence rate of *O. volvulus* infection to be 8.2% in the rain forest and 6.0% in the savannah area.[6] Antigenic differences have been demonstrated between *O. volvulus* of African and American strains and even between savannah and rain forest filarial strains in Africa. The savannah type is predominantly associated with ocular lesions and blindness.[7]

Clinical Features

A patient with onchocerciasis could present with pruritus, onchocercal dermatitis, onchocercomata, swelling of a limb, and blindness.

There is a broad spectrum of clinical presentation in onchodermatitis. The clinical types depend on geographic location, immune status of the host, and chronicity of infection.

The commonest complaint is pruritus, which may not be associated with a dermatitis. The pruritus is usually generalized but may be localized to one limb and is usually worse at night. Onchocercal pruritus may be minimal in some patients, but frenzied in the majority. Such is the maddening pruritus that the disease is locally called "Ina-orun" which literally means "hell fire."

The dermatitis is a nonspecific papular eruption worsened by scratching. Examination reveals erythematous or skin-colored papular eruption, invariably excoriated, leaving numerous tiny depigmented scars surrounded by an erythematous or pigmented halo, and excoriation marks. Favored sites are the back, shoulders, upper arms, buttocks, and thighs (Fig. 37.5). Only one of these regions may be affected, such as one thigh, or there may be a combination of various noncontiguous sites. The face is usually spared in onchodermatitis of forested Africa, but is commonly involved in Central America. However, the face may also be affected in savannal onchocerciasis.[7]

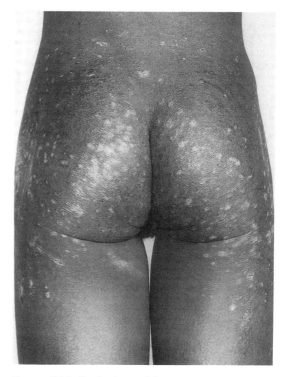

FIGURE 37.5. Onchodermatitis.

Traumatic scratching may eczematize the lesion. The skin becomes thickened, wrinkled, and dry, like a lizard's skin.

Firm, nontender lymphadenopathy is a common feature of onchocerciasis; the nodes involved usually drain areas of onchocercal dermatitis (Fig. 37.6). The nodes progressively get sclerosed, the groin glands being frequently involved—sclerosing hypertrophic inguinocrural lymphadenopathy. "Hanging groin" is characterized by a loose atrophic skin sac containing large fibrotic nodes. Sometimes there is extensive lichenification of the scrotal skin from prolonged scratching and elephantiasis of the scrotum. Postinflammatory depigmentation could occur, especially on the scrotum and the pretibial areas ("leopard skin") (Fig. 37.7), in a long-standing onchodermatitis in Africans.

The skin eruption is associated with the presence of microfilariae (embryo worms) in the skin and nodules (onchocercomata) that are

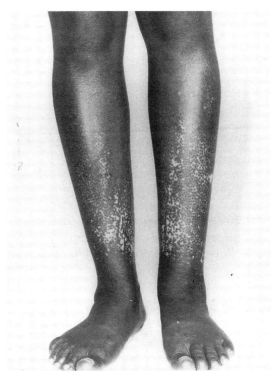

FIGURE 37.7. The "leopard shins" in late onchodermatitis.

formed by collections of adult worms grouped together within fibrous tissue. These are in the subcutaneous tissue, and in the early stages, they have to be identified by palpation. Particular areas to palpate are the regions over the iliac crests, the greater trochanters, the coccyx, the scalp, and the ribs. The nodule feels like a hard pea, is mobile, and the skin can be moved over it. Apart from site of bony prominence, nodules may also be found on other parts of the skin. In the Central American variety, nodules are found on the face and scalp, probably due to the different biting habits of the vector, simulide. Occasionally, a patient may present with one or more nodules in the absence of a dermatitis or pruritus, and in such a case, the diagnosis can only be established by removing a nodule for sectioning.

Chronic swelling of one arm, in the absence of dermatitis and irritation, has been reported as a manifestation of onchocerciasis.[8]

The presence of microfilariae in the eyes can give rise to a number of ocular complications such as iridocyclitis, sclerosing keratitis, and

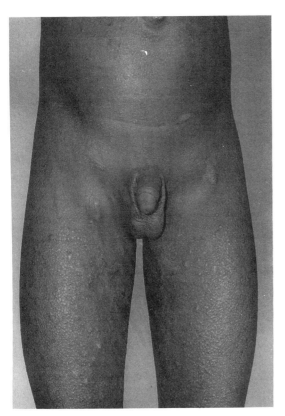

FIGURE 37.6. Onchodermatitis with lymphadenopathy.

superficial punctate keratitis. The latter is observable with the naked eye if the light of a torch is directed from one side and the observer inspects from the opposite side. The tiny opacities in the superficial portion of the cornea, resembling tiny drops of candle grease, are better seen with the aid of a torch and loupe.

Diagnosis

A definitive diagnosis can be made by demonstrating microfilaria in the skin snips or by removing a nodule and examining sections for the presence of onchocercal worms. Unlike the other forms of filariasis, microfilariae are not present in the blood in onchocerciasis, but eosinophilia is invariably present.

The above tests are not always positive in clinical practice. Only 3.7% of clinically suspected patients with onchocerciasis examined at the Lagos University Teaching Hospital were found to be positive for *O. volvulus* on laboratory examination.[9] Clinically, the diagnosis is usually evident, but scabies must be excluded.

Finally, the Mazzotti test can be used in cases where the diagnosis is difficult to establish. A sharp accentuation of the complaint after one dose of Banocide is often used as a diagnostic test for the disease. Banocide is very toxic to microfilariae, and one tablet is quite enough to kill large numbers within a couple of hours. It has been suggested that the local and systemic reactions that appear after the administration of diethylcarbamazine (Mazzotti reaction) are the results of anaphylactic phenomena due to the interaction of microfilarial antigens with IgE antibodies.[10–12]

Caution is necessary in patients with ocular onchocerciasis, as a severe Mazzotti reaction could cause severe deterioration of ocular involvement that may result in blindness.

Treatment

Diethylcarbamazine citrate (Banocide, Hetrazan) is effective against the microfilaria. The recommended method of starting with a low dose of Banocide and increasing gradually to avoid severe Mazzotti reaction has seldom been found to be necessary in clinical practice in Lagos as the Mazzotti reactions are often mild and ocular manifestations are uncommon (rain forest type).

The patient may start with the full dose of 150 mg, 3 times daily for 1 month, plus an antihistamine tablet to suppress reactions. Very severe cases may need corticosteroid eye drops during Banocide therapy, and sometimes even systemic corticosteroid may be necessary for the occasional patient with severe Mazzotti reaction. The course of treatment is repeated after 3–4 months or when symptoms reappear after months or years.

Suramin (Antrypol) kills both the adult worms and the microfilariae. A dose of 0.5–1 g is given intravenously weekly for 4–6 weeks. The urine should be examined weekly for protein, red cells, and casts before each injection because suramin is nephrotoxic. Severe morbilliform or bullous drug eruption is also a possibility.

Nodules should be removed surgically (nodulectomy) where practicable.

Ivermectin,[13] the new potent microfilaricide, is a macrocyclic lactone antibiotic derived from Streptomyces avermitis. It has recently been evaluated in onchocerciasis and found to be effective in single oral dose regimes of 0.1–0.2 mg/kg. It has a long duration of action of about 9 months; hence, a single dose per year suffices. Ivermectin has the added advantage of producing only a mild Mazzotti reaction compared with diethylcarbamazine.

Loiasis

Loa loa (the eye worm) occurs only in the rain forests of West and Central Africa. Tabanid flies of the genus *Chrysops* are the intermediate host insect vectors. In Africa, *Chrysops silacea* and *C. dimitiata*, commonly called mangrove flies, are the principal vectors, and unlike mosquitoes they are biters by day.

Argyll-Robertson in 1895[14] removed two worms (one of each sex) from the eyes of a woman who had lived in Old Calabar. He vividly described the worms and the clinical presentation of loiasis and the fugitive swelling—hence Calabar swelling. Argyll-Robertson was, however, not the first to describe the disease. It is believed that Pigafetta probably saw the disease first along the Congo River in 1598.[15]

Clinical Features

The patient may present with urticaria, but more often the patient presents with a diffuse, firm, nonpitting swelling, usually on the wrist or forearm, giving the impression that the limb has been sprained (Fig. 37.8). This is called a Calabar or fugitive swelling because they are transient, may regress in several hours, or last for several days. The swellings usually continue to recur in the same or a different location at intervals of days to months. It is of normal skin color but may be erythematous. There may be pain or pruritus. The swelling is invariably single; other sites that may be affected are face, ankles, and dorsa of feet.

Eye involvement may result in recurrent periorbital edema. There may be pain, irrita-

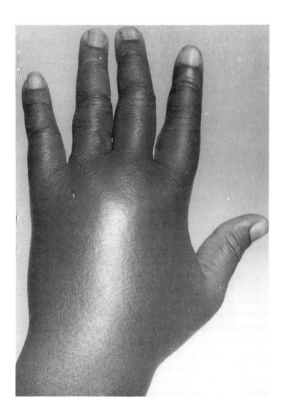

FIGURE 37.8. Calabar swelling in Loiasis.

tions, impaired vision, paraesthesia, or local weakness. Calabar swellings are localized allergic reactions to adult worms in sensitized individuals.

The worms may be seen crossing under the conjunctiva or migrating subcutaneously wherever the skin is thin, such as under eyelids. This can be demonstrated by asking the patient to shut the eyes in a relaxed manner; the wrinkles on the eyelid can then be manually straightened out by pulling the lid downward with a finger tip.

Diagnosis

Diagnosis is based on clinical features and is confirmed by a finding of microfilariae of loa loa in the blood sample taken during the daytime, and eosinophilia. In only about one-third of affected patients is microfilaria demonstrable in blood. In practice, diagnosis is more often based on clinical history and findings.

Treatment

Diethylcarbamazine effectively kills both microfilariae and adult worms, unlike onchocerciasis.

Elephantiasis (Filarial Lymphedema)

Filarial lymphedema is caused by *Wuchereria bancrofti* and *Brugia malayi* in Nigeria.

The clinical phases of the disease may be divided into inflammatory and obstructive; symptoms of both may coexist.

The early inflammatory stage is characterized by recurrent febrile attacks and is associated with symptoms of acute lymphangitis and regional lymphadenitis. Lymphadenitis may occur independent of lymphangitis. Although the lower extremity is predominantly involved, the upper extremity may occasionally be affected. The lesion usually starts in one leg and later involves the other extremity. The lymphadenitis may be associated with orchitis, funiculitis, epididymitis, or urticaria.

At the beginning of the obstructive stage, swelling of the extremity is present only toward the end of the day (gravitational) and may be slightly pitting. Chronic edema stimulates growth of dermal connective tissue. With chronicity, there is thickening of the lymphatic walls fibrosis, hyalinization, calcification, and obliterated lymphatic channels. The edema becomes nonpitting at this stage.

In the late chronic stage, there may by lymphatic varices. The genitalia show lymph scrotum, edematous skin, and hydrocoel.

In very long-standing cases of lymphedema, there is verrucous hyperplasia of the skin like that of an elephant, hence the name "elephantiasis" (Fig. 37.9).

Secondary chronic lymphedema from other causes is, however, more prevalent than that due to filariasis. Secondary lymphedema could be inflammatory or obstructive in nature; both frequently coexist because edema fluid is rich in proteins and is an excellent culture medium. Any defect in the integrity of the skin is a potential entry point for recurrent bacterial infections, usually hemolytic streptococci (but may be mixed—streptococci or staphylococci). These recurrent erysipelas and cellulitis cause lymphangitis, lymphadenitis, and phlebitis. Healing is by fibrosis, and the insults, if recurrent, will eventually lead to obstructive syndrome. The infective type is the commonest type in our environment. The foci for recurrent infections are usually guinea worm ulcers and other chronic leg ulcers (e.g., tropical and sickle cell ulcers), tungiasis, tinea pedis, chronic dermatitis, and plantar fissures.

Other less common causes of chronic lymphedema are deep mycoses (mycetoma), neoplasma—Kaposi's sarcoma in particular, tuberculosis lymphadenitis, and surgical extirpation of nodes. Chronic lymphedema often antedates the appearance of the nodules in Kaposi's sarcoma.

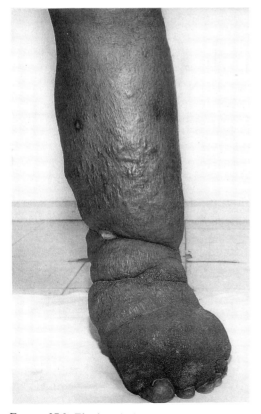

FIGURE 37.9. Elephantiasis.

Larva Migrans (Creeping Eruptions)

Larva migrans (Fig. 37.10) is frequently seen among children, particularly children of market women who leave their children to crawl and play about naked on the bare market grounds. The droppings of cats and dogs often abound in such places. The skin of patients who harbor *Strongyloides stercoralis* in the intestine may be autoinoculated by the larvae. This type is usually localized to the back, abdomen, buttocks, or thighs. The larva moves fast and may cover about 30 cm in 12 h, hence the name "larva currens" or racing larva.

Treatment

Freezing the advancing end of the tunnel with ethyl chloride, dry ice, or liquid nitrogen is effective. The affected site later exfoliates. Topical application of thiabendazole is very effective. We simply instruct the patient to rub on mintezol syrup. Thiabendazole orally for 2–4 days has the added advantage of taking care of

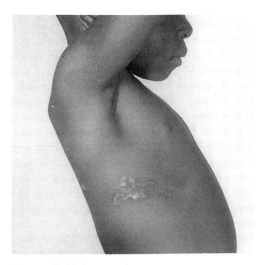

FIGURE 37.10. Larva migrans.

concurrent intestinal worms. Secondary bacterial infection introduced from scratching should be treated with topical antibiotics.

Myiasis

This is an infection of man by larvae (maggots) of dipterous (two-winged) insects. Primary myiasis occurs when the larvae are capable of burrowing into normal skin, and secondary (traumatic) myiasis occurs when an antecedent wound, ulcer, or draining lesion invites occupation by maggots.

Myiasis is more common near cattle-grazing regions. Cattle rearers and shepherds are most vulnerable. In Nigeria, it is caused by the larvae of a botfly (tumbu fly, mango fly) known as *Cordylobia anthropophata.*

Children appear to be more susceptible to primary myiasis. The eggs are laid on human skin or on clothing (e.g., diapers, vests) and the emerging larvae burrow into the skin. Secondary myiasis is usually found in elderly and neglected individuals.

Clinically, this condition should be suspected if a patient presents with a painful or stinging furunclelike papule or papules on any part of the body. On examination with a magnifying lens, a small aperture will be seen at the summit

of the lesion through which the larva obtains air. Before the larva emerges, severe pain or stinging sensation may be caused by movements of the spiny larva. Pruritus is also common. After 2–3 months of comfortable development within the skin, the larva (now considerably fatter and larger) emerges from the lesion and drops to the ground to pupate. This is followed by spontaneous involution of the lesion.

The traditional method of freezing the larva with ethyl chloride, dry ice, or liquid nitrogen tends to result in an intradermal dead larva, which later is complicated by a foreign-body granulomatous reaction or calcified larvae or an abscess. Though a horrifying sight, if the lesions are multiple, it is better to leave the larvae to mature and crawl out. Solitary lesions may be incised and removed with forceps.

At times, the patient presents when the lesion is "ripe" and the summit of the lesion is exposed, but the larva remains buried in situ. An atraumatic extrusion of the larva can be achieved thus: Two wooden spatulas (one held in each hand) are used to simultaneously compress the bottom of the lesions on two opposing edges as demonstrated in Fig. 37.11. The larva simply pops out en mass like a grain of rice (without being crushed). Postextrusion topical antibiotic is all that is necessary. The lesion heals within a few days.

If the lesions are multiple, a systemic antimicrobials may be necessary to prevent or treat secondary bacterial infections. Antibiotic ointments or other oily preparations should not be applied before the maggot matures and crawls out. The patient should be advised against forcibly squeezing out the larva, as this could result in intraderma, rupture of the larva and cellulitis.

Dracontiasis (Guinea Worm Disease)

Guinea worm disease is endemic in tropical and subtropical countries without an adequate source of pipe-borne water. It is caused by a nematode, *Dracunculus medinensis*, and contracted through drinking water contaminated

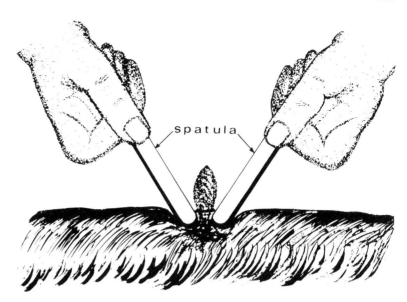

FIGURE 37.11. Extrusion of
the larva in myiasis.

with a small crustacean or water fleas (cyclops) in which the dracunculus is parasitic.

In the stomach, the larvae leave the cyclops and penetrate into the mesentery, and finally mature in the loose connective tissue under the skin, especially that of the legs and feet. The male worm is small and dies after copulation. The female requires up to a year to become gravid. The female worm then burrows to the cutaneous surface to deposit her larvae. As the worm approaches the surface, it may be felt as a cordlike thickening and forms an indurated papule on which a blister later forms. This blister breaks down to form an ulcer about 1 cm across, and the anterior end of the worm protrudes into this ulcer (Fig. 37.12). On contact with water, the head of the worm ruptures, and the uterus periodically discharges the larvae infective to the cyclops.

The diagnosis cannot always be made from a casual question on the current source of drinking water. The patient may have contracted the disease when he or she visited his village, which lacked potable water, and because of the long incubation period, the ulcer may manifest itself when the patient is residing in a place with pipe-borne water.

Guinea worm disease could be associated with extreme morbidity and loss of several working days because of incapacitating guinea worm arthritis and associated cellulitis. A large percentage of community may be so incapacitated as to adversely affect the agricultural labor force in a community where guinea worm is endemic. Progressive lymphedema could complicate the recurrent erysipelas and cellulitis from secondary bacterial infections of the wound. Clostridium tetani may contaminate the wound and tetanus may result.

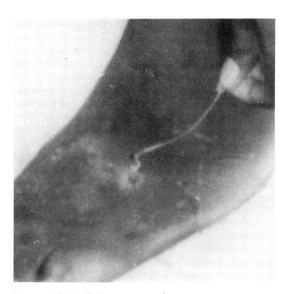

FIGURE 37.12. Guinea worm ulcer.

Treatment

The threadlike female worm measures up to 1 m long. Gradually winding the worm out of the ulcer by turning it on a stick (match or broom stick) a few centimeters a day is still common practice. As the worm is positively hydrotropic, the natives have learned to immerse the affected part in water to attract the emergence of the worm. Extraction must be done with care, for in the event of rupture of the worm, it escapes into the tissues and produces fulminating inflammation.

Three drugs have been documented as useful in the treatment of guinea worm disease.[16] These are niridazole (usually given in doses of 25 mg/kg body weight daily for 10 days), thiabendazole (50 mg/kg daily for 3 days), and metronidazole (400 mg for an adult daily for 10–20 days). All the drugs have similar effects. None of the drugs has been found to be lethal to the worm, but it is believed that they simply act as anti-inflammatory agents, thereby facilitating a less traumatic removal of the worm.

My observation in clinical practice is that the frequency of allergic reactions to niridazole is rather disturbing in patients with guinea worm, and some patients on their own discontinue the drug after the first few doses. The drug does not kill the worm, as it is not uncommon to find another worm emerging from another site while a patient is on niridazole.

Letting the patient gradually roll out the worm the traditional way, while under appropriate antimicrobial cover, appears to suffice. In any case, the worm dies after delivering all her larvae. Very important aspects of the treatment are combating the cellulitis and preventing permanent disability from ankylosis of joints or contracture of limbs as well as prevention of a complicating tetanus.

A course of systemic antibiotic is almost always necessary because of the concomitant bacterial cellulitis. Appropriate antitetanus prophylaxis is always necessary as well as adequate nursing of the wound.

Guinea worm disease confers no immunity and reinfestation readily occurs with continued exposure. The community should be educated to boil the drinking water and to filter it with a clean white cloth. There is, however, no superior substitute to the provision of clean pipe-borne water.

Kwashiorkor Dermatitis

Kwashiorkor is a form of protein-energy malnutrition in children. It is usually manifested during weaning or post weaning periods or after a severe debilitating illness like measles. Various interpretations have been given to the origin of the term "kwashiorkor." It comes from the Ga language of Ghana and it is sometimes reported that Cicely Williams coined the term which means "the sickness of the deposed baby."[17] In a more recent report, Handa[18] claims that it is a distorted version of a name used by the Ga tribe of Ghana: 'Kwashie' is the traditional name for the first child in a family, and 'ko' means 'go' or 'gone,' meaning that when the second child arrives, the first child, who is Kwashie, goes or is gone, i.e. dies of malnutrition (kwashioko). This name became distorted over the years into 'kwashiorkor' and acquired the symbolic meaning of "the illness of the deposed one."

A child with kwashiorkor has retarded growth and may also exhibit psychomotor changes. He is irritable and apathetic. He has a moon face and is pale. The pallor may be due as much to thinning and distension of the skin as to actual loss of pigment and associated anemia. The hair is fine and sparse and has a reddish-brown tinge. The face looks miserable, but bloated because of prominent buccal fat pads and bilateral parotitis. There is a patchy dirty brownish pigmentation particularly on the face. Lanugo hair is prominent, especially on the face and posterior aspect of the neck. The eyelashes are sparce, having a broomstick appearance. The child is usually pot-bellied. The classical dermatosis of kwashiorkor has been described as 'crazy pavement,' 'crackled skin,' 'mosaic skin,' 'enamel paint,' and 'flaky paint.' The crackled skin is usually associated with a localized (hands and feet) or generalized edema (which may mask the muscle wasting). Some of these features are demonstrated in Fig. 37.13. Other associated findings are angular stomatitis,

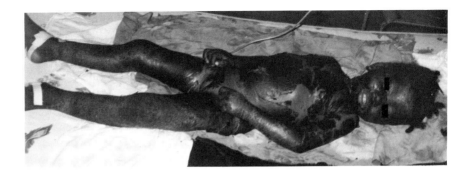

FIGURE 37.13.
Kwashiorkor
dermatitis.

glossitis, hypoalbuminemia, and manifestations of immune depression. All these features respond dramatically to a corrective high-protein diet.

Phrynoderma and Infundibulo-Folliculitis

Phrynoderma is due to vitamin A deficiency and is largely seen among children of school age. The lesions are hyperkeratotic follicular papules distributed mainly on the extensor surfaces of the trunk, elbows, and knees (Fig. 37.14). Mildly scaly hypopigmented patches often accompany the follicular keratosis. The patients improve dramatically on keratolytics, for example, Tretinoin cream or 2–5% sulfur-salicyclic acid cream, and simple dietary measures to augment vitamin A intake from palm oil, cod-liver oil, carrots, and vegetables, for example.

Disseminated infundibulo-folliculitis (Fig. 37.15) is a condition of unknown etiology.[19] It

is not associated with a history of atopy. It is a recurrent follicular eruption predominantly affecting the trunk; it may be asymptomatic or mildly pruritic. The papules are skin colored. Each attack lasts for several weeks to months. The histology is a superficial follicular spongiotic dermatitis. It is self-limiting and responds to keratolytics and topical corticosteroid ointment.

Pellagra

This is due to a deficiency of niacin or tryptophan. It is predominantly seen among the

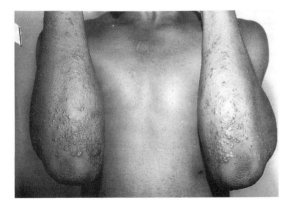

FIGURE 37.14. Phrynoderma.

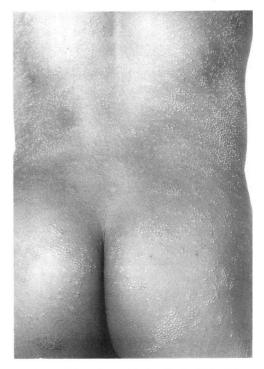

FIGURE 37.15. Disseminated infundibulo-folliculitis.

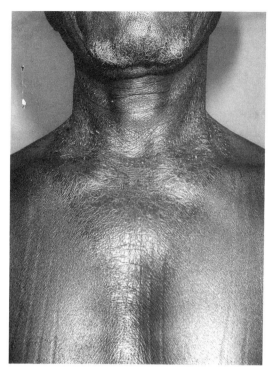

FIGURE 37.16. Pellagra.

Hausa tribe in the northern part of Nigeria because this is a population whose major dietary intake is maize and millet (sorghum), which may interfere with tryptophan metabolism because of its high leucine content.

Pellagra classically is manifested by dermatitis, diarrhea, and dementia; however, diarrhea and dementia are later features of advanced pellagra. The cutaneous manifestation is therefore the common presentation. It is a characteristic dermatitis of the exposed parts (Fig. 37.16) associated with a stomatitis and glossitis.

As it is impracticable for affected individuals to change their culinary habit, they are simply placed on 500 mg of nicotinic acid daily for several weeks and then maintained on 50 mg daily indefinitely.

Contact Dermatitis

Nickel jewelry, shoes, and clothing are the most common causes of contact dermatitis.[20,21] Allergens readily bleed out from these sources by sweat, which is often profuse because of the

prevailing heat and humidity. Nickel jewelry, rubber and plastic shoes, and polyester (crimplene) fabrics are inexpensive, hence they constitute the most common sources of contact dermatitis.

Housewives' hand dermatitis is not common in Nigeria. This is due to 'hardening,' because domestic chores are normally done with ungloved bare hands from childhood. One common source of occupational hand eczema in women is the orange peel—the sensitizer being the essential oils in oranges.[22] Such patients usually give a positive patch test response to 'fragrance mix.' The most common cause of exfoliative dermatitis (erythroderma) is a herbal concoction dispensed by a herbalist to prevent or treat diseases. Such a concoction is either taken orally or used during a bath.

Marginal Alopecia

Marginal alopecia is due to two factors: traction from tight braiding and plaiting and friction and pressure from the heavy head ties that regularly accompany the traditional costume. It is, therefore, exclusively found in women (Fig. 37.17).

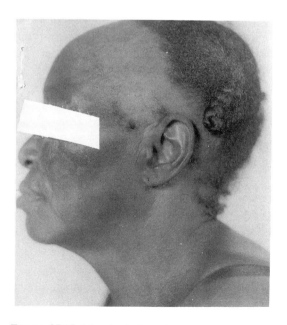

FIGURE 37.17. Marginal alopecia.

Hydroquinone-Induced Exogenous Ochronosis

Hydroquinone is a regular active ingredient in cosmetic skin-lightening creams. Findlay et al.[23] first reported exogenous ochronosis and formation of pigmented colloid milia from use of skin-lightening creams containing hydroquinone. The etiopathogenesis has been well documented.[24]

The clinical appearance has also been described.[25,26] The affected sites are predominantly the sun-exposed area. The morphologic appearance depends on the duration of the lesion.

Initially, it may present as a facial hyperpigmentation with a butterfly distribution. Later, the affected areas appear polished (shiny and smooth), thickened, firm, and difficult to pinch. Later yellow-brown, dome-shaped, discrete, translucent 1–2-mm papules (colloid milia) develop (Fig. 37.18). These later fuse to form nodules of various sizes. With further induration, the grayish-brown macules become slightly raised, smooth, irregularly shaped plaques. With progression, the skin takes on a rippled, reticulate, or shagreen pattern. Finally, after

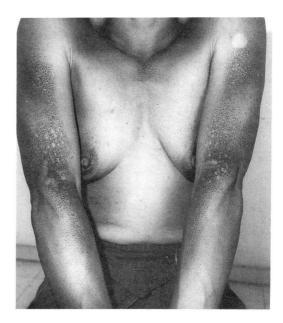

FIGURE 37.19. Hyperkeratotic hydroquinone-induced ochronosis (late stage).

prolonged photodamage, the skin becomes hypertrophic and hyperkeratotic (Fig. 37.19).

These changes are irreversible even after cessation of the use of hydroquinone-containing cosmetics.

Hydroquinone-induced ochronosis needs to be differentiated from melasma, drug-induced hyperpigmentation, and the erythema abigne on the face of local cooks.[26]

Hypertension and diabetes are two very common diseases in Nigeria; hence, thiazide diuretics and chlorpropamide are commonly consumed photosensitizing drugs that cause hypermelanosis. Proguanil (paludrine) is also a common antimalarial consumed for prophylaxis, particularly among sickle cell patients. In these later conditions, there is no change in the texture of the skin apart from the discoloration; the color change is also reversible after withdrawal of the causative drug. The occupational history would suggest the cause of the pigmentation; the texture of the skin is also unaltered.

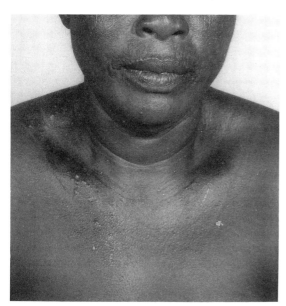

FIGURE 37.18. Hydroquinone-induced ochronosis with colloid milia (early stage).

Steroid Acne

Topical corticosteroid preparations are also
used as skin-lightening cosmetics. Hence, recalcitrant acne, folliculitis, and striae are
common sequelae. The folliculitis are frequently
seen on the posterior axillary folds (Fig. 37.20),
whereas the striae are found largely on the
axillary folds, shoulder, upper trunk, and thighs
(Fig. 37.21). Facial hypertrichosis is also a
frequent accompaniment of steroid acne.

Dermatitis Cruris Pustulosa et Atrophicans (Oil Acne, Sychosis Cruris, Vaselinoderma)

Clark[26] in 1952, lucidly described a pustular
dermatosis on the pretibial region among
Nigerian patients, and descriptively called it
dermatitis cruris pustulosa et atrophicans
(DCPA). Various reports have subsequently
emerged.[27,28] The exact etiopathogenesis is not
certain, but it is attributed to the regular use of
very oily pomades like petroleum jelly (Vaseline)
brilliantine, coconut oil, palm kernel oil, or shea
butter. When these oils block the hair follicles,
a chain of events (similar to acne vulgaris) sets

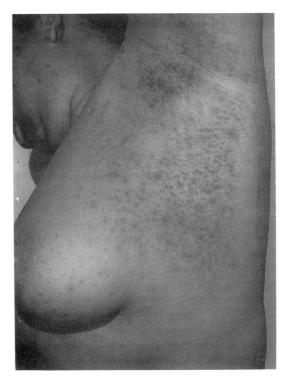

FIGURE 37.20. Corticosteroid-induced folliculitis.

in; pathogenic organisms, if found, are probably
secondary invaders. The shins appear to be more
vulnerable because of the erect nature of the
hairs on this part of the body, but there appears
to be individual predisposition to the develop-

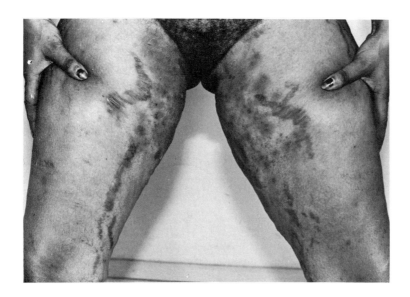

FIGURE 37.21. Corticosteroid-induced striae.

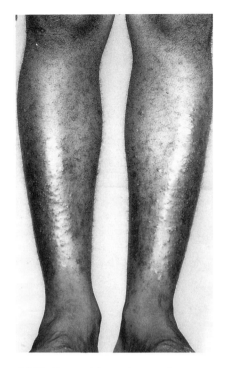

FIGURE 37.22. Dermatitis cruris pustulosa et atrophicans.

ment of this type of acne as the majority use them without adverse effects.

Clinically, the skin of the affected shins appears shiny and taut with loss of skin markings. There are follicular papules and pustules (Fig. 37.22). At times it is pruritic. With healing, there is postinflammatory dyschroia. The condition is notoriously chronic, but some patients respond to low-dose, long-term broad spectrum antibiotics and topical preparations used for acne vulgaris.

Irritant dermatitis from various brands of antiseptic soaps is common. There is an erroneous belief that all skin diseases are caused by germs, a belief largely promoted by manufacturers of assorted brands of "medicated" or "antiseptic" soaps. The people also believe that the longer the soaps stay on the skin, the more effective they are in cleansing the skin, so the soaps are simply rubbed on the skin and left on overnight; some people actually rub the soaps sparingly on the skin after daily bath to prevent skin disease. Some of the soaps contain

mercury, and pigmentation from cumulative toxicity sometimes develop.

Photodermatitis from assorted herbal concoctions, which are taken orally or used for a bath, is a common occurrence. Herbal concoctions invariably contain psoralen-type photosensitizers. The Fagara species and the genus *Citrus* (C) belong to the Rutaceae family which contains photosensitizing furocoumarins. The Fagara wood and *C. aurantifolia* (lime) are fairly constant ingredients of herbal concoctions in Nigeria. Other common photosensitizers are topical antihistamines and buclosamide.

Dermatophytid is frequently seen because of the widespread use of penicillin topically and systemically. Penicillin ointment is erroneously regarded as a panacea for skin diseases by the people and is one of the first-line drugs for self-medication in skin diseases.

Patients who patronize the herbalists for skin diseases are given sulfur paste, fresh garlic paste, or herbal concoctions. If it is a fungal infection, sulfur paste or garlic often suffice, but the frequency of contact dermatitis to these preparations and poor cosmetic acceptability make them not universally acceptable.

Sulfur or garlic (Allium sativum) have been used as folk medicine. The herbalist often instructs the patients to use a razor blade or sandpaper or abrasive sponge to scrape the lesion before applying the above preparations. This may account for the frequency of contact dermatitis, and "id" reactions.

Ampicillin is the most commonly prescribed antibiotic by general medical practitioners. It is, hence, the commonest cause of drug eruption. Patients with pityriasis rosea are particularly intolerant to ampicillin.[30]

Pseudofolliculitis Barbae (Barber's Rash)

This condition affects essentially men with tight coiling, kinky hair. When the free end of the hair is sharpened by the shaving process, it acts like a hook and penetrates the epidermis. This results in foreign-body inflammatory reaction in the dermis. The role of bacteria is secondary.

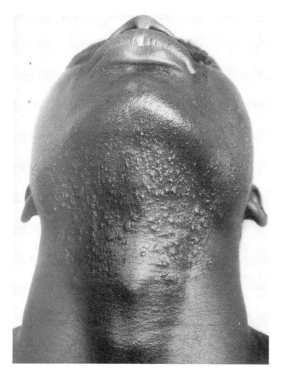

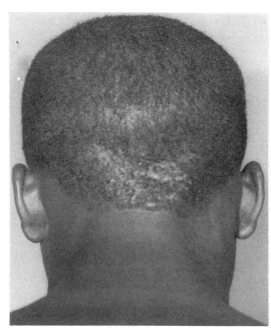

FIGURE 37.24. Folliculitis keloidalis nuchae (early lesion).

FIGURE 37.23. Pseudofolliculitis barbae.

Clinically, it is characterized by 1–2-mm papules and sometimes papulopustules (Fig. 37.23). The lesion may be slightly pruritic, painful, and bleeds easily with shaving. A postinflammatory hyperpigmentation results. Hypertrophic or keloidal scarring may result.

Folliculitis Keloidalis Nuchae (Sycosis Nuchae; Acne Keloidalis; Dermatitis Capillaris Capillittii)

This is a fairly common condition affecting young adult men and appears to have the same pathogenesis as pseudofolliculitis barbae, that is, a foreign body reaction to ingrown hair. The effect of the barber's blade and constant friction from stiff collars are trigger factors on the predisposed individual with kinky hair.

This condition regularly affects the nape of the neck. It begins as large comedons which become follicular papules and pustules pierced by hairs (Fig. 37.24). Keloid formation slowly appears at

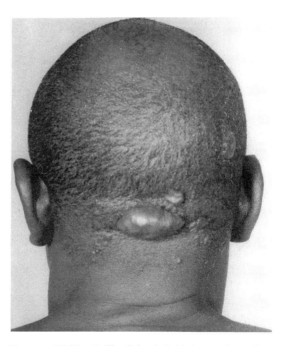

FIGURE 37.25. Folliculitis keloidais nuchae (late lesion).

the base of the papule and invades the papulopustule. The coalescence of lesions forms irregularly shaped, hard, keloidal masses, located transversely across the nape (Fig. 37.25). Abscesses and draining sinuses may occur. The development of large masses takes several years. At the onset, it may be asymptomatic, but later it becomes pruritic and tender.

The treatment of this condition is not very satisfactory. Intralesional triamcinolone injection is not easily achieved through the hard keloidal lesion as most of the drug is spilled. A better result is achieved if the keloidal lesion is first pared down with a scalpel blade before attempting the intralesional injection. A dermo-jet is ideal for the intralesional injection. As an adjuvant, a potent topical corticosteroid–antibiotic ointment could be applied twice daily during the intervals between the weekly intralesional injections. The prekeloidal pseudo-folliculitis are treated like acne vulgaris with long-term low-dose antibiotic and benzoyl peroxide.

Seborrheic Dermatitis

The infantile and adult type of seborrheic dermatitis are frequently seen. Erythema is not a prominent feature as in Caucasians. There is marked postinflammatory hypopigmentation (Figs. 37.26 and 37.27). This pigment loss and the associated scaling are the dominant clinical features. In the adult, a "butterfly" hypopigmentation on the face (Fig. 37.28) is a common presentation, particularly in men. The infantile type is frequently complicated by candidal infection.

Dermatosis Papulosa Nigra

This is a nevoid condition unique to the black race. Dermatosis papulosa nigra (DPN) is quite common among Nigerians and tends to be familial. The lesions are small, firm, discrete,

FIGURE 37.26. Infantile seborrheic dermatitis with complicating candidiasis.

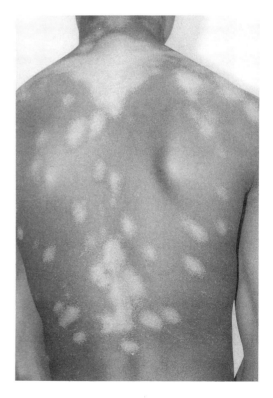

FIGURE 37.27. Seborrheic dermatitis in the adult.

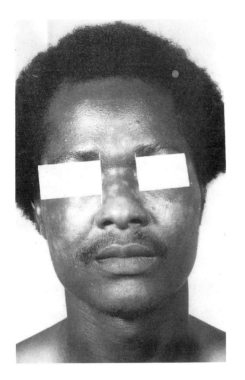

FIGURE 37.28 "Butterfly" hypopigmentation in adult seborrheic dermatitis.

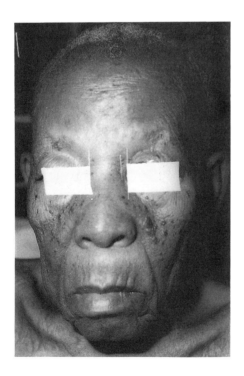

FIGURE 37.29. Dermatosis papulosa nigra.

smooth, globoid, black papules and nodules (Fig. 37.29) distributed mainly on the malar and lateral orbital areas. They may extend to the upper back and chest. At times, it may be disseminated. The lesions usually start to erupt just before puberty and rapidly increase in number over several months or years and then become static and remain for life.

Histologically, they are akin to seborrheic keratosis,[31] but clinically they are distinct from lusterless, greasy verrucous seborrheic keratoses, which are rarely seen among Nigerians.

The majority has recognized the nevoid and familial nature of DPN, and most of those affected do not seek medical attention. Some who are disturbed because of its cosmetic appearance do consult, but are simply advised to leave them alone, as locally available methods of surgical removal tend to leave unsightly scars.

Sarcoidosis

The various presentations of sarcoidosis in Nigeria have been documented.[32–35] Scar sarcoid, manifested by enlargement of scarification marks or tribal marks, is the commonest and earliest cutaneous manifestation (Figs. 37.30 and 37.31). Cutaneous scarification with razor blades is a therapeutic procedure used by native herbalists in Nigeria before the application of herbal concoctions. Recent tumifaction of these old scarification scars is a noteworthy sign.

None of our patients had lupus pernio. Because this is partly temperature dependent, it is unlikely to be seen in a hot tropical country like Nigeria.

Erythema nodosum is also rarely seen. The presence of erythema nodosum in association with sarcoidosis has been linked to HLA-B8, but the incidence of this haplotype among Nigerians is unknown. Cook and Carter[35] have observed that erythema nodosum from whatever cause is generally rare among West Africans. Several reports on sarcoidosis among various black populations[36,37] (except West Africa) have consistently observed that blacks have more

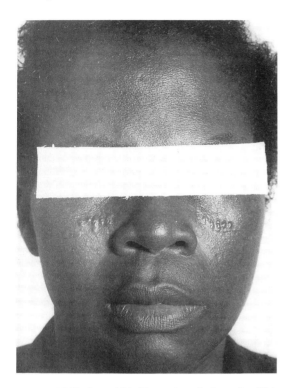

FIGURE 37.30. Sarcoid infiltrate in tribal marks. This patient also had facial palsy from parotid gland involvement.

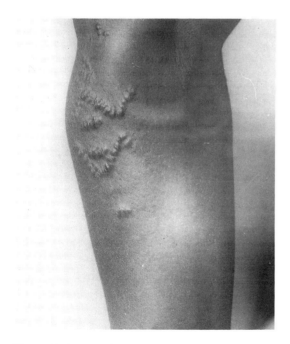

FIGURE 37.31. Sarcoid infiltrate in tribal tattoo marks.

atypical cutaneous expressions and also experience a more fulminant course. These aggressive types are not seen among Nigerians.

References

1. Clarke GHV: Skin diseases in a developing tropical country. *Br J Dermatol* 1962;**74**: 123–126.
2. Shrank AB, Harman RRM: The incidence of skin diseases in a Nigerian teaching hospital dermatology clinic. *Br J Dermatol* 1966;**78**:235–241.
3. Okoro AN: Skin diseases in Nigeria. *Trans St John's Hosp Dermatol Soc* 1973;**59**:68–72.
4. Fekete E: The pattern of diseases of the skin in the Nigerian guinea savanna. *Int J Dermatol* 1978;331–338.
5. Olumide YM: A Pictorial Self-instructional Manual on Common Skin Diseases. Ibadan, Nigeria, Heinemann, 1990.
6. Soyinka F, Hossain MZ, Abayomi IO: Epidemiology of Onchocerciasis in the Savannah and Rainforest Areas in Nigeria. Proceedings of the First Pan African Congress of Dermatology. African Association of Dermatology. Dar Es Salaam, Tanzania, 1981: 45.
7. Bryceson AAM, Van Veen KS, Oduloju AJ, et al. Antigenic diversity among Onchocerca vulvulus in Nigeria, and immunological differences between onchocerciasis in the savanna and forest of Cameroon. *Clin Exp Immunol* 1976;**24**:168–176.
8. Jopling WH: Onchocerciasis presenting without dermatitis. *Br Med J* 1960;**1**:861.
9. Acholonu ADW: Onchocerciasis in Nigeria. Proceedings of the First Pan African Congress of Dermatology. African Association of Dermatology. Dar Es Salaam, Tanzania, 1981: 46.
10. Ngu JL, Blackett K: Immunological studies in onchocerciasis in Cameroon. *Trop Geogr Med* 1976;**28**:111–120.
11. Henson PM, Mackenzie CD, Spector WG: Inflammatory reactions in onchocerciasis: a report of current knowledge and recommendations for further studies. *Bull WHO* 1979;**57**: 667–682.
12. Yarzabal L: The immunology of onchocerciasis. *Int J Dermatol* 1985;**24**:249–258.
13. Brown KR, et al: Clinical trial and treatment schedules in onchocerciasis. *Acta Leiden* 1990;**59**: 169–175.
14. Argyll-Robertson D: Case of Filaria loa in which the parasite was removed from under the conjunctiva. *Trans Ophthal Soc UK* 1989;**15**: 137–167.

15. Marriott WRV: Loiasis. *Int J Dermatol* 1985;**24**: 329–332.
16. Muller R: Control and treatment of guinea worm disease. *Postgrad Doctor (Africa)* 1981;**3**:292–295.
17. Williams CD: Kwashiorkor. *JAMA* 1953;**153**: 1280–1285.
18. Handa PK: Meaning of 'Kwashiorkor.' *Medi Dig* 1992;**18**:53–54.
19. Hitch J, Lund H: Disseminate and recurrent infundibulofolliculitis. *Arch Dermatol* 1972;**105**: 580–583.
20. Olumide YM: Contact dermatitis in Nigeria. *Contact Dermatitis* 1985;**12**:241–246.
21. Olumide YM: Some studies on contact dermatitis and occupational dermatoses in Lagos. MD thesis, University of Ibadan, 1990.
22. Olumide YM: Contact dermatitis in Nigeria 1. Hand dermatitis in women *Contact Dermatitis* 1987;**17**:85–88.
23. Findlay GH, Morrison JGL, Simson IW: Exogenous ochronosis and pigmented colloid milium from hydroquinone bleaching creams. *Br J Dermatol* 1975;**93**:613–622.
24. O'Donoghue MN, Lynfield YL, Derbes V: Ochronosis due to hydroquinone. *J Am Acad Dermatol* 1983;**8**:123.
25. Olumide YM, Elesha SO: Hydroquinone induced exogenous ochronosis. *Nigerian Med Practit* 1986;**11**:103–106.
26. Olumide YM, Odunowo BD, Odiase AO:

27. Clarke GH: A note on dermatitis cruris pustulosa et atrophicans. *Trans R Soc Trop Med Hyg* 1952;**46**:558–559.
28. Jacyk WK: Clinical and pathological observation in dermatitis cruris pustulosa et atrophicans. *Int J Dermatol* 1978;**10**:802–807.
29. Olumide YM, Odunowo BD, Odiase AO: Regional dermatoses in the African black. III. Pretibial lesions. *Int J Dermatol* 1991;**30**:186–189.
30. Olumide YM: Pityriasis rosea in Lagos. *Int J Dermatol* 1987;**26**:234–236.
31. Hairston MA Jr., Reed J, Derbes VJ: Dermatosis papulosa nigra. *Arch Dermatol* 1964;**89**:655–658.
32. Ogunlesi TO, Rankin TB: Sarcoidosis in West Africa. *J Trop Med Hyg* 1961;**64**:318–320.
33. Femi-Pearse D, Odunjo EO: Sarcoidosis in the Nigerian. A report of five cases. *Trop Geogr Med* 1973;**25**:130–138.
34. Olumide YM, Bandele EO, Elesha SO: Cutaneous sarcoidosis in Nigeria. *J Am Acad Dermatol* 1989;**21**:1222–1224.
35. Cook G, Carter R: Sarcoidosis in the West African: a report of 3 cases. *Br J Dis Chest* 1960;**60**:23–27.
36. Irgang S: Sarcoidosis in the Negro. *Cutis* 1969;**5**:823–829.
37. Sartwell PE: Racial differences in sarcoidosis. *Ann NY Acad Sci* 1976;**278**:360–370.

Regional dermatoses in the African. I. Facial hypermelanosis. *Int J Dermatol* 1991;**30**:186–189.

38

Rwanda

Eric Van Hecke

The Country and the People

Rwanda is a small country in Central Africa with an area of 26,000 km^2. It has a high population density: 290 habitants/km^2. The population has grown very fast in recent years: from 4.8 million at the 1978 census to an estimated 7.5 million in 1991.

Most Rwandese live in huts disseminated over the land. They live on their ancestral land and eat the crops they grow, mainly yams and beans. The cattle they herd is not for food consumption but is considered an investment, not unlike Westerners investing in bonds, shares, and gold. These people wear traditional clothing, the children often school uniforms; they walk barefoot. They have no schooling after primary school and speak only Kinyarwanda, the national language. They are considered farmers. We refer to this social group as rural population.

Cities are of recent venues in Rwanda. Only 4% of the population live in cities; nevertheless, they grow rapidly but are still rather small. The university city of Butare had 12,000 inhabitants in 1979 and now has a population of 30,000. In the cities, a substantial number of the inhabitants earn an income in the public service, the army, the university, in small private enterprises, and in commerce. These people dress in European fashion, wear shoes and glasses, use soap and cosmetics, and drive cars, motorcycles, or bicycles. The live in brick-built houses. They have had schooling after primary school and speak a European language, usually French. We refer to this social group as the urban population.

The Medical Organization and the Pharmaceutical Dilemma

The University of Rwanda is located in Butare. The faculty of medicine runs the University Hospital. It has an entire Rwandese staff. The dermatologic section is headed by a European-trained Rwandese dermatologist. It is housed since 1980 in a separate building with a facility for hospitalization (16 beds) and with an outpatient clinic. There is running water, electricity, and telephones. Bacterial and mycological examination including culture can be performed, a biopsy specimen can be taken, and small tumors can be treated. The general laboratory of the hospital carries out blood tests including serology for syphilis. HIV serology is done in a separate laboratory. The hospital's pharmacy delivers dermatologic preparations for a symbolic fee; however, flaws in supply are many, and often the patients do not obtain the prescribed medication or in insufficient quantity. Efforts are made to provide basic dermatologic preparations such as Whitfield's lotion and ointment, salicylic acid ointment, benzylbenzoate solution, lindane ointment, eosine and gentian violet solutions, a shake lotion, a corticosteroid cream, an antimicrobials cream, and a liquid for wet dressings. Oral and parenteral medication is limited to inexpensive antimicrobials such as penicillin, tetracycline, sulfonamides, and dapsone. Griseofulvin, corticosteroids, and modern antifungals and antimicrobials are virtually unobtainable.

Wealthy citizens can get their prescriptions filled by the private pharmacies at a cost. Most people cannot afford this. Moreover there is a black market of highly sophisticated drugs of the Western pharmaceutical companies. These are sold by the unit for high prices, for example, one pill of fluconazole costs 8 US$. This practice does not contribute in any way to the health of the buyer because only a few pills can be bought.

Most patients rely initially on traditional medicine. Traditional healers (umuvuzi) use, in addition to incantations and charms, a variety of topical and oral preparations of vegetal origin. Attempts have been made to separate active ingredients from endogenous plants used in traditional medicine. Two pharmacologically active preparations are marketed for dermatological use, one as treatment for scabies and one as treatment for pityriasis versicolor.[1,2] These medications have, in addition to their putative activity, the advantage of being produced within Rwanda at low cost. This contributes substantially to the economic development of the country.

Diseases of the Skin

There have been reviews on skin disease in Rwanda by Dockx and Ntabomvura,[3] Van Hecke and Bugingo,[4] by Dockx et al.,[5] and Harelimana and Bugingo.[6] The author also had information on the hospital statistics for 1989.[7] Because a civil war broke out in Rwanda in 1990, more recent information is lacking.

These surveys are not entirely comparable because they include different sections of the population. Nevertheless, they teach us that dermatological disease is essentially the same as in any other part of the world. However, in all surveys, a majority of skin disease is infectious (Table 38.1). Another constant fact is a different disease pattern in the rural and the urban population (Table 38.2).

Parasitic Disease

Among parasitic infection scabies is extremely prevalent. It is often widely impetiginized. Often, all members of the family are affected because they live together in intimate contact in small huts. Treatment failure is the rule, one of the reasons being that the patients do not succeed in treating the whole family because of the shortage of medication in the pharmacy. Tungiasis is very common and treated by the

TABLE 38.2. Common skin disease in Rwanda according to socioeconomic situation.

| Urban population |
| Venereal disease |
| HIV disease |
| Tinea pedis |
| Contact dermatitis |
| Aggressive Kaposi's sarcoma |
| Rural population |
| Tinea capitis |
| Tinea versicolor |
| Symptomatic keratoderma of the feet |
| Endemic Kaposi's sarcoma |

TABLE 38.1. Infectious Dermatologic Disease in Rwanda over a Period of Twenty Years.

	Dockx and Ntabomvura[3]	Van Hecke and Bugingo[4]	Harelimana and Bugingo[6]	Bugingo[7]
Year	1971	1980	1988	1989
All infections	74%	67%	26.5%	51.6%
Scabies	15.1%	29.9%	8.44%	14.4%
Mycoses	34.2%	22.45%	7.67%	9.26%
Tinea capitis	29.75%	13.3%	2.8%	3.7%
Tinea Versicolor		8.6%	3.24%	1.8%
Impetigo	7.3%	3.8%	5.14%	5.4%

people themselves. Pediculosis capitis is rare in black children. Onchocerciasis is very rare.

Mycoses

Mycoses are very prevalent. Most important are tinea capitis and versicolor. Tinea capitis is very common in children. The differences in frequency of tinea capitis in the surveys is dependent on the inclusion of school visits. The cause of microsporic tinea capitis is *Microsporum langeroni*, whereas the cause of trichophytic tinea capitis is *Trichophyton violaceum*.[8,9] Variation of prevalence of the fungi has been noted by Dockx:[8] the higher the patients lived in the hills, the more *T. violaceum* was found, whereas *M. langeroni* prevailed in the plains Trichophytic tinea capitis is not only found in children but also in adult women. No effective treatment is given because oral antifungals are scarce or not available at all.

Tinea versicolor is a common skin disease in young adults in the countryside. They complain most of light brown depigmented finely scaling macules of the face, neck, chest, and arms, clearly visible on the black skin. This is most conspicuous because they walk barechested.

Tinea versicolor is a common skin disease in young adults in the countryside. They urban population. Treatment of these superficial mycoses is done with Whitfield's lotion and ointment.

Deep mycoses are exceptional in Rwanda. There have been reports of sporotrichosis, histoplasmosis, blastomycosis and chromoblastomycosis.

Bacterial Infection

Bacterial infections are very common in Rwanda as in the rest of the world; however, impetigo occurs often as a widespread pyoderma with crusts and pustules. Very often, scabies is the underlying cause. Topical antiseptics, antibiotic creams, and parenteral penicillin are the available treatments. Leprosy does not contribute substantially to dermatological disease in the surveys. Since 1971, "Father Damian's Friends," the charitable organization with headquarters in Brussels, has organized the detection and follow-up of leprosy patients. As a result, the number of registered leprosy patients has gradually declined from the original 1000 in 1971.

Yaws (frambesia tropica) has been reported from marshlands. A few cases of gangosa have been reported.

Viral Infection

Viral diseases contribute to 7% of the dermatologic clinics at the university hospital of Butare. Remarkable is the occurrence of widespread common warts not only on the hands or feet but also on the arms and legs. Mollusca contagiosa equally shows widespread involvement.

Clinicians have noticed that during the eighties, the number of some viral diseases has risen. These diseases present in a more severe form, do not respond well to therapy, and relapse often. This is most evident with herpes zoster. In 1980, in 2819 patients, Van Hecke and Bugingo[4] did not have one case of herpes zoster. In 1989, Bugingo[7] noted 48 or 1.7% of herpes zoster in 2806 patients.

In 1990, Harelimana and Bugingo[10] found that 90% of all patients presenting with herpes zoster are HIV antibody positive. Among 617 HIV antibody positive patients, 240 or 39% had herpes zoster as primary manifestation of immune impairment. They conclude that herpes zoster is a common and early manifestation of HIV infection in Rwanda. They proposed using herpes zoster as an indicator of HIV infection prevalence.

HIV antibody positivity is also very high in other viral diseases of the skin such as herpes simplex, molluscum contagiosum, and condylomata accuminata (see Table 38.3).

In Rwanda, HIV infection is a most important health problem. Surveys on HIV antibody prevalence in the population show a very high percentage of seropositivity. There is a marked difference between the rural and the urban population.

Bugingo et al.[11] conducted a representative survey over the entire country and found 1.7%

TABLE 38.3. Dermatologic disease and HIV infection in Rwanda 1985–1990.

	n	HIV antibody positive
Herpes zoster	401	367 (92%)
Herpes simplex	58	51 (88%)
Molluscum contagiosum	38	32 (84%)
Condylomata acuminata	170	119 (70%)
Prurigo	205	185 (90%)
Seborrheic dermatitis	54	49 (91%)
Tinea corporis	59	50 (85%)
Oral candidiasis	40	38 (95%)
Aggressive Kaposi's sarcoma	34	34 (100%)
Urticaria	42	22 (52%)
Generalized pruritus	32	22 (69%)
Furunculosis	59	46 (78%)

Source: Reference 16.

prevalence in the rural population and a 18.1% prevalence in the urban population. The capital cities of the 10 provinces and 2 more cities were considered to be urban. In some boroughs of Kigali, the nation's capital, seropositivity ranks as high as 1 out of 3 inhabitants. Butare, the university city, has a 16% seropositivity. Most affected is the age group between 22 and 45, men and women equally. The mode of infection is mainly heterosexual contact, but transfusions of infected blood and injections with infected needles contribute to the spread of the HIV virus.

Clinically, HIV infection presents with viral infections as herpes zoster, nonhealing herpes simplex, and widespread molluscum contagiosum. Seborrheic dermatitis, widespread pruriginous lesions (Fig. 38.1), and relapsing forms of folliculitis are also very common. In contrast, oral candidiasis, hairy leukoplakia, and aggressive Kaposi's sarcoma are less common than in comparable HIV antibody positive patients in America and Europe.

Sexually Transmitted Diseases

Veneral disease ranks high in all surveys. It is diagnosed more frequently in the urban population than in the rural population. Syphilis is rather common, with 0.7% of the diagnoses in 1971, 1.9% in 1980, and 2.6% in 1989. Gonorrhea is equally common: 5.9% in 1980 and 0.6% in 1990. Chancroid was not mentioned in the 1971 survey, but an epidemic was reported in 1976.[12] The 1980 survey found 2.9% in the urban population, whereas the 1989 survey only comes to 0.24%. These figures suggest a wave of infection starting in the early seventies but gradually declining later. A most important phenomenon is the appearance of HIV infection in the beginning of the eighties. As early as 1982, wealthy Rwandese came to Belgian hospitals with AIDS. Since then, HIV infection has spread to large sections of the urban population.

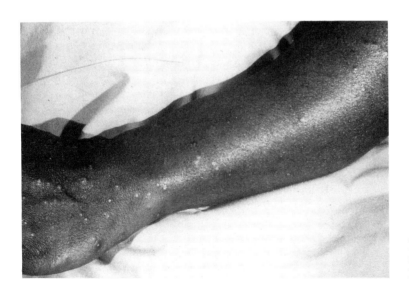

FIGURE 38.1. Kaposi's sarcoma in a 30-year-old Rwandese man.

Dermatitis

Dermatitis is a common diagnosis in dermatology in Rwanda; in the surveys, some 10–15% of patients have this diagnosis.

Contact dermatitis is very common. The cause is often traditional medication of botanical origin externally applied or highly allergenic topical medication such as penicillin ointment and neomycin-containing preparations. Contact dermatitis is much more common in the urban population.

Seborrheic dermatitis was recognized in the past as a rather uncommon condition [4 in 2819 patients[4]]. Recently, it has become much more common [51 in 2806 patients[7]]. Because 91% of the patients with seborrheic dermatitis are HIV antibody positive, most of the present cases can be considered an expression of HIV disease.

Symptomatic keratoderma of the feet is a very common disorder of adult women living in the countryside. These people do not wear shoes and do most of the labor in the fields. The mechanical factors are considered to be the cause of the hyperkeratosis with often painful fissures.

Tumors

Skin tumors are quite important in the pathology statistics. Most skin tumors are squamous cell carcinomas, often occurring in long-lasting leg ulcers. Basal cell carcinomas and melanomas are seldom found.

The pathology laboratory of the University of Butare reports 653 biopsies of malignant tumors for the years 1976–1978;[13] 112 or 17.5% are skin tumors and 35 or 5.4% are Kaposi's sarcoma. The proportional rate of Kaposi's sarcoma in 1979–1982 was 6.3% and in 1983–1986 was 6.5%.[14] Kaposi's sarcoma in Rwanda is thus much more prevalent than in Western or Arab central and eastern Africa such as Zaire, Burundi, and Uganda. Several types of the African endemic Kaposi's sarcoma have been described.

In a survey of 119 cases of Kaposi's sarcoma diagnosed in the pathology department of Butare, 89% had skin lesions and 11% were extracutaneous, mainly with involvement of the

TABLE 38.4. Anatomical locations of 119 cases of Kaposi's sarcoma.

Skin involvement	106 (89%)
Localized	
Lower extremities	66 (55.5%)
Upper extremities	11 (9.2%)
Lower and upper extremities	7 (6%)
Back	1
Scrotum	1
Eyelid	1
Generalized	15 (12.6%)
Extracutaneous	13 (11%)
Lymph nodes	10
Mouth	1
Gastrointestinal tract	2

Source: Reference 14.

lymph nodes (Table 38.4). In this series, HIV serology was done in 18 patients. The 8 HIV antibody positive patients all had generalized aggressive Kaposi's sarcoma. The 10 HIV antibody negative patients all had localized skin involvement.[14]

Harelimana and Bugingo[15] reviewed 44 cases of Kaposi's sarcoma between 1985 and 1990. Serology for HIV antibody was done in all. Seropositivity was found in 34. These patients had aggressive Kaposi's sarcoma, belonged to the higher socioeconomic class of the urban population, and had a mean age of 52 years. They had a mean survival of 2 years (Fig. 38.2). The seronegative patients had slowly growing Kaposi's sarcoma of the extremities, belonged to the lower socioeconomic class of the rural population, and had a mean age of 52 years. They survived for many years.

Conclusions and Recommendations

The characteristics of the dermatological situation in Rwanda can be summarized as follows:

1. Presence of all types of dermatological disease with preponderance of infectious disease.
2. Shortage of skilled personnel, apparel, and drugs to make correct diagnoses and to treat even readily curable disease.

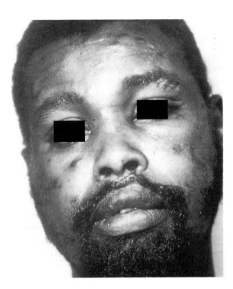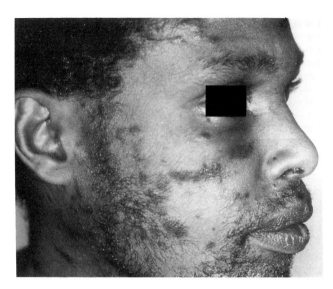

FIGURE 38.2. Pruriginous disease. Chronic pruriginous disease in a 39-year-old black man, HIV antibody positive.

From the medical point of view, it is obvious how to intervene:

1. Health care personnel should be trained in recognizing and treating scabies, tinea, syphilis, and other common diseases.
2. Simple adequate and cheap medication should be provided.
3. Programs aimed at one particular health problem may be more fruitful than individual care. A good example is the leprosy program. It seems easy to conduct programs for venereal disease, scabies, and tinea capitis. The industrial cities of Europe and America were able to control tinea capitis in schoolchildren long before griseofulvin was introduced. Syphilis had decreased a great deal even before the development of Salvarsan.
4. An especially great threat to the Rwandese society of today is the HIV infection. A whole section of the young adult population faces eradication. The propagation of the virus is intimately linked to sexual behavior and secondarily to insufficient knowledge of aseptic medical care. There is a need for a large-scale program aimed at the education of the population to understand the ways of infection of the HIV virus including the free distribution of condoms.

Medical care is not only a matter of a patient and a health worker; it is a matter of the whole society. The Rwandese society becomes poorer and poorer every year and the standard of medical care decreases proportionally.

The population explosion is uncontrolled. There is no reason to believe it will be under control in the near future. Economical progress is thus not to be expected and this is the necessary support for developing medical care. As a consequence, a reservoir of infectious human disease will persist in central Africa. This is a threat to the health of all human beings on the globe.

References

1. Van Puyvelde L, Hakizayezu D, Bogaerts J, De Vroey C: Activité anti-Pityrosporum ovale d'un extrait des racines de Pentas longiflora. Colloque international sur la recherche et al production de médicaments à base de plantes medicinales, Kigali (Rwanda), February 26–March 3, 1990.
2. Van Puyvelde L, Heyndrickx G, Brioen P, et al: Development of an anti-scabies drug from the roots of Neorantanenia mites. International Joint Symposium on Biology and Chemistry of Active

Natural Substances, Bonn (Germany), July 17–22, 1990.

3. Dockx P, Ntabomvura V: Incidence des maladies cutanées dans la préfecture de Butare. *Rev Med Rwandaise* 1971;**3**:5–7.

4. Van Hecke E, Bugingo G: Prevalence of skin disease in Rwanda. *Int J Dermatol* 1980;**19**:526–529.

5. Dockx P, De Brauwere D, De Weert, J, et al: Maladie cutanées. In: Meheus A et al, eds. *Santé et maladies au Rwanda.* Wilrijk, Belgium: Universitaire Instelling Antwerpen, 1982:657–669.

6. Harelimana F, Bugingo G: Traitement des dermatoses les plus fréquentes à l'hôpital Universitaire de Butare. *Rev Med Rwandaise* 1988; **20**:102–109.

7. Bugingo G: Personal communication, 1990.

8. Dockx P: The clinical picture of dermatophytoses in Rwanda and Burundi. *Ann Soc Belg Med Trop* 1969;**49**:457–464.

9. Bugingo G: Dermatrophic infection of the scalp in the region of Butare (Rwanda). *Int J Dermatol* 1983;**22**:107–108.

10. Harelimana F, Bugingo G: Herpes zoster and HIV infection in Rwanda. Abstract Th B 448, Volume 1 Abstracts, Sixth International Conference on AIDS, San Francisco, June 20–24, 1990.

11. Bugingo G, Ntilivamunda A, Nzaramba D, et al: Etude sur la séropositivité liée à l'infection au virus de l'immunodéficience humaine au Rwanda. *Rev Med Rwandaise* 1988;**20**:37–42.

12. De Weert J: Ulcus molle: Klinische studie van een epidemie in Butare. *Ned Tijdschr Geneesk* 1976;**120**:2021.

13. M. Bonyingabo P: Service d'anatomo-pathologie. In: Santé et maladies au Rwanda. Meheus A, et al, eds. Wilrijk, Belgium: Universitaire Instelling Antwerpen, 1982;780–782.

14. Ngendahayo P, Mets T, Bugingo G, Parkin DM: Le sarcome de Kaposi au Rwanda: aspects clinico-pathologiques et épidémiologiques. *Bull Cancer* 1989;**76**:383–394.

15. Harelimana F, Bugingo G: Kaposi's sarcoma and AIDS in Rwanda. Abstract 128, Seventeenth International Congress of Chemotherapy, Berlin, June 23–28, 1991.

16. Harelimana F, Bugingo G: Can some skin disease serve as sentinel signs for HIV epidemic in Rwanda? Abstract MB 2244, Abstract Book Volume 1, Seventh International Conference on AIDS, Florence, June 16–21, 1991.

39

South Africa

E. Joy Schulz

The Republic of South Africa is known for its generally temperate climate and abundance of sunshine. It consists of four provinces, the Cape, Orange Free State, Natal, and Transvaal (Fig. 39.1). Along the western coast, the country is arid and sparsely populated. The more densely populated eastern coastal belt has a more humid climate that becomes subtropical toward the north. The central part of the country is generally flat and dry. To the north, the land rises to form a mountainous plateau known as the Transvaal Highveld. One-third of the urban population of the country is concentrated in the Transvaal. The largest city, Johannesburg, is situated 6000 ft above sea level at a latitude of 26°S and has on average 8.6 h of sunshine daily.

The population comprises four main groups —black, white, mixed race (so-called colored) and Asian. The black population consists of several ethnic groups with different languages and customs. The largest group consists of the Nguni-speaking tribes (Zulu, Xhosa, and Swazi) who constitute more than half of the black population. The second largest group consists of the Sotho and Tswana, whereas the Tsongo (Shangaan) and Venda form two additional groups that are much smaller. The first white immigrants came from the Netherlands when the Dutch East India Company established a settlement at the Cape of Good Hope in 1652. These were followed by French, British, and Germans. The South African Dutch established the Protestant Dutch Reformed Church and developed a language of their own. Known as Afrikaners, they form 54% of the white

population. The coloreds have a mixture of European, Hottentot, and Malay ancestry. The Asian population consists mainly of descendents of emigrants from India who first came to work in Natal in the 1860s.

In 1992, the total population of South Africa was estimated to be about 390 million, comprising 75% blacks, 14% whites, 10% coloreds, and 2% Asians. The population ranges from a developing black rural community living under poor socioeconomic third world conditions to an urbanized white community with a first world standard of living. Rapid, explosive urbanization and population growth with a great need for employment, housing, and infrastructure are features of present-day black society. Although most have access to modern medicine, a large proportion of both the rural and urban black population first consults traditional healers ("witch doctors") with the result that many patients are seen with advanced, florid disease.

Common Skin Disorders

The relative frequency of common skin disorders according to comparable recent surveys is shown in Table 39.1.[1–5] Dermatitis is by far the commonest skin diseases in all races, its incidence being particularly high in Indians. Seborrheic dermatitis is diagnosed twice as frequently as atopic dermatitis. Photosensitive seborrheic dermatitis occurs in all races but seems to be most common in Indians, in whom

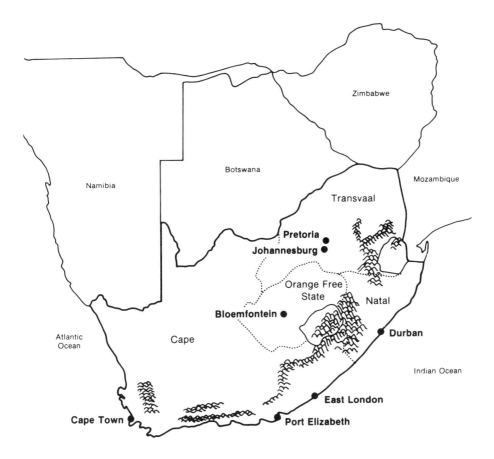

FIGURE 39.1. Map of South Africa.

photosensitizing foodstuffs are sometimes suspected to play a role. Chronic actinic dermatitis
of the actinic reticuloid type and hydroa
aestivale are rarely, if ever, diagnosed. Polymorphic light eruption occurs only in whites.

Notable racial differences are seen in some
skin disorders. Black patients have an incidence
of pityriasis rosea double that of other races,
often with more florid and widespread eruptions. Erythema multiforme and its severe forms,
Stevens-Johnson syndrome and toxic epidermal
necrolysis, also occur more frequently in
blacks. The incidence of psoriasis in blacks is
half that in other races. The incidence and
severity of psoriasis is greatest in Indians. In a
recent survey, the incidence of lichen planus was
found to be much higher in blacks than in other
races.[1] In black patients with lichen planus,
buccal involvement is rarely encountered, but

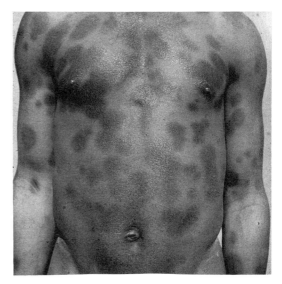

FIGURE 39.2. Fixed drug eruption due to phenolphthalein. Multiple residual slatey macules.

the lips tend to be involved. Some cases of cheilitis initially diagnosed on biopsy as lichen planus eventually turn out to be lupus erythematosus. Lichen planus tropicus is seldom diagnosed.

The incidence of drug eruptions, urticaria, and discoid lupus erythematosus is similar in all races. Vitiligo occurs more frequently in Indians.[5] Fixed drug eruptions due to phenolphthalein are common in blacks (Fig. 39.2). Lichenoid drug eruptions, mainly due to antihypertensive drugs, are seen in all races. A common skin disorder that does not appear in Table 39.1 is exogenous ochronosis due to creams containing hydroquinone.[6] Sooty pigmentation and black caviar-like papules occur on the sun-exposed parts of the face and neck (Figs. 39.3 and 39.4). Dermatitis due to bleaching creams accounted for 6.5% of dermatological consultations in a survey done in 1982.[1] Subsequently, the amount of hydroquinone allowed in bleaching creams was restricted to 2% and the incidence and severity of exogenous ochronosis is declining. Contact dermatitis due to industrial and household allergens appears to be similar in incidence and type in all races. The commonest cause of plant dermatitis is an indigenous shrub unique to South Africa,

TABLE 39.1. Common skin disorders in various races in South Africa, percentage of dermatological outpatients.

Disease	Black	White	Colored	Asian
Dermatitis	29.0[a]	28.8[b]	22.4[d]	39.0[e]
	22.7[c]	17.7[d]		
Acne	11.3[a]	10.0[b]	9.1[d]	9.0[e]
	6.0[c]	11.4[d]		
Bacterial	4.8[a]	2.5[b]	8.2[d]	11.0[e]
infections (coccal)	11.4[c]	3.1[c]		
Superficial	5.5[a]	3.7[b]	8.1[d]	7.0[e]
fungal infections[f]	4.6[c]	5.3[d]		
Scabies	4.3[a]	1.0[b]	12.8[d]	2.0[e]
	11.0[c]	5.5[c]		
Pityriasis rosea	2.4[a]	1.0[b]	0.9[d]	1.0[e]
	2.0[c]	1.0[d]		
Erythema multiforme	2.3[a]	1.0[d]	1.4[d]	0.3[e]
	2.0[c]			
Psoriasis	1.8[a]	4.0[b]	5.3[d]	5.0[e]
	0.7[c]	4.3[d]		
Warts	1.8[a]	4.0[b]	8.5[d]	2.0[e]
	2.0[c]	5.3[d]		
Lichen planus	1.7[a]	0.7[b]	0.6[d]	0.1[e]
	0.7[c]	0.6[d]		
Drug eruptions	1.5[a]	0.8[b]	1.4[d]	0.1[e]
	1.0[c]	1.2[d]		
Urticaria	1.3[a]	2.0[b]	2.3[c]	2.0[e]
	1.0[c]	1.9[d]		
Lupus erythematosus	1.2[a]	0.8[b]	1.1[d]	0.4[e]
(mainly discoid)	1.0[c]	0.9[d]		
Vitiligo	0.8[a]	0.8[b]	1.6d	2.0[e]
	0.5[c]	0.9[d]		

[a] From Ref. 1.
[b] From Ref. 2.
[c] From Ref. 3.
[d] From Ref. 4.
[e] From Ref. 5. Values are extrapolated.
[f] Includes candidosis, tinea versicolor, and dermatophyte infections.

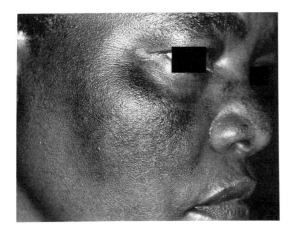

FIGURE 39.3. Cosmetic ochronosis. Hyperpigmentation and small black papules in a relatively mild case.

Smodingium argutum, which belongs to the same family as poison ivy. Like poison ivy, the plant has attractive multicolored autumn foliage, and the dermatitis it causes is usually severe. It has caused several outbreaks of dermatitis among school children.[7]

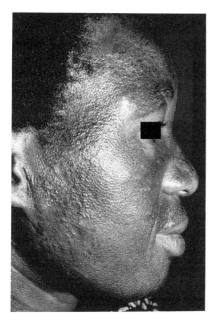

FIGURE 39.4. Cosmetic ochronosis. More severe involvement with larger papules.

Connective Tissue Disorders

The incidence of discoid lupus erythematosus (LE) is similar in blacks, whites, and coloreds[1–4] but appears to be less in Indians, at least in the Transvaal.[5] Systemic LE is common in all races,[8–10] but the incidence is lowest in whites.[8] In Johannesburg, LE accounts for 80% of all systemic connective tissue disorders in black patients. Acute fulminating forms of systemic LE and lupus profundus appear to be more common in blacks.

Morphea and generalized scleroderma are relatively uncommon in all races. Systemic scleroderma with diffuse involvement is the type most often seen in blacks.[11] An occupational form of systemic sclerosis related to exposure to silica-containing dust occurs in gold miners.[12] It is characterized by the presence of interstitial lung disease and by the rarity of Raynaud's phenomenon, dysphagia, and renal involvement.

Dermatomyositis has been estimated to be 10 times more common in blacks than in whites, at least in the Transvaal.[13] In blacks, most cases occur in early- and mid-adult life and there is no association with carcinoma.[13]

Bullous Disorders

Bullous disorders appear to be more common in black South Africans than in other races. In the Johannesburg area, 44% of bullous disorders in blacks are due to bullous pemphigoid and 26% to the pemphigus group. Pemphigus vulgaris and pemphigus foliaceus are diagnosed with equal frequency, but some cases show transitional forms and are not easily classifiable. Linear IgA dermatosis is seen in both adults and children, but dermatitis herpetiformis has not yet been diagnosed in black patients in Johannesburg. Linear IgA dermatosis of childhood is common in black children in Natal.[14]

Nutritional Disorders

Maize, which is deficient in essential amino acids, is the staple diet of most black South Africans and kwashiorkor is still seen regularly in infants. Pellagra in adults is now seen mainly in black male alcoholics, who occasionally also develop alcoholic neuropathic changes in the feet that need to be differentiated from leprosy. In leprosy, the upper limbs are involved first and show evidence of advanced motor and sensory disturbance by the time both feet are affected.

Infections

Sexually Transmitted Diseases

Venereal disease is particularly common in the black population in whom chancroid is the main cause of genital ulceration, followed by syphilis. Congenital syphilis is seen regularly in black neonates. Endemic syphilis occurs mainly in the arid impoverished parts of the Orange Free State.[15] Granuloma inguinale is endemic in South Africa, most cases occurring in the Eastern Transvaal and Natal.[16] Lympho-granuloma venereum is uncommon, at least in the urban population.

By the middle of 1992, 1186 cases of AIDS had been reported in South Africa of which 53% were due to heterosexual contact. The African type of HIV infection is increasing, most cases presenting with pulmonary tuberculosis. Herpes zoster is the initial manifestation in three quarters of patients presenting with dermatological disease.[17]

Fungal Infections

Tinea versicolor is more common in blacks and Indians than in whites.[1,3,5] Dermatophyte infections show some racial and geographical differences, which were reviewed by Vismer and Findlay in 1988.[18] Tinea capitis is most common in black children, mainly due to *Trichophyton violaceum*. Usually visible only as a mild scaling, it is often undiagnosed and untreated and spreads easily among household contacts and at school. Scalp ringworm due to *Microsporm audouini* is uncommon, occurring only in black children. Favus due to *T. shoenleini* is extremely rare today. Almost all cases of tinea capitis in white children are due to *M. canis*. *T. rubrum* is the predominant organism found in other dermatophyte infections, at least in Natal and the Transvaal. *T. rubrum* infections, tinea pedis, and tinea cruris are extremely rare in blacks.

Of the deep fungal infections, sporotrichosis is by far the commonest, most cases occurring in the Transvaal and Natal. Sporotrichosis previously occurred in epidemic form in the gold mines of the Witwatersrand due to contaminated timber props,[19] but it is now mainly due to occupational and recreational exposure to soil and plants. It occurs mainly in the lymphatic form and less often as a single warty or ulcerated granulomatous plaque. Disseminated cutaneous forms and bony involvement are extremely rare. Chromomycosis is seen mainly in Natal and much less frequently in the Transvaal and eastern Cape.[20] Cases of mycetoma are relatively rare. Most are of the soft grain type due to *Nocardia asteroides*; the hard black grain mycetoma due to *Madurella mycetomatis*[21] is less common. Blastomyces dermatitidis infections are rare in South Africa. The granulomatous ulcers, sinuses, and underlying lung involvement are usually mistaken for tuberculosis.[22]

Tuberculosis

Pulmonary tuberculosis is rife in the black population with over 70,000 new cases reported per year. In comparison, cutaneous tuberculosis and tuberculides are relatively rare. Of the true infections, lupus vulgaris and scrofuloderma are commonest; warty tuberculosis and tuberculosis gummas are seldom diagnosed.

Most cases of tuberculosis skin disease consist of papulonecrotic tuberculides.[1] Starting as firm papules, they soon form pustules and crusts and heal to leave round to oval atrophic scars (Fig. 39.5). Lesions are characteristically multiple and symmetrical, with a tendency to be grouped over the buttocks, knees, elbows, shins, and on the ears. The tuberculin test is strongly positive and an underlying tuberculous focus is often found. Papulonecrotic tuberculides have been seen in association with so-called idiopathic gangrene of the extremities in Africans, which is likely to be of tuberculous origin.[23] Nodular vasculitis and erythema induratum are frequently encountered on the lower legs in healthy, often obese young women. In spite of a strongly positive tuberculin

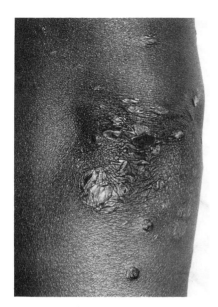

FIGURE 39.5. Papulonecrotic tuberculides. Crusted papules and atrophic scars over elbow.

test, no underlying infection is demonstrable, but the skin lesions respond to anti-tuberculous treatment. This observation, made by Scott in 1972,[24] is still true today. Abdominal or genitourinary tuberculosis is often suspected in these young women but seldom confirmed. Lichen scrofulsorum is occasionally seen, either alone or together with papulonecrotic tuberculides. Lesions consist of small firm papules in a grouped or diffuse distribution on the trunk and limbs, and tuberculoid granulomas are seen on biopsy.

Leprosy

In 1992, about 200 new cases of leprosy were diagnosed in the Republic of South Africa, an incidence of 0.5 per 100,000 of the population. At Westfort Hospital, Pretoria, the sole remaining institution specializing in leprosy, half of the newly diagnosed patients were classified as lepromatous or borderline lepromatous. Some observations made at Westfort are of general interest. Alopecia, either patchy or diffuse, is seen regularly in lepromatous leprosy. Rare cases of Lucio's phenomenon have been observed in both nodular and diffuse forms of advanced, untreated lepromatous leprosy. Pa-

tients with widespread, well-circumscribed, depigmented macules that show only mild, nonspecific histological changes and no bacilli on skin biopsy are usually classifiable as borderline lepromatous leprosy on nerve biopsy. A few South African cases of pure neuritic leprosy have been confirmed on nerve biopsy at Westfort.

Viral and Rickettsial Diseases

South African tick bite fever is a common rickettsial disease due to *R. conori* var. *pijperi*. Veld rodents are the natural reservoir, and the infection is transmitted to man by ixodid ticks. The infection is usually mild in young persons but may run a fulminating fatal course particularly in elderly patients.[25] It is characterized by fever, photophobia, severe headache, and a generalized maculopapular rash that involves the palms and soles. A black eschar is usually visible at the site of the bite, accompanied by enlarged regional lymph glands. The disease responds well to tetracycline within 48 h.

Three arbovirus infections—Sindbis, West Nile, and chikungunya fever—are known to cause human outbreaks in the northern parts of the country. They occur when mosquitoes are abundant after periods of unusually high rainfall. All three are associated with widespread maculopapular rashes on the trunk and limbs, including the palms and soles. Sindbis and West Nile infections cause a mild disease with transient joint and muscle stiffness.[26] Chikungunya fever is accompanied by polyarthritis equally affecting large and small joints which may be intensely painful and stiff. Patients with long-standing symptoms develop positive serological findings indicative of rheumatoid arthritis.[27]

Insects and Parasites

Papular urticaria is common in the summer months, particularly in the humid, subtropical, northern, and coastal regions. It is mainly due to fleas, less often to mosquitoes, and rarely to ticks and bedbugs. Dermatitis from caterpillars and beetles, spider bites and long-lasting, intensely itchy granulomas following tick bites are far less common, occurring mainly in visitors to rural areas and game parks. Cutaneous myiasis due to the larvae of *Cordylobia anthropophaga* is seen in Natal and the northern Transvaal. Sandworm (larva migrans) infestations, due to the dog and cat hookworm *Ankylostoma brasiliense* are commonly acquired on beaches in Natal but are also encountered in other parts of the country.

Schistosomiasis is endemic in Natal and most parts of the Transvaal and eastern Cape. Occasionally, ectopic ova cause itchy granulomas in the skin, mainly in the perineal area. In an occasional patient with chronic urticaria, positive serological tests for schistosomiasis have been found and the urticaria has cleared after treatment with praziquantel. Amoebic dysentery is common in Natal, but skin lesions, which consist of chronic granulomatous ulcers in the perineal region, are extremely rare.

Skin Tumors

Skin cancer accounts for 36% of all cancers in whites and 15% in blacks.[28] The white population has a high incidence of sun-induced skin lesions with an incidence of solar keratoses and basal and squamous cell carcinoma similar to that of Australia.[29] Although basal cell carcinomas account for over half of skin cancers in whites,[28] they are seldom diagnosed in the other races. Rare cases of basal cell carcinoma in blacks are regarded as nevoid in origin. Squamous cell carcinoma is relatively common in blacks, mainly related to burns or chronic ulcers and infections but are sun-induced in albinos.

The incidence of malignant melanoma and the sites involved in whites are similar to those in other parts of the world. Malignant melanoma is 2.5–6 times more common in blacks than in whites and is rare in the other racial groups.[30] In blacks, most melanomas occur on the soles and palms and are usually diagnosed at a late stage. These melanomas may be related to the presence of racially determined pigmented macules, which are found in these sites in about 60% of black South Africans.[31]

Kaposi's sarcoma of the classic endemic type involving the extremities has always been relatively common in black South Africans particularly in the Transvaal and Natal. Dermatofibrosarcoma is far more common in blacks than in whites.[28]

The occurrence of benign tumors in the various racial groups is similar to that in other parts of the world. Dermatosis papulosa nigra is common in blacks, coloreds, and Indians. Nevocellular nevi are found in about 70% of the black population in Johannesburg but are never a presenting complaint. Eruptive syringomas on the eyelids are notably more common in young black women than in any other group.

Miscellaneous Disorders

Sarcoidosis

The incidence of sarcoidosis per 100,000 population in the Cape peninsula has been estimated at 23.2 in blacks, 11.6 in coloreds, and 3.7 in whites.[32] In black patients, erythema nodosum due to sarcoidosis is uncommon, but direct skin involvement is six times more common than in whites.[33] Severe necrotizing and mutilating forms with ulceration of skin lesions and bony destruction of hands and feet have been described in black patients.[34] Even in the absence of ulceration, skin biopsies in black patients with sarcoidosis may show significant histological evidence of necrosis, which is mistakenly interpreted as being due to tuberculosis. The tuberculin test remains the most useful means of differentiating between the two diseases.

Pityriasis Rotunda

Pityriasis rotunda is a well-known incidental finding in black patients undergoing investigation for debilitating diseases such as tuberculosis. Recent observations have shown that in South Africa hepatocellular carcinoma is the commonest cause, followed by tuberculosis and chronic benign hepatic disease.[35] Lesions are asymptomatic, usually occur on the trunk, and consist of large, round, well-circumscribed,

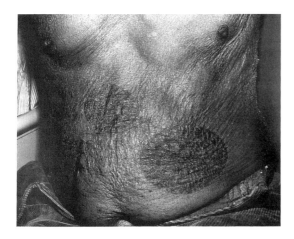

FIGURE 39.6. Pityriasis rotunda.

hyperpigmented macules with a superficial ichthyosiform scale (Fig. 39.6).

Pyoderma Gangrenosum

Pyoderma gangrenosum has been reported in black patients in association with Crohn's disease and ulcerative colitis. The later is being recognized with increasing frequency in this group of the population.[36]

Genetic Disorders

Genetic disorders are common in all races due to inbreeding, and in whites also to the so-called founder effect. This is seen when limited numbers of ancestors have been responsible for large numbers of descendants with a prevalence of certain diseases higher than in the original stock. Notable among these are familial hypercholesterolemia in Afrikaners and Jews and diabetes mellitus in Indians. The Afrikaners have so far remained a well-defined group with a unique genetic constitution and genealogical studies in this population are facilitated by the fact that birth and marriage registers have been kept by the Dutch Reformed Church since 1675.

Porphyria

Porphyria cutanea tarda (PCT), due to liver damage, is most common in blacks. In the past, it was mainly the result of iron overload due to

the consumption of liquor home-brewed in iron pots. Its incidence has decreased considerably since the 1970s when blacks were first allowed to buy "white" liquor. In whites, the commonest type is porphyria variegata (PV), an autosomal dominantly inherited disorder that has been traced back to a pair of Dutch settlers who married in the Cape in 1688.[37] Porphyria variegata may be asymptomatic or associated with intermittent acute attacks of abdominal and neuropsychiatric complaints, often precipitated by drugs, particularly barbiturates and sulphonamides. Skin changes in PV resemble those of PCT, with skin fragility and the formation of subepidermal blisters after minor trauma occurring mainly on the backs of the hands and fingers. In PV, the tendency to blister on sun-exposed skin first becomes evident in early adult life and decreases in late middle age. Slatey hyperpigmentation on sun-exposed parts and hypertrichosis involving the temples, forehead, and cheeks are seen in both PV and PCT (Fig. 39.7). Erythropoietic protoporphyria (EPP) is seen in white patients, although much less frequently than PV. The scarred, waxy appearance of the skin found in the late stage resembles

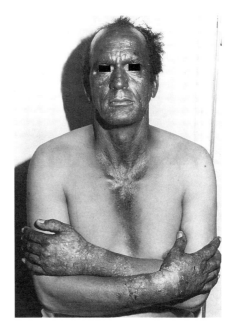

FIGURE 39.7. Porphyria cutanea tarda. Hyperpigmentation on sun-exposed parts. Blisters and scars on face, backs of hands, and arms.

lipoid proteinosis.[38] However, in EPP the skin changes are relatively mild and self-limiting and mucous membranes are not involved.

Lipoid Proteinosis

Due to the founder effect, South Africa has the highest prevalence rate of this autosomal dominantly inherited condition in the world. It occurs among Afrikaner whites and coloreds and no cases have been reported in blacks.[39] The characteristic hoarseness due to infiltration of the larynx is usually noticed soon after birth. Minor trauma and recurrent infections result in a worm-eaten appearance of the face and patchy alopecia of the scalp (Fig. 39.8).

Keratolytic Winter Erythema (Oudtshoorn Skin)

This autosomal dominantly inherited disorder appears to be unique to South Africa, occurring mainly in the Afrikaner population.[40] It is named "Oudtshoorn skin" after the district in the cape province that was the ancestral home to many of the affected families. Locally, it is also known as "Mostertvel" (Mostert skin), Mostert being a common surname among affected families. Keratolytic winter erythema (KWE) shows features similar to the genodermatose en cocarde of Degos and its likely origin was a French immigrant to the Cape Province.[40]

In KWE, only the skin is involved and the rash causes only mild discomfort. The sexes are equally affected with onset between early infancy and adulthood. Recurrent cyclical attacks of annular erythema and peeling always affect the palms and soles symetrically. In rare severe cases, the limbs and trunk are also involved, but the head is never affected. Individual lesions start as red macules that enlarge, coalesce, and spread peripherally in waves, often developing new central spots with the formation of concentric rings. The outer skin layers dry to form a firm elastic scale that peels off to leave a peripheral collarette placed within the erythematous advancing edge (Fig. 39.9). Individual lesions last 6–8 weeks after which the cycle is repeated. Two striking features are the seasonal occurrence, with attacks starting in early winter, and associated palmo-plantar sweating. Attacks are precipitated by cold weather, trauma, and fever. The condition improves after the age of 30 years and also during pregnancy. Treatment gives equivocal results, tar baths and ultraviolet light being perhaps the most effective. The effects of topical retinoic acid are yet to be evaluated.

Oculocutaneous Albinism

This autosomal recessively inherited disorder has a particularly high prevalence rate in black South Africans.[41] There is a great difference in prevalence between the two main black ethnic groups in South Africa (Sotho/Tswana and Nguni/Zulu). This is ascribed to different

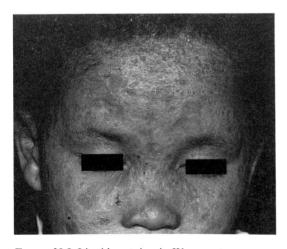

FIGURE 39.8. Lipoid proteinosis. Worm-eaten scars on face of a young colored girl.

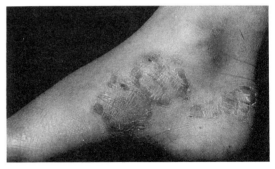

FIGURE 39.9. Keratolytic winter erythema. Plaques on side of foot with centrifugal scaling. (Photo courtesy of Dr. JGL Morrison.)

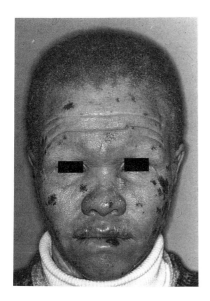

FIGURE 39.10. Tyrosinase positive albino with freckles.

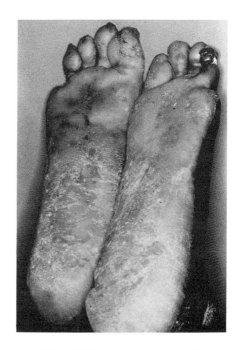

FIGURE 39.11. Diffuse plantar keratoderma with ainhum of toes.

customs regarding intermarriage, which is encouraged in the former but taboo among the latter.[41]

Tyrosinase positive OCA is by far the commonest type of albinism in South Africa. The tyrosinase positive albino, who has straw colored hair and brown eyes, often develops large arborescent, darkly pigmented freckles on sun-exposed skin (Fig. 39.10). Chronic solar damage with marked elastosis is apparent from an early age and multiple keratoses and skin cancers develop on sun-exposed parts. The risk of developing skin cancer appears to be less in patients with freckles.[42]

Other Genetic Disorders

Keratoderma involving the extremities is relatively common in black South Africans. Linear, punctate, and diffuse palmo-plantar types occur, the last sometimes associated with ainhum (Fig. 39.11). A fourth, rare type consists of pebbly papules on the sides and extensor surfaces of the hands and feet, often extending proximally onto the limbs. The punctate type of palmo-plantar keratoderma is the commonest (Fig. 39.12). It is often associated with hyperhidrosis. Lesions on the soles are often misdiagnosed and treated as plantar warts.

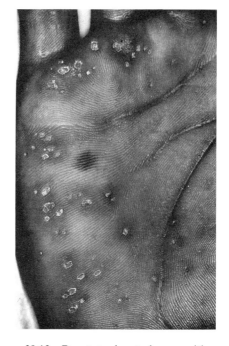

FIGURE 39.12. Punctate keratoderma with racial palmar pigmentation.

A type of lamellar ichthyosis with a distinctive distribution is seen in blacks.[43] The trunk, proximal part of the extremities, scalp, and temples are involved with almost complete sparing of the face, limbs, and buttocks. Two main types of epidermolysis bullosa are found in blacks in the Transvaal: dominant dystrophic and recessive lethal.[44] The recessive lethal type is commonest and about 10 cases are seen yearly in neonates in the Transvaal. Pseudoxanthoma elasticum is seen mainly in the Afrikaner population but also occurs in blacks.[45] Ehlers-Danlos syndrome is uncommon, occurring predominantly in Afrikaners. A single black patient is on record.[46] Xeroderma pigmentosum is rare, most known cases being in black children from rural districts in the Transvaal.

References

1. Schulz EJ: Skin disorders in Black South Africans. A survey of 5000 patients seen at Ga-Rankuwa Hospital, Pretoria. *S Afr Med J* 1982;**62**:864–867.
2. Findlay GH: The age incidence of common skin diseases in the white population of the Transvaal. *Br J Dermatol* 1967;**79**:538–542.
3. Park RG: The age distribution of common skin disorders in the Bantu of Pretoria, Transvaal. *Br J Dermatol* 1968;**80**:758–761.
4. Flöter W: Nume statistiese oorsig van velsiektes in die Wes-Kaap. *S Afr Med J* 1978;**53**:214–216.
5. Findlay GH, Park RG: Common skin diseases in the Transvaal: An analysis of 22,000 dermatological outpatient cases. *S Afr Med J* 1969;**43**:590–595.
6. Findlay GH, Morrison JGL, Simson IW: Exogenous ochronosis and pigmented colloid milium from hydroquinone bleaching creams. *Br J Dermatol* 1975;**93**:613–622.
7. Whiting DA: Plant dermatitis in the southern Transvaal. *S Afr Med J* 1971;**45**:363–367.
8. Jessop S, Meyers OL: Systemic lupus erythematosus in Cape Town. *S Afr Med J* 1973;**47**:222–225.
9. Dessein PHMC, Gledhill RF, Rossouw DS: Systemic lupus erythematosus in black South Africans. *S Afr Med J* 1988;**74**:387–389.
10. Seedat YK, Pudifin D: Systemic lupus erythematosus in Black and Indian patients in Natal. *S Afr Med J* 1977;**51**:335–337.
11. Pudifin DJ, Dinnematin H, Duursma J: Antinuclear antibodies in systemic sclerosis. Clinical and ethnic associations. *S Afr Med J* 1991;**80**:438–440.
12. Cowie RL, Dansey RD: Features of systemic sclerosis (scleroderma) in South African goldminers. *S Afr Med J* 1990;**77**:400–402.
13. Findlay GH, Whiting DA, Simson IW: Dermatomyositis in the Transvaal and its occurrence in the Bantu. *S Afr Med J* 1969;**43**:694–697.
14. Aboobaker J, Wojnarowska FT, Bhogal B, Black MM: Chronic bullous dermatosis of childhood—clinical and immunological features seen in African patients. *Clin Exp Dermatol* 1991;**16**:160–164.
15. Scott FP, Lups JGH: Endemiese sifilis. *S Afr Med J* 1973;**47**:1347–1350.
16. Freinkel AL: The enigma of granuloma inguinale in South Africa. *S Afr Med J* 1990;**77**:301–303.
17. Karstaedt AS: AIDS—the Baragwanath experience. Part III. HIV infection in adults at Baragwanath Hospital. *S Afr Med J* 1992;**82**:95–97.
18. Vismer H, Findlay GH: Superficial fungal infections in the Transvaal. *S Afr Med J* 1988;**73**:587–592.
19. Findlay GH: The epidemiology of sporotrichosis in the Transvaal. *Sabouraudia* 1970;**7**:231–236.
20. Findlay GH: Chromoblastomycosis caused by the Simson species of Hormodendrum. *S Afr Med J* 1957;**31**:538–540.
21. Findlay GH, Vismer HF: Black grain mycetoma. *Br J Dermatol* 1974;**91**:297–303.
22. Berkhowitz I, Diamond TH: Disseminated Blastomyces dermatitidis infection in a nonendemic area. A case report. *S Afr Med J* 1987;**71**:717–719.
23. Morrison JGL, Fourie ED: The papulonecrotic tuberculide from Arthus reaction to lupus vulgaris. *Br J Dermatol* 1974;**91**:263–270.
24. Scott FP: Skin diseases in the South African Bantu. In: Marshall J, ed. Essays in Tropical Dermatology, Vol. 2. Amsterdam: Excerpta Medica, 1972:1–17.
25. Gear JHS, Miller GB, Martins H, et al: Tick-bite fever in South Africa. The occurrence of severe cases on the Witwatersrand. *S Afr Med J* 1983;**63**:807–810.
26. Findlay GH, Whiting DA: Arbovirus exanthem for Sindbis and West Nile viruses. *Br J Dermatol* 1968;**80**:67–74.
27. Fourie ED, Morrison JGL: Rheumatoid arthritic syndrome after chikungunya fever. *S Afr Med J* 1979;**56**:120–132.
28. Rippey JJ, Schmaman A: Skin tumours of

Africans. In: Marshall J, ed. Essays on Tropical Dermatology, Vol. 2. Amsterdam: Excerpta Medica, 1972:98–115.

29. Whiting DA: Skin tumours in White South Africans. Part I. Patients, methods and incidence. *S Afr Med J* 1978;**53**:98–102.

30. Rippey JJ, Rippey E: Epidemiology of malignant melanoma of the skin in South Africa. *S Afr Med J* 1984;**65**:595–598.

31. Freinkel AL, Rippey JJ: Foot pigmentation in blacks. *S Afr Med J* 1976;**50**:2160–2161.

32. Benatar SR: Sarcoidosis in South Africa. A comparative study in Whites, Blacks and Coloureds. *S Afr Med J* 1977;**52**:602–606.

33. Smith C, Feldman C, Reyneke J, et al: Sarcoidosis in Johannesburg—a comparative study of black and white patients. *S Afr Med J* 1991;**80**:523–427.

34. Morrison JGL: Sarcoidosis in the Bantu. *Br J Dermatol* 1974;**90**:649–654.

35. Berkowitz I, Hodkinson HJ, Kew MC, Di-Bisceglie AM: Pityriasis rotunda as a cutaneous marker of hepatocellular carcinoma: a comparison with its prevalence in other diseases. *Br J Dermatol* 1989;**120**:545–549.

36. Smith EH, Essop AR, Segal I, Posen J: Pyoderma gangrenosum and ulcerative colitis in black South Africans. *S Afr Med J* 1984;**66**:341–343.

37. Dean G, Barnes HD: Porphyria in Sweden and South Africa. *S Afr Med J* 1959;**33**:246–253.

38. Findlay GH, Scott FB, Cripps DJ: Porphyria and lipid proteinosis. A clinical, histological and biochemical comparison of 19 South African cases. *Br J Dermatol* 1966;**78**:69–80.

39. Heyl T: Lipoid proteinosis. I: The clinical picture. *Br J Dermatol* 1963;**75**:465–472.

40. Findlay GH, Morrison JGL: Erythrokeratolysis hiemalis—keratolytic winter erythema or 'Oudtshoorn Skin.' A new epidermal genodermatosis with its histological features. *Br J Dermatol* 1978;**98**:491–495.

41. Kromberg JGR, Jenkins T: Prevalence of albinism in the South African Negro. *S Afr Med J* 1982;**61**:383–386.

42. Kromberg JGR, Castle D, Zwane EM, Jenkins T: Albinism and skin cancer in Southern Africa. *Clin Genet* 1989;**36**:43–52.

43. Scott FP, Lups JGH: Badbak-distribusie van lamellere igtiose in die Bantoe. 'n Nuwe entiteit. *S Afr Med J* 1974;**48**:2449–2453.

44. Menter MA, Patz IM: The pattern of epidermolysis bullosa in the Transvaal Bantu. *Br J Dermatol* 1971;**85**(suppl 7):32–36.

45. Jacyk WK, Lodder JV, Dreyer L: Pseudoxanthoma elasticum in South African black patients. A report on 7 cases. *S Afr Med J* 1988;**74**:184–186.

46. Winship IM: Ehlers-Danlos syndrome in the Western Cape. *S Afr Med J* 1985;**67**:509–511.

Japan

Yoshiki Miyachi

Variations observed in skin diseases in Japan result from several factors that make them occasionally quite different from those seen in other areas of the world. This chapter is devoted to how skin diseases are affected by climate, geography, genetics, nationality, and socioeconomic factors in Japan.

Climate

Japan is located in the temperate region with the typical four seasons as well as a rainy season. In summer, the days are very muggy, which keeps the intertriginous skin regions moist. This may be why many patients present fungal infections. Many foreigners, especially from Western countries, suffer from tinea cruris and pedis for the first time in Japan. On the other hand, the past four decades after World War II witnessed the remarkable development of air-conditioning network systems both at home and in the office. Thus, the skin is kept dry with subsequent occurrences of dry skin and so-called asteatotic dermatitis of the aged, especially in winter. This phenomenon also results from the excessive use of soap and friction from nylon towels (see friction melanosis). Actinic skin damages such as photoaging and photo-carcinogenesis have drawn public attention in recent years. Because of our photoprotective skin type, the incidence of skin cancers in sun-exposed area still remains much lower than in Caucasians. There exist sun worshipers who appreciate tanned skin, and the incidence of actinic skin cancers is increasing year by year. It is very important even in Japan to educate the public about the dangers of sun exposure.[1]

Geography

Major geographic skin diseases in Japan include the following conditions.

1. Adult T-cell leukemia (ATL). ATL is a new disease entity of T-cell malignancy with characteristic cutaneous and hematologic features and is geographically distributed in southwestern Japan, the Caribbean region, and the southeastern United States. In the most prevalently affected area of Japan, almost 15% of the population are reported to be carriers of human T-cell lymphotropic virus type I (HTLV-I).[2] Cutaneous-type ATL is proposed[3] and should be diagnosed by dermatologists.

2. Tsutsugamushi disease (Scrub typhus). This disorder is a type of rickettsiosis mediated by *Leptotrombidium* and characterized by fever, skin eruption, and the history of insect bites. Minocycline is used as a first-choice drug.

3. Japanese spotted fever. This belongs to the group of spotted fever rickettsioses and the symptoms consist of fever and skin eruption. Tetracyclines are also effective.

4. Izumi fever. This is a *Yersinia pseudotuberculosis* infection and shows characteristic scarlet-fever-like symptoms. Differential diagnosis includes Kawasaki disease (mucocutaneous lymph node syndrome) and drug eruption. ABPC is a choice for treatment.

Genetics

Because Japan is an island country surrounded by the ocean and has a rather monoclonal race, the incidence and characteristics of some cutaneous disorders are different from other parts of the world, presumably due to the genetic difference.

Table 40.1 summarizes world-wide accepted dermatologic conditions found by Japanese. Most of them are reported mainly in Japan, which may reflect the genetic background. Recent available review articles are cited.[4-7] As for the difference in commonly encountered skin diseases, the following comments are possible.

1. Psoriasis. The incidence of psoriasis in Japanese is much lower than in Caucasions, but the number of patients who visit dermatologic clinics is increasing to 2% of the total outpatient population, although psoriatric arthritis is rare. The drastic changes in life style, especially with the introduction of Western cuisine, must have contributed to the dramatic increase of patients with psoriasis after World War II. Administration of eicosapentaenoic acid, which might provide improvement of psoriasis, is now seriously considered even in Japan.[8]

2. Behçet's disease. Behçet's disease is unusually common in Japan, probably in association with HLA B51. Of interest is the high incidence of Behçet's disease in the region around the Mediterranean Sea and the countries along the Silk Road. Although unique treatments such as colchinine and cyclosporin A have been developed, it still remains a refractory disease.

3. Malignant melanoma. The number of patients with malignant melanoma in Japan is increasing recently, however, the most common type is acral lentiginous melanoma (47.4%). Nodular melanoma and superficial spreading melanoma account for 32.5% and 13.3%, respectively. Lentigo maligna melanoma accounts for only 6%. This proportion is quite different from Caucasoids. In addition, over 30% of malignant melanoma occurs on the soles though the total incidence of cutaneous melanoma is much lower than in Caucasoids.

4. Skin types. Japanese skin types for sun exposure belong to types III–V, that is, the degree of erythema reaction (sunburning) is milder, but the ability to tan and to stimulate melanin pigmentation is deeper than for Caucasoids. This fortunate skin type results in lower incidence of actinic keratosis in the elderly people in Japan. Japanese skin types are proposed by Satoh et al.[9] accordingly. As far as the subgroups of xeroderma pigmentosa are concerned, Japan has more patients with group A, F, and variant than other countries.

5. Dermatitis herpetiformis. Duhring's disease is quite rare in Japan and linear rather than granular IgA deposition is common. The well-known complication of gluten-sensitive enteropathy is rarely observed and the common association with the HLA-B8 is not found in Japanese cases.

TABLE 40.1. World-wide accepted dermatologic conditions reported by Japanese.

Nevus fuscoceruleus ophthalmomaxillaris (Nevus of Ota)
Incontinentia pigmenti achromians (Hypomelanosis of Ito)
Acropigmentatio reticularis (Kitamura)
Eosinophilic pustular folliculitis[4]
Lipodystrophia centrifugalis abdominalis infantilis[5]
Prurigo pigmentosa[6]
Papuloerythroderma[7]
Eosinophilic lymphoid granuloma (Kimura's disease)
Mucocutaneous lymph node syndrome (Kawasaki's disease)

---

4. Nationalistic Considerations

Japanese people have imported Chinese and other Oriental cultures for the past 1200 years and, thus, they are still deeply affected by Chinese medicine. After the Meiji Restoration (1868), Japan learned much from German medicine and then, after World War II, from American medical science. This explains why the ordinary people still trust Oriental medicine, whereas younger physicians are enthusiastic about modern medical science. This gap in understanding the background of the diseases occasionally produces misunderstandings.

Effects of Oriental Culture

People still believe that most cutaneous disorders are induced by allergic or toxic reactions of foods. They always ask what is wrong with their foods. Even in atopic dermatitis, the significant role of food allergy is overestimated. They pay keen attention to natural products and Chinese herbs and use natural cosmetics even for the treatment of several skin diseases. They also believe that any skin eruption has something to do with internal diseases, especially with hepatic diseases. Over 90% of patients with urticaria wish to check their liver functions on their first visit to clinics. These phenomena never change despite the remarkable scientific progress in medical knowledge and technology.

Effects of Japanese Nationality

Japanese people are sticklers for cleanliness and, thus, they want to keep their skin very clean, resulting in the overuse of soap and a friction nylon towel. Because they are indifferent to the need for skin care to counteract dryness, there are many patients with dry skin and so-called friction melanosis.[10] A similar skin condition is also reported in the United States as nylon brush macular amyloidosis.[11]

Japanese people are very shy, and they hate to present genital skin lesions to dermatologists. It is believed that the reason for the poor prognosis of genital Paget's disease can be partly explained by their late consultation with specialists.

Effects of Western Culture

Japanese people used to desire a very pale coloring; however, the younger generation now worships sun-tanning. This trend may attribute to a possible increase in skin cancer induced by actinic damage in the future, in combination with ozone depletion. Dermatologists have organized the Japanese Committee for Solar UV Protection and have warned the public of the harmful effect of sunbathing.

Socioeconomic Factors

Drastic industrial and economic development in the past 40 years in Japan brought about several changes in socioeconomic facets of dermatological disorders. Many kinds of infectious skin diseases are now rarely observed due to improved public hygiene; however, skin diseases such as atopic dermatitis are increasing. Acute exanthems are frequently seen after adolescence and old-fashioned infectious diseases such as scabies and pediculosis are found as sexually transmitted diseases.

The proportion of the elderly people has been increased and, thus, skin diseases in old age are commonly seen in the clinic. These include not only malignant cutaneous disorders but also cosmetic or aesthetic dermatoses. Because of the newly developed costly drugs, older and less expensive drugs are not commonly used or even not available. For example, dapsone is very difficult to obtain, presumably due to the fact that pharmaceutical companies find it difficult to produce it profitably, even though dermatologists still want to use it.

Presentation of a Disease: Transfusion-Associated Graft-Versus-Host Disease

Synonyms

Postoperative erythroderma, post-transfusion GVHD.

Clinical Features

Transfusion-associated graft-versus-host disease (GVHD) is a rare complication after surgery for which blood transfusion has been required. Erythroderma as well as fever, pancytopenia, hepatic insufficiency, and diarrhea inevitably occur several days after the operation even in immunocompetent patients. Skin eruptions are nonspecific and it is impossible to make a differential diagnosis from drug eruptions by clinical appearance alone (Fig. 40.1). In spite of every effort of treatment, the outcome for patients remains almost always fatal. In Japan, a high incidence (1 in 300–400 in open heart

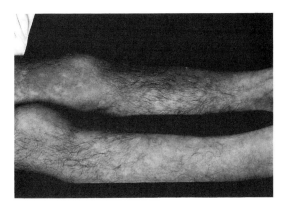

FIGURE 40.1. Clinical appearance of so-called postoperative erythroderma. Note nonspecific erythema on the legs.

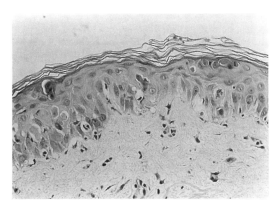

FIGURE 40.2. Typical lichenoid tissue reaction observed in the biopsy specimen (HE, × 200).

surgery) is reported. The etiology is assumed to be a type of GVH reaction caused by transfused lymphocytes.[12]

Variations in Japan

A retrospective Japanese survey identified 96 cases of GVHD in immunocompetent patients who underwent cardiac surgery. The incidence is 1 in 658.9 with a 90% mortality rate.[13] Although the disease is reported in Western countries,[14] the incidence in Japan is unusually high. Because the Japanese population is homogeneous, it is possible that blood transfusion (a lymphocyte graft) from a person homozygous for a certain HLA haplotype is given to a heterozygote for the same haplotype.

The host accepts the graft, the graft rejects the host, and GVHD ensues.[15]

Another reason for this high incidence in Japan seems to be attributable to the use of fresh, immediate-family blood donors. This increases the incidence of the dangerous HLA combination.

Diagnosis

Transfusion-associated GVHD is characterized by erythroderma, fever, liver dysfunction, diarrhea, and pancytopenia and develops in apparently immunocompetent patients who are transfused with fresh blood during surgery.[16] Because the skin eruptions are nonspecific, it is

absolutely required to make an exact diagnosis by skin biopsy. When frozen sections are stained with hematoxylin and eosin, typical lichenoid tissue reactions are observed showing a liquefaction denervation, exocytosis, and epidermal cytoid bodies (Fig. 40.2). Immunohistochemical studies demonstrate the predominant CD8$^+$ cytotoxic T-cell infiltration in the upper dermis (Fig. 40.3) and the disappearance of Langerhans cells. HLA-DR antigens are strongly expressed on the epidermal cell surface (Fig. 40.4). More direct diagnoses could be made by proving the replacement of the patient's peripheral lymphocytes by donated lymphocytes. This HLA phenotype examination may provide hard

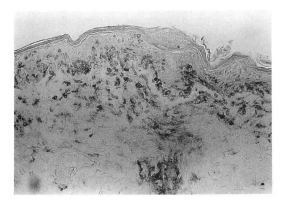

FIGURE 40.3. Infiltrating cells in the epidermis and upper dermis are CD8$^+$ cytotoxic T-cells (PAP, × 200).

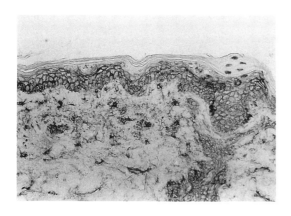

FIGURE 40.4. HLA DR antigens are strongly expressed in the epidermal cell surface (PAP, × 200).

evidence that postoperative erythroderma is a type of GVHD.[17]

Treatment

No successful treatment for transfusion-associated GVHD is available at present; it must be prevented either by using irradiated blood products or by using blood that has been stored for more than 10 days to allow lymphocytes to lose immunocompetence.

References

1. Miyachi Y, Yoshioka A, Imamura S, et al: The cumulative effect of continual oxidative stress to the skin and cutaneous aging. In: Kligman AM, Takase Y, eds. Cutaneous Aging. Tokyo: University of Tokyo Press, 1988:435–447.
2. Hinuma Y, Komada H, Chosa T, et al: Antibodies to adult T-cell leukemia virus associated antigen (ATLA) in sera from patients with ATL and controls in Japan. A nationwide seroepidemiologic study. Int J Cancer 1982;29:631–635.
3. Takahashi K, Tanaka T, Fujita M, et al: Cutaneous-type adult T-cell leukemia/lymphoma. Arch Dermatol 1988;124:399–404.
4. Ofuji S: Eosinophilic pustular folliculitis. Dermatologica 1987;174:53–56.
5. Imamura S, Yamada M, Yamamoto K: Lipodystrophia centrifugalis abdominalis infantilis. A follow-up study. J Am Acad Dermatol 1984;11:203–209.
6. Joyce AP, Horn TD, Anhalt GJ: Prurigo pigmentosa. Arch Dermatol 1989;125:1551–1554.
7. Ofuji S, Furukawa F, Miyachi Y, Ohno S: Papuloerythroderma. Dermatologica 1984;169:125–130.
8. Kojima T, Terano T, Tanabe E, et al: Long-term administration of highly purified eicosapentaenoic acid provides improvement of psoriasis. Dermatologica 1991;182:225–230.
9. Satoh Y, Kawada A: Action spectrum for melanin pigmentation to ultraviolet light and Japanese skin typing. In: Fitzpatrick TB, Wick MM, Toda K, eds. Brown Melanoderma. Tokyo: University of Tokyo Press, 1986:87–95.
10. Tanigaki T, Hata S, Kitano Y, et al: Unusual pigmentation on the skin over trunk bones and extremities. Dermatologica 1985;170:235–239.
11. Hashimoto K, Ito K, Kumakiri M, et al: Nylon brush macular amyloidosis. Arch Dermatol 1987;123:633–637.
12. Mori S, Kudo H, Ino T, et al: Postoperative erythrodermia, a type of graft-versus-host reaction? Pathol Res Pract 1989;184:53–59.
13. Juji T, Takahashi K, Shibata Y, et al: Post-transfusion graft-versus-host disease in immunocompetent patients after cardiac surgery in Japan. N Engl J Med 1989;321:56.
14. Decoste SD, Boudreaux C, Dover JS: Transfusion-associated graft-vs-host disease in patients with malignancies; report of two cases and review of the literature. Arch Dermatol 1990;126:1324–1329.
15. Ray TL: Blood transfusions and graft-vs-host disease. Arch Dermatol 1990;126:1347–1350.
16. Hidano A, Yamashita N, Mizuguchi M, et al: Clinical, histological and immunohistological studies of postoperative erythroderma. J Dermatol 1989;16:20–30.
17. Ito K, Yoshida H, Yanagibashi K, et al: Change of HLA phenotype in post operative erythroderma. Lancet 1988;1:413–414.

41

India

Patrick Yesudian

From the towering peaks of the Himalayas in the north to land's end down south at Cape Coumarin and between the fertile shore lines from the eastern to western ghats, there are nearly a billion people inhabiting the Indian subcontinent. Always pouring into India, from the dawn of history, were different kinds of people at completely different levels of culture, different colors—black, white, and yellow—and different religions, the vast majority of whom are followers of Hinduism but with a good number of Christians, Moslems, Jains, and Buddhists. The climate varies enormously—the biting cold of the Himalayan mountains, the cruel sun blazing down in the south, and the torrential rains and floods that affect the coastal areas. There are innumerable languages and dialects. There are conflicting contrasts in the economic front also, from the enormously rich living in palatial houses to the poorest living on pavements in semi-starvation and half-nudity. India is a country steeped in ancient traditions and folklore with even the highly educated resorting to traditional medicine when afflicted with chronic illnesses.

Some of the problems encountered by a practicing dermatologists in India are the extreme variations in color and culture. They must also contend with illiteracy with its attendant ignorance. Given the population explosion, overcrowding and poor nutritional state, infections, and infestations head the list of common skin diseases afflicting the majority of the population throughout the country. They are parasitic, bacterial, fungal, viral, protozoal, and helminthic, in that order of decreasing frequency.

Scabies

The itch-mite is undoubtedly the commonest parasite encountered in hospital practice in every part in India. In the Tamil Nadu (formerly Madras) State in the south, the incidence of scabies among the skin outpatient population is between 20 and 30%. The incidence is much lower among the affluent private-paying patients, evidently due to better personal hygiene, bathing facilities, and good nutrition. Though the diagnosis is made clinically with ease in most cases, at times problems arise in recognizing the disease—when patients have used corticosteroids topically, when they present with extensive crusted lesions, and when, as in the case of meticulously clean patients, the lesions are minimal and confined to the genital areas only. Scabies in the very young is also a diagnostic problem due to involvement of the scalp, face, palms, and soles. A high index of suspicion is required in correctly diagnosing scabies in developing countries.

The two important differential diagnoses are animal scabies and papular urticaria, because most slum dwellers have pet dogs that are infested with mites, ticks, and fleas.

Treatment is easy in individual cases, but it is at times a virtual impossibility to eradicate it from a family, a slum, a school, or a community because people are reluctant to apply medications when their skin is apparently normal. In addition, infected children, though successfully treated, quickly become re-infected at school and bring the parasite back into their homes.

The answer to this therapeutic frustration would be for a medical team with paramedical support to visit the schools, orphanages, hostels, or slums and supervise the treatment of the entire community. Brief talks on the importance of daily baths, washing of the clothes, and the value of personal hygiene should form part of the treatment protocol. Scabies, like leprosy, can be considered to be a thermometer of civilization.

Pyoderma

This constitutes nearly 15% of outpatients. Most cases of pyoderma are secondary to underlying scabies, insect bite, fungus, or eczema. However, primary pyodermas are common among children of the poor, the factors favoring prevalence being the same as that for scabies. The usual organism isolated from both primary and secondary pyodermas is *Staphylococcus aureus*. Occasionally beta-hemolytic *Streptococcus* can be the cause of the pyoderma, and it could be nephritogenic. Unlike most countries in the West, in India, glomerulohephritis in children often results from skin lesions colonized by the *Streptococcus*.

Because most hospitals cannot afford to hand out antibiotic creams due to financial constraints, the old treatment with dyes, particularly genetian violet and methylene blue, are still employed in hospital practice.

Tropical Ulcer

These appear commonly on the lower extremities, with etiologic factors being "filth, food, friction, and fusospirillosis." Most cases have occurred among slum dwellers. Following minor trauma, the ulcer appears usually over the skin and spreads rapidly, and is painful and foul smelling with copious discharge of serosanguineous secretion (Fig. 41.1). If left untreated, the

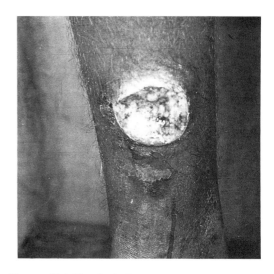

FIGURE 41.1. Tropical ulcer.

ulcer may last for several months and eventually will heal with a thin scar. Rarely will carcinomatous changes supervene. Bed rest, good food, and antimicrobials bring about a rapid cure of ulcers.

Though the incidence of tropical ulcers is not high when compared to other pyodermas, epidemics tend to occur during times of floods and storms.

Culture from the ulcers has shown a variety of bacteria,[1] but the predominant role of the anerobes cannot be ignored because of their regular presence in the ulcer and the prompt response to treatment with metronidazole.[2]

Dermatitis Cruris Pustulosa et Atrophicans

Under the name dermatitis cruris pustulosa et atrophicans (DCPA), Clarke, in 1952, reported this condition among the Negroes in Nigeria. Since then, DCPA has been reported in blacks from other tropical climes like Ghana, Trinidad, and India. The incidence of DCPA at the General Hospital, Madras, is about 0.5%.

DCPA occurs in a wide variety of patients, but its appearance in hairy women is exceptional. It also occurs mostly in the lower socioeconomic class of patients. The characteristic features of this disease are a superficial but chronic and recurrent pustular folliculitis appearing symmetrically on the legs between the knee and the ankle, mainly on the anterior surfaces and, hence, is also known as the "shin disease." Itching of variable intensity is present in most cases, but pain is absent. Crops of pustules keep appearing over months or years, leading to chronicity (Fig. 41.2). Eventually the skin becomes atrophic, shiny with loss of skin markings and hairs, at which point spontaneous cure results.

Staphylococcus aureus is grown from the pustules, which is susceptible to most standard antibiotics, but fresh crops appear as soon as the drug is stopped.

Histopathologically, events occur mostly around hair follicles. There is mild to moderate hyperkeratosis with parakeratosis. Acanthosis and spongiosis are constantly present.[3] A neutrophil-containing blister is present subcoreally, centered around a hair. In the dermis, surrounding the hair follicle and independent of

its plasma cells, eosinophils and neutrophils can be seen.

The exclusive occurrence of DCPA in blacks in the tropics is explained on the basis of the custom of massaging coconut or mustard oil, not a very satisfactory explanation. There are many other inexplicable facts about this disease—why it is such a chronic malady among the economically poor and why it leads to atrophy of the skin clinically and histologically although the pustules are only superficial. The answer may be found in the future.

Leprosy

This disease continues to be a major problem in India, nearly one-third of the world's leprosy cases being found in this country, particularly along the eastern coast of India. With the help of multidrug therapy (MDT) the prevalence of leprosy has been decreased in most of the states, but its eradication from the country by the turn of the century remains a dream. There is no doubt that the incidence of deformities due to the disease has been significantly reduced with MDT. The serious drawbacks to the eradication program are the prejudice and ignorance, because most patients including the educated believe that

(a) leprosy is a hereditary disease;
(b) it is caused by bad habits;
(c) it is a curse of God;
(d) it is highly infectious;
(e) it is incurable;
(f) it always leads to physical deformities.

Hence, patients resort to quack treatment.

Mass education and propaganda are being carried out to counteract these misconceptions through media and other means. Mobile units comprising of a doctor and paramedical workers survey, educate, and treat (SET units) cases of leprosy in remote villages. Vaccinations have been launched at various endemic areas in a phased and controlled manner, but the effectiveness of these measures will be known only after a decade.

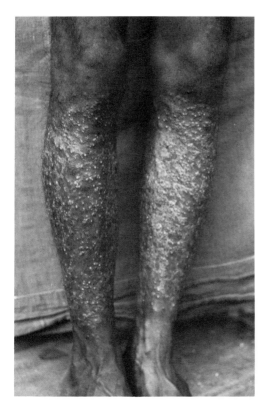

FIGURE 41.2. Dermatitis cruris pustulosa et atrophicans.

Tuberculosis Cutis

Though not a major problem, tuberculosis cutis is still seen in its various forms. On average, about 100 cases a year are seen at the General Hospital, Madras, out of a total of about 40,000 new cases attending the outpatient clinic.

The commonest form is tuberculosis verrucosa cutis and this mostly occurs on the soles of the feet due to walking barefoot and the habit of pulmonary tuberculosis patients spitting indiscriminately on the pavements.

Lupus vulgaris is the next common form of skin tuberculosis (TB) and the site most frequently affected is the gluteal region followed by the face. Scrofuloderma cases mostly attend the surgical outpatient clinic and, hence, are not seen often in the skin department. Tuberculosis cutis orificialis is only rarely seen because attention is focused on the primary site from which the skin ulcers originated.

Among the tuberculides, the type seen most often is papulonecrotic tuberculide, which presents as indolent nodules that appear in crops, undergo central necrosis, and heal with scars. Fresh crops appear over several months or even years. In the majority of patients, the primary site of TB cannot be located and the diagnosis is based on clinical morphology, positive tuberculin test, histopathology, and the prompt response to antituberculous treatment. Only rarely lichen scrofuloscorum and erythema induratum are encountered. The commonest cause of erythema nodosum in India is tuberculosis.

Mycoses

Mycoses account for 10–16% of all dermatoses seen in hospital practice. The predisposing factors for such a high incidence in Madras could be overcrowding, high environmental temperature and humidity, and low annual rainfall. The major group involved is males between 10 to 30 years, but tinea capitis affects children below 10 years.

Of the various mycoses, superficial mycoses, particularly dermatophytoses and pityriasis versicolor, predominate. Among dermatophytoses, tinea cruris and tinea corporis constitute the majority of cases.

The common dermatophytes that prevail in India include *Trichophyton rubrum*, *T. mentagrophytes*, and *Epidermophyton floccosum*, mainly in the glabrous skin and nails, whereas *T. violaceum* and *T. tonsurans* predominate in the scalp.

Tinea nigra, white piedra, and black piedra are rare mycoses. Cutaneous trichosporosis of the genitocrural and perianal regions are frequent[5] in man, particularly during summer, and may cause pruritus.

Deep mycoses are less common (0.14%) in skin departments and are mostly cases of mycetomas and entomophtharomycoses, the former being the more common. Others such as chromomycosis, sporotrichosis, and mucormycosis have been occasionally seen. Rhinosporidiosis, though a predominantly nasopharyngeal infection, has been rarely seen on the skin where it may resemble a verruca.[6]

Mycetomas are common in farmers between 18 and 50 years and occur in both sexes. The sites involved include the feet, legs, thighs, buttocks, upper trunk, hand, and scalp in that order of decreasing frequency.[7] The common causative agents have been *Actinomadura madurae*, *A. pellatierii*, *Nocardia brazieliensis*, and *N. asteroides*. Medical treatment with judicious surgical intervention has been invaluable in most cases.

Viral Infections

These constitute about 2% of the outpatients. The commonest viral infection is verrucae and the clinical appearance and therapeutic problems are the same as in other parts of the world.

Protozoal Infections

Cutaneous leishmaniasis caused by *L. tropica* is endemic in some of the northern states of India, whereas in Tamil Nadu dermatologists still encounter, albeit rarely, cases of post kalazar dermal leishmaniasis (PKDL) caused by *L. donovani*. This latter condition is unique in its extremely close resemblance to leprosy in all its forms. If skin smears are negative in a clinically diagnosed multibacillary type of leprosy or if sensory changes are absent in a presumptive borderline tuberculoid leprosy, PKDL should be suspected and skin smears are then taken in the same way as for leprosy but should be stained by Giemsa or Leishman methods. The slightly oval Leishman-Donovan bodies will be found within macrophages.

The treatment of choice is pentavalent antimonials. In recalcitrant cases, amphotericin-B has given good results in our experience.[8]

Helminthic Infections

Filariasis caused by *Wuchereria bancrofti* is endemic in most parts of India. These patients occasionally present at the skin department either for infections and eczema associated with lymphoedema, for urticaria, or for lymph scrotum.[9] Onchocerciasis caused by *O. volvulus* is not seen in India.

Larva migrans is not uncommon in Madras. In children, it is seen on the feet and buttocks. Sometimes multiple larvae may gain entry into the skin. The commonest larva is that of *Ankylostoma brazieliensis* excreted by the innumerable stray dogs on the beaches and other public places.

Treatment consists of freezing the larvae with liquid nitrogen. Oral albendazole has been recently claimed to be effective if given for 3 consecutive days.

Pigmentary Disorders

Indians, particularly the generally dark-complexioned South Indian Dravidians, are extremely color-conscious and the women are constantly falling prey to quack preparations claiming to lighten skin color. Paradoxically, when depigmentation occurs in the form of vitiligo, it can have devastating cosmetic results. Further, in the local Tamil language, vitiligo is known as "Ven Kushtam," meaning white leprosy and this increases the social stigma attached to this disease.

Vitiligo is an acquired loss of pigment of unknown etiology. It is not fatal but constitutes a major sociopsychological problem in dark-skinned races. The term vitiligo might have been derived from the Latin word "Vitium," which means a blemish.

Although the etiopathogenesis remains obscure, various hypotheses have been put forward, the accepted ones being genetic, autoimmune, neurogenic, and melanocyte self-destruction hypothesis. Recently, it has been suggested that the depigmentation could be due to a reduction in certain growth factors locally and in circulation, which normally have a mitogenic effect on the melanocytes.[10]

In India, the prevalence of vitiligo is about 4%. Clinically, it is characterized by milky-white macules of different sizes and shapes that gradually spread peripherally and often exhibit a pigmented border. There are no textural changes on the surface of the affected skin. Depending on the pattern of involvement, we recognize vitiligo areata, zosteriformis, mucosae, acrofacialis, vulgaris, and universalis. Gray hairs may be found emerging from the depigmented patches.

The course of vitiligo is highly unpredictable. Generally it progresses gradually with periods of quiescence. Spontaneous spotty repigmentation does occur. When occurring on the mucosae and the distal parts of the extremities, the prognosis is poor.

PUVA therapy is still the treatment of choice. Topical clobetasol dipropionate used judiciously can repigment some patches, particularly those on the face. Recently, melagenina, an alcoholic extract obtained from the placenta of healthy women, when applied externally and exposed to infrared light has been claimed to be superior to previously reported methods of treatment. But more scientific trials need to be carried out before its efficacy can be accepted. The administration of phenylalanine combined with UVA exposure has also been found effective.

When medical treatment fails, surgical methods can be undertaken such as placing a new source of pigment cells to reinitiate melanogenesis within the affected areas. Thin Thiersch grafts, epidermal grafts obtained from suction blisters, minigrafts using punch grafts, and, recently, transplantation of in vitro cultured epidermis or melanocytes have all been used to repopulate the vitiliginous skin with viable melanocytes.

If vitiligo is very extensive and fails to respond to therapy, depigmenting the remaining normal skin with 10% monobenzyl ether of hydroquinone may be attempted.

There are two other conditions producing depigmentation of the skin that are not uncommon in India—chemical leukoderma and idiopathic guttate hypomelanosis (IGH). The former is usually seen under the straps of cheap rubber or plastic chappals (Fig. 41.3). The probable depigmenting chemical is paratertiary butyl phenol (PTBP). Conventional patch tests are negative at 48 h, but if the patch is left on for 7 days, depigmentation may occur at the patch-test site.

Idiopathic guttate hypomelanosis is found in more than 60% of the Indian population above 40 years of age. It consists of multiple small achromic macules, sharply defined with angulated or circular borders. The size is 2–5 mm in diameter and there may be from few to numerous macules. It occurs mainly on the extensor aspects of the lower extremities. There is no spontaneous repigmentation. Fear of vitiligo or leprosy brings the patient for consultation. Histologically, lack of melanin in

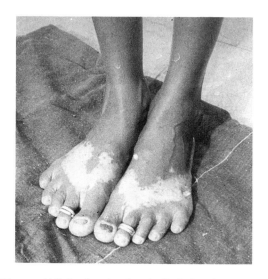

FIGURE 41.3. Leukemia, chemically induced.

the basal cell layer and decreased number of melanocytes have been reported. No treatment is required other than reassurance.

Dermatitis

It is an erroneous belief that most types of dermatitis are relatively uncommon in the black races. Both in hospital as well as private practice, next to infections and infestations, eczemas constitute a major problem to the dermatologist—15% of the daily outpatient attendance.

By the time the patient reaches the dermatologist he would have already tried home remedies or alternative forms of treatment with Siddha, Ayurvedha, or homeopathy. The patterns and problems posed by contact dermatitis, both irritant and allergic, are the same as in the rest of the world. Peculiar to India are two forms of allergic contact dermatitis: parthenium dermatitis and bindi or kumkum dermatitis.

Kumkum Dermatitis

Kumkum is also known as bindi or tilak and it is a mark worn on the center of the forehead both by Hindu men and women for socio-religious reasons but it is deemed compulsory for married women. Only widows do not use this mark. In the "olden" days, kumkum was prepared at home by mixing turmeric powder with lime juice and then adding alum and dye. But, of late, the market is flooded with commercially made kumkum under different trade names. Most of them have a vermillion color and are available as powder, liquid, or paste. The composition cannot be obtained from the manufacturer because it is considered a trade secret. But evidently it contains an azodye such as scarlet red or rhodamin-B and also, at times, red sulfide of mercury called "Sindhoor." A more recent innovation is to use colored disks with adhesive backs. Some women also use red lipstick. With the frequent sweating in the tropics, conditions are ideal for chemicals to be leeched out of the kumkum and brought into intimate contact with the skin.

Three patterns of dermatoses[11] are recognized as being caused by vermillion marks.

Contact Dermatitis

This can be both of the irritant or allergic type. The former can be caused by either the alum or by the alkalinity of the homemade kumkum and presents with an acute dermatitis resembling contact with escharotics. It can appear within a few hours of application, accompanied by a burning sensation. It leaves behind a post-inflammatory pigmentation or depigmentation. Allergic contact dermatitis presents with itching and oozing with crusting. Although usage material adequately diluted often gives a positive patch test, the specific allergen probably varies in individual patients. As mentioned earlier, the composition cannot be obtained from the manufacturers. A patient allergic to one brand of kumkum often reacts to other trade marks as well, indicating a common allergen. In our experience, a few patients with kumkum dermatitis also have leather footwear dermatitis. If there is a common allergen, it has yet to be identified.

Hyperpigmentation

Some women develop pigmentation under the kumkum after years of usage without preceding dermatitis. From this starting point, a greyish-black or bluish-black pigmentation spreads to involve the sides of the forehead, cheeks, neck, forearm, and waist area, all of which are sun-exposed areas in saree-wearing South Indian women and, rarely, even the covered areas. The clinical appearance resembles ashy dermatosis or lichen planus pigmentosus more than the pigmented cosmetic dermatitis (PCD) or Riehl's melanosis[12] described in Japan or Sweden. Patch tests and photopatch tests are negative. Histology of the pigmented patch shows a lichenoid appearance. Provocative tests are not possible because of the insidious onset of the pigmentation, but that it is related to the kumkum cannot be disputed because in the few patients who strictly avoided using kumkum, the pigmentation gradually faded although it may be 3–4 years before resolution occurs. The most probable offending agent is the azodye, as with the Japanese cases of PCD where lithiol red[13] was suspected to be the cause in some.

Depigmentation

This can occur as a postinflammatory phenomenon, but it happens mostly de novo without preceding inflammation. The latter is invariably due to using plastic bindis with an adhesive back. Many of these patients also develop depigmentation under their plastic chappals. Patch testing with PTBP is negative at the conventional 48–72 h, but if the patch is left on for 7 days, some patients develop depigmentation at the site. All forms of kumkum dermatitis are difficult to treat because most Indian women are married and even unmarried women are loathe to appear in public without the red dot on the forehead. Widowhood brings on spontaneous cure when the use of kumkum ceases.

Parthenium Dermatitis

Parthenium hysterophorus, after its initial introduction into the Maharashtra state on the west coast of India with food grains imported from the southern part of United States,[14] has virtually invaded the Indian peninsula and is now so prevalent that few parts of India are free of this scourge. It belongs to the Compositae family and cross-reactions may occur with *Helenium dahila and Chrysanthemum*. Parthenin and ambrosin are the two major allergens that are carried on the trichromes—small organelles found on the leaf surface, phyllaries, and achenes.

The dermatitis mostly affects men who are agricultural workers and seen in the age range 40–50 years. Initially, the dermatitis is restricted to the growing season but soon becomes perennial with seasonal exacerbations. The feet and legs may be involved early in agricultural workers who wade barefooted through Parthenium-infested fields. The primary lesions are papules or papulo-vesicles that coalesce to involve the entire face, forearm, neck, and upper back. After the initial phase of acute eczematous dermatitis, pronounced lichenification sets in and almost the entire skin becomes involved, but lesions are always more severe on exposed areas of the skin. The lichenification is the hallmark of the disease and may be

associated with hyperpigmentation or hypopigmentation, fissuring, oozing, and secondary
infection. The nails may have a polished
appearance due to the intense pruritus. An
apparent photodistribution suggests sun sensitivity and, indeed, a few patients complain of
burning sensation on exposure to sunlight, but
photopatch tests have given unequivocal results.

In the differential diagnosis, contact dermatitis to other airborne allergens, atopic dermatitis,
seborrheic dermatitis, and actinic reticuloid
should be considered.

Treatment of the condition is most frustrating
as long as the patient continues to live in the
Parthenium-infested areas. Even if he is willing
to pull up his roots and settle elsewhere, there
are few places he can choose for this
resettlement, as the plant's distribution is
widespread in India. A few patients contemplate
suicide.

Conclusion

The problems faced by dermatologists in
developing countries seem almost insurmount-
able, but as mentioned by the late Orlando
Canizares, this calls for a crusade, a crusade to
combat the infective parasitic dermatoses and
the age-old traditions and customs that prove
to be obstacles in the fight against odds.

Acknowledgments. The Dean of Government
General Hospital, Madras, gave permission to
publish hospital statistics and Dr. A. Kamalam
provided the section on mycoses.

References

1. Adriaans B: Tropical Ulcer. In: Champion RH, Rye RJ, eds. Recent Advances in Dermatology No. 9, New York: Churchill Livingstone, 1992.
2. Yesudian P, Thambiah AS: Metronidazole in the treatment of tropical phagedenic ulcers. *Int J Dermatol* 1979;**18**:755–757.
3. Tiwari VD, Ramji C, Tutakne MA, et al: Dermatitis cruris pustulosa et atrophicans. *Indian J Dermatol Venereol Leprol* 1987;**53**:116–177.
4. Kamalam A, Thambiah AS: Tinea capitis in South Indian families. *Mykosen* 1979;**22**:251–254.
5. Kamalam A, Senthamilselvi G, Ajithads A, Thambiah AS: Cutaneous trichosporosis. *Mycopathologia* 1988;**101**:167–175.
6. Yesudian P: Cutaneous rhinosporidiosis mimicking verruca vulgaris. *Int J Dermatol* 1988;**27**:47–48.
7. Kamalam A, Thambiah AS: A clinicopathological study of Actinomycotic mycetoma caused by Antinomadura madurae and Actinomadura Pellitieri. *Mycopathologia* 1987;**97**:151–163.
8. Yesudian P, Thambiah AS: Amphotericin B in dermal leishmanoid. *Arch Dermatol* 1974;**109**:720–722.
9. Yesudian P, Kumaraswami V: Filiariasis—the scourge of India. *Int J Dermatol* 1989;**28**:192–194.
10. Ramiah A, Puri N, Mojamdar M: Etiology of vitiligo—a new hypothesis. *Acta Dermatol Venereol (Stockh)* 1989;**69**:323–326.
11. Kumar AS, Pandhi, RK, Bhutani LK: Bindi dermatoses. *Int J Dermatol* 1986;**25**:434–435.
12. Rorsman H: Riehl's melanosis. *Int J Dermatol* 1982;**21**:75–78.
13. Nakayama H, Matsuo S, Hayakawa K, et al: Pigmented cosmetic dermatitis. *Int J Dermatol* 1984;**23**:229–305.
14. Lonkar A, Mitchell JC, Calnan CD: Contact dermatitis from Parthenium hysterophorus. *Trans St John's Hosp Dermatol Soc* 1974;**60**:43–53.

42

Lebanon

Ramsay S. Kurban and Amal K. Kurban

Lebanon is one of the smallest countries in the Middle East, measuring 135 miles in length and 30 miles in width. The entire length of the western border is the Mediterranean, the north and east borders are shared with Syria, and the southern border is shared with Israel. Many of Lebanon's cities are on the coastline. Two parallel mountain ranges running along the length of Lebanon bound the fertile Bekaa Valley, through which courses the Litani River. Because of the geographic location and terrain, Lebanon enjoys a moderate climate. Summers are hot and humid on the coastal plain, hot and dry in the Bekaa Valley, and much cooler on the mountains. Winters are wet and cold on the mountains, and cool on the plains. The spring and fall seasons are mild. On an average, there are 300 sunny days in a year. The economy of the country relies heavily on tourism, agriculture, and light industry.

The factors that have affected the spectrum of skin diseases in Lebanon are the racial admixture, consanguinity, and immigration to Lebanon. These factors emerge by examining Lebanon's history that spans more than 7000 years. As early as 5000 B.C., city states on the Lebanese coast were developing into flourishing commercial centers trading with the pharaohs of Egypt and the rest of the Mediterranean world. Those Phoenician cities maintained their independence until they were overrun by a succession of conquering armies, including the Assyrians, Persians, Greeks, Romans, Arabs, Crusaders, and Ottomans. Many of these people intermarried, and settled in the country.

Following World War I, Lebanon became a French mandate, gaining its independence in 1946. Lebanon prospered well, especially in the 1960s and early 1970s. In 1975, internal and external conflicts triggered a civil strife, which lasted until 1991 when peace came to the troubled land. Over the span of these centuries, the Lebanese population witnessed a fascinating admixture of races with a resultant spectrum of skin color ranging from the fair-skinned Celtic to tan-brown and olive-colored skin, to dark brown skin. Such a spectrum of skin color underlies the relative high incidence of actinic-induced sun damage and resultant dermatoses.

Within the background of wide genetic admixture, consanguineous marriages, albeit on a decline, are still prevalent in Lebanon and may account for a higher incidence of congenital disorders.

Because of its location at the crossroads between East and West, Lebanon has attracted numerous visitors who would stay for varying periods of time, bringing with them diseases not usually encountered in Lebanon. Moreover, the Lebanese are avid travelers and immigrants. The latter head mainly toward Saudi Arabia and the Gulf states, Africa, and the Americas. When they return to the homeland, they bring with them the diseases of their adopted countries.

The pattern of skin diseases in the Middle East, in general, and in Lebanon, in particular, resembles that observed in Europe and North America. Certain epidemiological and demographic deviations peculiar to that area exist. Although many of the studies conducted on the prevalence and distribution of dermatological diseases in Lebanon predate the devastating 15-year-old war, such figures probably remain representative of the current cutaneous disease pattern. Interestingly, dermatology was one of the few disciplines whose ranks remained unchanged or even increased during the war.[1]

In this chapter, emphasis will be placed on the disorders that seem to be at variance from what is usually seen in North America and Europe.

Genetic Skin Diseases

In a survey of 2652 ambulatory dermatologic patients seen over an 18-month period in the early 1960s, 12 patients (0.4%) had congenital diseases, including the ichthyotic dermatoses, congenital ectodermal dysplasia, acrodermatitis enteropathica, xeroderma pigmentosum, Ehlers-Danlos syndrome, and pseudoxanthoma elasticum.[2,3] The relatively high incidence and prevalence of genetic diseases is ascribed to consanguineous marriages in certain communities. Rare disorders like prolidase deficiency,[4] a hitherto undescribed entity (odontoonychodermal dysplasia)[5] have been reported from those communities.

Cutaneous Infections

One-third of all outpatient visits to dermatology clinics are related to infectious etiologies.[2] Superficial fungal infections account for 9% of the total outpatient load seen at the skin clinics of a major medical center[6] and tinea versicolor accounts for an additional 3%. Of the fungal infections, *T. violaceum* is the main cause of tinea capitis, *E. floccosum* of tinea cruris, and *T. mentogrophytes* of tinea pedis.[6] Interestingly, *Microsporum* sp. is only very rarely encountered.[6,7] Similarly, favus, due to *T. schoenleini* is only seen in patients from outside Lebanon. *Candida albicans* accounts for 24% of superficial fungal infections[7] and involves intertriginous areas, paronychial tissues, and mucocutaneous sites. Subcutaneous and deep fungal infections are unknown in Lebanon. Two cases of blastomycosis have been reported, but

the infection was probably contracted outside the country.[8,9]

Cutaneous leishmaniasis is endemic in the Middle East, especially in Syria, Iraq, the Jordan Valley, Kuwait, and eastern Saudi Arabia. Very few cases originate in Lebanon. However, many patients who have contracted the infection in one of the endemic foci mentioned earlier seek medical care in Lebanon. The high number of patients with cutaneous leishmaniasis seen at the major medical centers in Lebanon has given rise to several studies and surveys on the subject.[10-16]

There are several endemic foci of leprosy in the Middle East. In Lebanon, there are two minor foci, one each in the north and south of the country. Several cases of leprosy have also been identified in immigrants returning from Africa. Cutaneous tuberculosis is very rare; and to date, there have been no cases attributed to other mycobacteria.

Sexually transmitted diseases in Lebanon were on the increase in the late sixties and early seventies[17] although chancroid, lymphogranuloma venereum, and granuloma inguinale were not encountered. There are no up-to-date surveys of this problem and the effect of the civil strife on the incidence of sexually transmitted diseases remains unknown. Several decades ago, patients were seen with nonsexually transmitted endemic syphilis, known as bejel, from northern Syria. Due to World Health Organization (WHO) efforts in identifying and treating endemic syphilis, this focus has been eradicated, though older patients who had contracted the disease in the prepenicillin era may be seen. A handful of patients with human immunodeficiency viral infection (HIV) have been recognized, but in each instance the infection was found to have been acquired outside the country.

Skin Cancer

The incidence of skin cancer in Lebanon has been reported to be around 17 per 100,000 in men and 10.6 per 100,000 in women.[18,19] Analysis of histopathological specimens during a 5-year period from the main pathology laboratories in Lebanon found a total of 1300 cases of basal and squamous cell carcinoma, 62% affecting males and 38% affecting females. Of these, 54% were basal cell carcinomas, and 46% were squamous cell carcinomas.[20] This ratio of almost 1:1 of basal and squamous cell carcinomas can be explained by the heterogeneous Lebanese population with a multitude of skin color. This falls intermediate between light-skinned populations in which basal cell carcinomas predominate and dark-skinned populations in which squamous cell carcinomas outnumber basal cell carcinoma. The importance of sun damage in the pathogenesis of basal cell carcinoma is well established.[21] The incidence of malignant melanoma is unclear, but the data on the distribution of the lesions show a preponderance of lesions on the head and extremities with relative sparing of the trunk.[22] This seems to be atypical when compared with data from the United States and Australia.[23]

Metabolic Diseases

Xanthomatosis comprised 0.75% of the diagnosed skin diseases.[2] This seemingly high prevalence could be accounted for by the consanguineous marriages. Another metabolic disease that seems to be seen more in the Middle East, including Lebanon, is primary cutaneous amyloidosis, especially the macular variety.[24]

Others

The incidence and prevalence of the majority of other skin disorders (e.g., the dermatitides, papulosquamous disorders, noninfectious bullous diseases, acne) is not different from that seen in Europe or North America.[2] The exception to that is actinic lichen planus with a prevalence of 14%.[25]

Conclusion

The great majority of skin disorders encountered in Lebanon is similar to that seen by dermatologists in western Europe and North America in their private offices or in medical school centers. The few diseases that may be unfamiliar to dermatologists outside Lebanon, or unexpected, fall into one of these groups:

1. Relative increased incidence of
   genodermatoses
   cutaneous leishmaniasis
   squamous cell carcinoma
   macular amyloidosis
   actinic lichen planus
2. Rarity or absence of infections due to *Microsporum*, subcutaneous and deep fungi, atypical mycobactaria, and HIV.

Acknowledgment. Dr. Howard Koh provided constructive review and criticism.

References

1. Kurban AK: Dermatology in a besieged community. *Int J Dermatol* 1989;**28**:407–409.
2. Chaglassian HT, Farah FS, Kurban AK: Epidemiology of cutaneous diseases in the Middle East. Excerpta Medica Int Congress 1962;**55**: 1141–1148.
3. Kurban AK: Genetic diseases of the skin. *Leb Med J* 1986;**36**:85–87.
4. DerKaloustian VM, Freij BJ, Kurban AK: Prolidase deficiency: an inborn error of metabolism with major dermatological manifestations. *Dermatologica* 1982;**164**:293–304.
5. Fadhil M, Ghabra TA, Deeb M, DerKaloustian VM: Odontoonychodermal dysplasia: a previously apparently undescribed ectodermal dysplasia. *Am J Med Genet* 1983;**14**:335–346.
6. Farah FS, Kurban AK, Chaglassian HT, Alami S: Survey of the pathogenic dermatophytes in Lebanon. *Leb Med J* 1962;**15**:75–79.
7. Farah FS, Kurban AK, Malak JA, Chaglassian HT: Superficial fungus infections in Lebanon. *Gazz Sanit* 1966;**15**:49–52.
8. Malak JA, Farah FS: Blastomycosis in the Middle East. Report of a suspected case of North American blastomycosis. *Br J Dermatol* 1971;**84**: 161–166.
9. Matta M, Farah FS: North American blastomycosis. Report of a case encountered in Lebanon and probably originating in Gambia. *Dermatologica* 1973;**146**:346–349.
10. Kurban AK, Farah FS, Chaglassian HT: Cutaneous leishmaniasis: analysis of the various therapeutic modalities used. *Leb Med J* 1965;**18**: 381–386.

11. Kurban AK, Malak JA, Farah FS, et al: Histopathology of cutaneous leishmaniasis. *Arch Dermatol* 1966;**93**:396–401.

12. Chaglassian HT, Farah FS, Kurban AK: The Leishmanid. *Dermatol Int* 1967;**6**:161–163.

13. Kurban AK, Malak JA, Farah FS, et al: Treatment of cutaneous leishmaniasis (Oriental sore) with a new repository antimalarial. *J Trop Med Hyg* 1969;**72**:86–88.

14. Farah FS, Malak JA: Late cutaneous leishmaniasis. *Arch Dermatol* 1969;**100**:773–774.

15. Farah FS, Malak JA: Cutaneous leishmaniasis. *Arch Dermatol* 1971;**103**:467–474.

16. Kibbi AG, Karam PG, Kurban AK: Sporotrichoid leishmaniasis in patients from Saudi Arabia: clinical and histological features. *J Am Acad Dermatol* 1987;**17**:759–764.

17. Kurban AK: Venereal diseases in Lebanon. *Leb Med J* 1973;**26**:489–493.

18. Abou-Daoud KT: Morbidity from cancer in Lebanon. *Cancer* 1966;**19**:1293–1300.

19. Azar HA: Cancer in Lebanon and the Near East. *Cancer* 1962;**15**:66–78.

20. Shbaklu Z, Kurban AK: Skin cancer in Lebanon. *Leb Med J* 1970;**23**:583–589.

21. Zaynoun S, Abi Ali L, Shaib J, Kurban AK: The relationship of sun exposure and solar elastosis to basal cell carcinoma. *J Am Acad Dermatol* 1985;**12**:522–525.

22. Rubeiz N, Zaynoun S: (unpublished data).

23. Balch CM, Shaw HM, Soong S-J, Milton GW: Changing trends in the clinical and pathologic features of melanoma. In: Balch CM, ed. Cutaneous Melanoma. Philadelphia: J.B. Lippincott, 1985:313–319.

24. Kurban AK, Malak JA, Afifi AK, Mire J: Primary localized macular cutaneous amyloidosis: histochemistry and electron microscopy. *Br J Dermatol* 1971;**85**:52–60.

25. Salman SM, Kibbi AG, Zaynoun S: Actinic lichen planus: a clinicopathologic study of 16 patients. *J Am Acad Dermatol* 1989;**20**:226–231.

43

United Arab Emirates

Ahmed Moh'd Abu Shareeah

The United Arab Emirates (UAE) was proclaimed in 1971. It is the result of the union between seven emirates, namely, Abu Dhabi, Dubai, Sharjah, Ajman, Umm Al Quwain, Ras Al Khaimah, and Fujeirah. It has a surface area of about 77,700 km² with the bulk of its territory being desert or semidesert. Abu Dhabi Emirate comprises 80% of UAE surface area and gives the federation its capital by the same name. The UAE is located in the heart of the Arabian Gulf region. It is bordered by Gulf water to the north and northwest, by Qatar and Arabia to the west, by Oman and Arabia to the south, and by Oman Gulf to the east. It is located between the two latitudes 22 and 26.5 degrees to the north and the two longitudes 51 and 56.5 to the east.

The population of the UAE is estimated to be approximately 2 million. The official language and the language of communications is Arabic and the state religion is Islam. The usual mode of dress is an Arabic dress called Candura (a long, loose white dress), and the head is usually covered with what is called a khotra. Racially, the people of the UAE are Caucasoids with moderate skin pigmentation.

The basis of the UAE economy is its oil production, which started to flow 25 years ago, Figures underline that UAE remains on a per capita basis among the richest countries in the world. The oil wealth has been wisely used to build a solid infrastructure that could well serve the future generations. A large-scale industrial base and booming agriculture and fisheries sectors are being given increased

attention as part of the efforts to diversify the national sources of income, which is still highly dependent on oil and gas revenues. The oil wealth has been also reflected in a modern and up-to-date educational, housing, hygienic, and health standards.

The climatologic year in the UAE differs from that reported from other regions in that there is no cold weather season. The year is usually divided in halves, a hot season from April to September (spring and summer) and a mild season from October to March (autumn and winter). Rain is rare. In the hot season, the temperature may reach 41–44°C with the relative humidity reaching up to the saturation point.

With the purpose of evaluating the pattern of skin diseases in the UAE, analysis of all new dermatological cases attending the outpatient clinics in Mafraq Hospital (the biggest hospital in the country, 33 km from the city proper) during a 2-year study was done (Table 43.1).[1,2] It was found that the incidence of skin diseases in the UAE constitutes 9.3% of all new cases seen in the country. A similar incidence was reported in England (8.3%)[3] and in Zambia (7%).[4] The problem of skin diseases in our country is perhaps much less than that reported from other third world countries. In India, for example, the incidence of skin diseases may reach 20–25%.[5] This high incidence not only reflects the influence of climate, but also the effect of socioeconomic and environmental factors. It is known that in developing countries the majority of the population belongs to the low-income group with inadequate hygienic environment, poor nutritional standards, and insufficient facilities for healthy living. The UAE has one of the highest per capita incomes in the world, and this has been reflected in advances both in medical services and in the peoples' standard of living.

Dermatoses Common in the UAE

The following discussion will be limited to the striking and particular aspects of the common skin diseases seen in the United Arab Emirates.

Dermatitis Group

The dermatitis group represents the highest incidence among patients where it constitutes about 21% of the new cases in the department (Table 43.1).

This incidence is comparable with those reported from some countries in the third world, and it is much less than those reported from the well-developed countries (Table 43.2).[4–10] This difference probably reflects the advanced industrialization of such communities resulting in

TABLE 43.1. Various dermatologic diagnosis recorded at the dermatology clinic at Mafraq Hospital (January 1987–December 1988).

Diseases group	Total no. of cases	% of each group
Dermatitis	2307	20.98
Acne vulgaris	997	9.07
Sup. fungus infection (incl. candidal & TV)	935	8.50
Viral infections	813	7.39
Pig. disorders	595	5.41
Psoriasis	494	4.49
STD	314	2.86
Pyoderma	280	2.55
Alopecia	249	2.26
Lichen planus	104	0.95
Pityriasis rosea	082	0.75
Others	3825	34.79
TOTAL	10,995	100.00

Note: TV: Tinea versicolor; STD: sexually transmitted diseases.

a high prevalence of industrial dermatitis and allergic contact dermatitis.

In our case, although all common types of dermatitis are found as described universally, atopic dermatitis is the commonest type seen, whereas allergic contact dermatitis and occupational dermatitis are seen less frequently. The clinical picture, diagnosis, differential diagnosis, and treatment are almost the same as those described elsewhere.

Acne Vulgaris Group

Acne vulgaris is common in the area. It constitutes about 9% of the patients seen in the dermatology department. This figure is apparently higher than what has been reported from other countries and could be explained either by the well-known effect of racial influence or the high standard of living and the easy availability of health services offered in the UAE, free of charge, which encourages people to seek medical advice even for minor problems.

Although the common types of acne vulgaris as described universally are seen in patients, inflammatory acne vulgaris with papulo-pustular lesions is the commonest type seen here. It affects both sexes of postpubertal age equally. Again, the clinical picture, diagnosis, differential diagnosis, and treatment are the same as those described universally.

Superficial Fungal Infections

Superficial fungal infections occur frequently in the UAE, accounting for 8.5% of new referrals to the dermatology outpatient clinic at Mafraq Hospital (Table 43.1). This figure is comparable with those reported from Zambia,[4] Kenya,[6] and Ethiopia,[8] but it is much less than that of India (15–20%)[5] and Mexico (13%).[7] Although both India (Calcutta) and Mexico have climatic characteristics like UAE (hot and humid weather) that facilitate survival and spread of the organisms that produce superficial fungus infections, the lower incidence in the UAE could be explained by the higher standard of living, which plays a major role in limiting such spread. Among the features of this high standard of living are the availability of good hygienic

TABLE 43.2. Comparative incidence in percentage of common dermatoses among different countries.

Skin diseases	Zambia[4]	Calcutta[5]	Kenya[6]	Mexico[7]	Ethiopia[8]	London[9]	Vancouver[10]	Abu Dhabi
Dermatitis	14.7	15–20	28.1	8–12	23.0	35.6	39.2	20.98
Acne vulgaris	2.1	3.5	3.9	3	5.0	5.6	7.3	9.07
Dermatophytosis Mycosis	10.8	15–20	9.5	13	7.8	3.2	4.3	8.50
Viral wart	1.6	2	2	5	NR[a]	7.4	6.8	5.47
Vitiligo	1.4	4	2.9	4	NR	NR	NR	3.18
Psoriasis	1.0	0.5–1.5	3.2	NR	NR	5.6	4.7	4.49
Pyoderma	20.3	30–40	6.4	6.5	7.1	4.6	5.7	2.55
Lichen planus	1.4	0.5–1.5	1.6	NR	NR	1.3	NR	0.95

Note: Number in parentheses denotes reference citation.

[a] NR: not received.

measures, absence of overcrowding, and presence of good preventative and therapeutic standards.

The frequency distribution of the different types of superficial fungus infections in the UAE is shown in Table 43.3. They are approximately similar to those reported from other places.[4,5,7] Deep or systemic fungus infections are very rare in this part of the world.

Dermatophytosis

Dermatophytic (tinea or ringworm) infection in the UAE has the same classification, manifestation, and treatment as those mentioned universally. Only the different incidences of dermatophyte species will be mentioned.

TABLE 43.3. Frequency of the different superficial fungus infections seen at the dermatology clinic at Mafraq Hospital (January 1987–December 1988).

Diseases group	Total no. of cases	% of each group
T. versicolor	411	43.96
Candidal infection	176	18.82
Toe web disease	113	12.09
T. cruris	97	10.37
T. corporis	81	8.66
T. capitis	41	4.39
Others	16	1.71
TOTAL	935	100.00

Tinea Capitis

Tinea capitis infection constitutes 4.39% of the total superficial fungus infection seen in clinics in the UAE. This incidence is much less than that reported from Rwanda,[11] Libya,[12] and Egypt.[13] *Microsporum canis* is the most prevalent organism isolated (68.8%), followed by *Trichophyton mentagrophytes* (9.4%) and *Trichophyton violaceum* (6.4%).[14] This incidence differs from those reported in Rwanda[11] and Egypt,[13] where *Trichophyton violaceum* is the most prevalent organism and from Libya[11] where *Trichophyton rubrum* is the commonest isolated organism. According to Lestringant et al.,[14] camels may be the reservoir for some zoophilic species in the UAE. Many of the inhabitants of the UAE keep camels, which are valued for their milk and for racing purposes.

Tinea Corporis and Tinea Cruris

Tinea corporis infection constitutes approximately 9% of the total superficial fungus infections seen in the UAE (Table 43.3). The commonest isolated organism is *Trichophyton rubrum*, followed by *Epidermophyton floccosum*.[15] This differs from those reported in Egypt,[13] where *Trichophyton violaceum* is the most common isolated organism.

Tinea cruris comprises 10% of the total superficial fungus infections seen in the UAE (Table 43.3). The commonest isolated dermatophyte species is *Epidermophyton floccosum*, followed by *Trichophyton rubrum.*[16] This is also in accordance with those reported from Egypt.[13]

Tinea versicolor and candida infections constitute approximately 43% and 19%, respectively, of the total superficial fungus infections seen in the UAE (Table 43.3). The etiology, clinical picture, diagnosis, differential diagnosis, and treatment are the same as those described elsewhere.

Viral Infection

Viral infections of the skin were diagnosed in 7.39% of the new cases attending the dermatology department. The frequent distribution of the different types of viral skin infections showed that human papilloma virus (HPV) infections is the commonest type seen and accounts for 71.96% of the total viral skin infections (Table 43.4). All the different clinical types of HPV infections are seen, although verruca vulgaris or common warts is the commonest type seen in our area. It is usually presented as multiple symmetrically distributed lesions varying in number, from solitary to a perfusion of 20–50, commonly affecting the children's distal extremities.

Pigmentary Disorders

Pigmentary disorders represent 5.4% of the new skin cases seen in the UAE. They include both hypomelanotic and hypermelanotic types of pigmentary disorders. The two most common

TABLE 43.4. Frequency of viral skin infections seen at the Dermatology clinic at the Mafraq Hospital (January 1987–December 1988).

Diseases group	Total no. of cases	% of each group
HPV infections	585	71.96
Moll. contag.	115	14.14
H. zoster	77	9.47
H. S. type-1 infection	19	2.34
Others	17	2.09
TOTAL	813	100.00

Note: HPV: human papillomavirus; H.S.: Herpes simplex.

disorders seen are melasma and vitiligo representing an incidence of 2.2% and 3.18%, respectively. Apparently, the racial background of the population with moderately pigmented skin is a predisposing factor for these disorders. Both disorders are presumably presenting the same manifestations as those described in other areas of the world.

Psoriasis

Psoriasis is a chronic disease with a worldwide occurrence; however, its prevalence varies with the different geographical regions. In the UAE, psoriasis constitutes about 4% of the new dermatological cases. Although this incidence is comparable with those reported from some countries,[6,9,10] it is still much higher than those reported in Zambia[4] and India[5] (Table 43.2).

Whereas psoriasis has the same manifestations as those described universally, still the majority of our patients experienced mild to moderate degree of itching, and there is no seasonal variations in the severity of the disease. Psoriatic arthropathy is very rarely seen in our cases.

Pyoderma

The UAE has a much lower pyoderma prevalence in comparison with developing countries in the third world (Table 43.2). Probably this lower incidence reflects and emphasizes the important role played by the high standard of living in the country in limiting chances for spread of infection. With a smaller population, and a relatively larger number of doctors and free health services in the country, prompt and effective delivery of medical care is obtained.

The etiology, clinical picture, diagnosis, differential diagnosis, and treatment of pyoderma in the United Arab Emirates is the same as those described universally.

References

1. Rook AJ, Savin JA, Wilkinson DS: The prevalence, incidence and ecology of diseases of

the skin. In: Rook A, Wilkinson DS, Ebling FJ, et al, eds. Textbook of Dermatology. Oxford: Blackwell Scientific Publications, 1986:39–53.

2. Abu Share'ah AM, Abdel Dayem H: The incidence of skin diseases in Abu Dhabi (United Arab Emirates). *Int J Dermatol* 1991;**30**:121–124.

3. Ratzer MA: Incidence of skin diseases in the west of Scotland. *Br J Dermatol* 1969;**81**:456–461.

4. Ratnam AV, Jayaraju K: Skin diseases in Zambia. *Br J Dermatol* 1979;**101**:449–455.

5. Banerjee BN, Datta AK: Prevalence and incidence pattern of skin diseases in Calcutta. *Int J Dermatol* 1973;**12**:41–47.

6. Verghan AR, Koten JW, Chaddah VK, et al. Skin diseases in Kenya: a clinical and histopathological study of 3,168 patients. *Arch Dermatol* 1968;**89**:577–586.

7. Canizares O: Geographic dermatology: Mexico and Central America. *Arch Dermatol* 1960;**82**:870–891.

8. West LG: Problems of tropical dermatology in Ethiopia. *Int J Dermatol* 1977;**16**:506–511.

9. Calnan CD, Meara RH: St. Johns Hospital diagnostic index. *Trans St Johns Hosp Dermatol Soc* 1957;**39**:56–68.

10. Mitchell JC: Proportionate distribution of skin diseases in a dermatological practice. *Can Med Assoc J* 1967;**97**:1346–1350.

11. Bugingo G: Dermatophytic infection of the scalp in the region of Butare (Rwanda). *Int J Dermatol* 1983;**22**:107–108.

12. Kanwar AJ, Belhaj MS: Tinea capitis in Benghazi, Libya. *Int J Dermatol* 1987;**26**:371–373.

13. Amer M, Taha M, Tosson Z, et al: The frequency of causative dermatophytes in Egypt. *Int J Dermatol* 1981;**20**:431–434.

14. Lestringant GG, Qayed K, Blayney B: Tinea capitis in the United Arab Emirates. *Int J Dermatol* 1991;**30**:127–129.

15. El Shiemy S, Abdel Dayem H, Sallam TH, et al: Tinea corporis in Abu Dhabi (UAE). *Egypt J Dermatol Venerol* 1981;**1**:55–59.

16. El Shiemy S, Sallam TH, Abdel Dayem, et al: Tinea Cruris in Abu Dhabi (UAE). *Egypt J Dermatol Venerol* 1982;**2**:125–128.

Part VI
Global Therapy

44

Therapeutic Considerations

Mohamed Amer

The diversity of presentations of skin disease from the global perspective is magnified even further by a broad range of therapeutic agents. Selected aspects of treatment are considered in certain chapters, but the primary role of this book is not directed toward therapy. Regional norms and variations would make the therapeutic approach to global dermatologic diseases an entirely separate volume of equal size. International variations in availability of topical agents and the broad variation in terminology, local usage, and regional indications all create a difficult area to cover adequately.

Background

The importance of microbial disease in the world population continues to be very great. Eczematous disease with secondary infections remains as one of the top tropical dermatological diagnoses. Complications of bacterial diseases, old and new, still remain a major problem, including toxic shock syndrome, glomerulonephritis, cellulitis, and lymphangitis with elephantiasis, just to name a few. Perhaps, even more significant for many people around the world is the chronic nature of some of these infections and the problem that multiple infections can have on the host.

Patients in parts of Africa have concurrent parasitic infestations and malaria, and additionally, bacterial infections, some intermittent and some chronic, such as mycobacterial infections. The end result in many of these instances is a serious decline in host immunity, which manifests itself in greater susceptibility to skin disease, and as we see in the present-day AIDS epidemic, unusual and extremely varied presentations of common skin diseases. Under these circumstances, standard treatments may fail because of the inability of the host to mount an adequate or appropriate immune defense to resolve the microbial attack.

Effective control and perhaps, in the future, eradication of many of these parasitic infections, deep fungal infections, and the more serious bacterial infections could have a profound impact on the longevity of people around the world and, hence, the importance of these newly developed or developing antimicrobials cannot be overemphasized.

Goals

This section on therapy has a more modest goal. If one looks at the morbidity and significance of dermatologic disease on a global aspect, infections, infestations, and parasitic disorders are of greatest therapeutic significance. Further, in these areas, there is more of a consensus in therapy. Antimicrobial therapy continues to grow in the research and development area, and newer groups of antimicrobial agents are providing significant breakthroughs across the world in providing better therapy for the treatment of the most serious aspects of skin disease, those primarily or secondarily of infective nature.

Because of this, the editors feel that dealing with principles and practices in antibacterial therapy, and with some reference to regional and national variations, would be useful. Similarly, superficial and deep fungal infections are appropriately treated with a core of a number of the newer antifungal agents. The imidazole, the allylamine, and other groups. They represent a dramatic breakthrough in the treatment of many of these infections that formerly throughout the world were the cause of extensive morbidity and mortality, especially in the more tropical environments. A newer core of safer and very effective agents is evolving to solve these therapeutic dilemmas, especially in the treatment of deep fungal infections.

Equally important have been the newer advances in effective treatment of parasitic diseases. This section provides an overview of this area which has slowly expanded in scope and therapeutic efficacy over the last two decades.

Conclusions

Other aspects of therapy for skin diseases are, in the editors' estimation, best left to regional journals and texts. The rapid evolution in dermatologicals, topical and systemic, also makes many texts outdated prior to or shortly after publication. Improved therapy for our patients has indeed been a most visible spin-off of the evolving science of dermatology.

45

Antimicrobial Therapy

J. Carl Craft

Cellulitis, infected wounds, abscesses, and other bacterial infections of skin and soft tissue account for a significant number of clinical visits to the dermatology, medicine, family practice, and pediatric clinics as well as emergency rooms worldwide. Before physicians in the many different countries can treat these infections, they must have a means of determining the causative bacteria. In the case of a primary bacterial infection produced by the invasion of normal skin by a single species of pathogenic bacteria, most infections will be due to Gram-positive organisms. Secondary infections develop in areas of already damaged skin and the infecting bacteria invasion and proliferation aggravate the underlying condition and prolong the disease. In contrast to the primary infections, secondary infections demonstrate multiple organisms including Gram-positive organisms, but Gram-negative organisms are not infrequently seen on culture. The majority of these infections are mild to moderate in severity and can be treated with either topical or oral medication. The etiological agents as shown in Table 45.1 vary little worldwide with *Streptococcus pyogenes* (Group A streptococcus) and *Staphylococcus aureus* accounting for greater than 90% of all skin infections. Even in those areas of the world where more exotic pathogens exist, the majority of infections are still caused by staphylococcus and streptococcus. This would suggest that treatment recommendations in any country would apply to all other countries.

Most textbooks recommend treatment of skin infections based on knowing the etiologic agent and recommend methods for examination and laboratory tests to assist the physician in making the correct diagnosis.[1–3] Thus, identification of bacteria from skin lesions provides this important information as to the cause of the cutaneous infections, and only by correlating the clinical appearance of the skin lesion with the culture data can one know the true cause of the dermatologic lesion. Waiting for the results of these tests can take several days and it would be unreasonable to expect patients to tolerate their symptoms until the exact etiology is determined. Because of this, the physician generally makes an assessment of the patient which includes a medical history and visual assessment of the lesions. These factors are evaluated based on local epidemiologic data, exposure history, patient factors, and microscopic examination of the smear of material sent for culture from the suspected skin infection; from this a presumptive diagnosis is made. Therapy is started, usually empirically. The initial therapy is not changed unless the treatment was not effective or culture data suggest a need to change the therapy.

Standard Therapy

Skin infections caused by Group A streptococci can be treated with penicillin. Penicillin is administered either as a single injection of long-acting benzathine penicillin or orally as penicillin VK. In penicillin-allergic patients, erythromycin orally is a suitable alternative.

TABLE 45.1. Bacterial pathogens causing cutaneous infections.

Gram-positive bacteria
  Staphylococcus aureus
  Streptococci
    Group A
    Other Groups B, C, D, G
    Anaerobic streptococci as part of mixed infections
    Streptococcus pneumoniae
  Bacillus anthracis
  Corynebacterium diphtheriae, minutissimum
  Propionibacterium acnes
  Clostridium perfringens, septicum, novyi, bifermentans,
    histolyticum, sporogenes, fallax, tertium
  Erysipelothrix rhusiopathiae (insidiosa)
  Borrelia burgdorferi
  Mycobacterium tuberculosis, marinum, fortuitum, chelonei,
    ulcerans, avium, leprae
Gram-negative bacteria
  Haemophilus influenzae
  Escherichia coli
  Proteus mirabilis
  Enterobacter aerogenes
  Pasteurella multocida
  Pseudomonas aeruginosa
  Nocardia asteroides, brasiliensis, caviae
  Actinomyces isrealii, naeslundii, viscosus, odontolyticus,
    proprionica
  Listeria monocytogenes
  Yersinia pestis
  Neisseria meningitidis
  Pseudomonas pseudomallei, mallei
  Bartonella bacilliformis
  Francisella tularensis

When the etiology is unknown and when *Staphylococcus aureus* is a possible pathogen, a semisynthetic penicillin (oxacillin, cloxacillin) should be used empirically because as many as 40% of isolates of *Staphylococcus aureus* are resistant to penicillin. Cephalosporins are used as an alternative to semisynthetic penicillins when the patient is intolerant or a question of penicillin allergy exists. In the truly allergic patient, erythromycin and clindamycin can be used as alternatives; however, the recent introduction of a variety of extremely potent oral antimicrobial agents has the potential for creating rather striking changes in the management of bacterial infections.[4] Indeed, with the availability of these broad-spectrum antimicrobial agents, the need to make a clinical decision is reduced to whether to treat or not.

The importance of knowing the etiological agent is reduced. Because of this, it is becoming common clinical practice in the industrial nations to use these newer agents with broad antibiotic spectrum for empiric outpatient treatment of mild to moderate soft tissue infections. Studies of the bacteriologic profile and clinical course of uncomplicated soft tissue infections indicate that treatment with a narrow-spectrum antibiotic would have the same result in nearly all cases.[5]

Global Therapy

Treatment of skin and soft tissue infections appears to be relatively straightforward and one would expect that global treatment would not differ substantially from one country to another. To investigate the treatment of skin infections globally, several methods were used to obtain an impression of the major trends in therapy. One method was to informally interview physicians who were attending international infectious disease or dermatologic conferences. Their options were recorded and used to get an impression of what they felt were the practices in their countries. Second, where available, commercial marketing tools used to track antibiotic use by indication were used. Thus, the information can be used to give a general impression regarding antimicrobial use worldwide.

In Tables 45-2 to 45-4 individual countries are listed by class (penicillin, cephalosporin, or macrolide) of antimicrobial agents and by the antimicrobial agents most frequently used to treat skin infections in that country. The majority of countries still use penicillin or a penicillin derivative as the drug of first choice. Cephalosporins are the next most widely used class of drug followed by macrolides. Macrolides are the drug of choice in only limited although very large markets. The quinolones are not the drugs of choice in any country, but in the countries with the expenditures for drugs they are rapidly replacing less expensive agents, causing the cost of treatment to increase.

TABLE 45.2. Countries where penicillins are the drug class most frequently used to treat skin and skin structure infections.

Country	Agent	Country	Agent
Argentina	Amoxicillin	India	Penicillin
Austria	Oxacillin	Hungary	Cloxacillin
Australia	Flucloxacillin	Mexico	Ampicillin
Bolivia	Penicillin	Norway	Penicillin
Brazil	Dicloxacillin	Pakistan	Penicillin
Canada	Penicillin	Paraguay	Amoxicillin
Central America	Amoxicillin	Peru	Amoxicillin
Chile	Amoxicillin	Poland	Penicillin
China	Penicillin	Russia	Penicillin
Colombia	Dicloxacillin	Switzerland	Amoxicillin/Clavicillinic acid
Czechoslovakia	Penicillin	Sweden	Penicillin
Denmark	Pivampicillin	Thailand	Dicloxacillin
Ecuador	Dicloxacillin	United Kingdom	Flucloxacillin
France	Oxacillin	Uruguay	Amoxicillin
Germany	Oxacillin	Yugoslavia	Penicillin

TABLE 45.3. Countries where cephalosporins are the drug class most frequently used to treat skin and skin structure infections.

Country	Agent	Country	Agent
*Africa	Cephadrine	Taiwan	Cephalexin
Egypt	Cephadrine	Turkey	Cephadrine
Greece	Cephadrine	United States	Cefadroxil
*Middle East	Cephadrine	Venezuela	Cefadroxil
South Africa	Cefadroxil		

* Combined results from several countries.

TABLE 45.4. Countries where macrolides are the drug class most frequently used to treat skin and skin structure infections.

Country	Agent	Country	Agent
Belgium	Roxithromycin	Netherlands	Roxithromycin
Finland	Erythromycin	Philippines	Roxithromycin
Italy	Miocamycin	Portugal	Erythromycin
Japan	Miocamycin	Spain	Roxithromycin

Penicillins

Penicillin was the ideal drug for skin infections when it was first discovered. It was highly effective, narrow spectrum, and well tolerated. Nearly 50 years later, it is still a very good drug, but some of the advantages have been lost. It is still highly active against the Group A *Streptococcus*, but the majority of strains of *Staphylococcus aureus* are now resistant. Rare strains of Group A *Streptococcus* have also become resistant to penicillin. The newer penicillin derivatives are active against the beta-lactamase-producing strains of *Staphylococcus aureus* but not to the methicillin-resistant strains. Penicillin is cost-effective even when a significant number of patients fail initial therapy. This strategy is acceptable when resources are limited, as skin infections are rarely fatal. It is not acceptable to the individual patient, and when the patients have a choice of physicians, they will choose the physician who gives them agents with little chance of failure. Penicillin use is limited to countries with government-controlled antibiotic usage. This can be in the form of a well-educated cooperative medical population that responds to the epidemiologic data, suggesting that the majority of patients will respond to the narrow-spectrum agents, which are also less expensive. In other cases, such as in Russia and China, the control is simply the lack of newer more expensive agents. In many areas, ampicillin and amoxicillin surpass penicillin not for any real advantage other than more marketing pressure and little difference in cost. The use of beta-lactamase-stable penicillins such as oxacillin are seen primarily in industrialized nations where there is a higher incidence of penicillin-resistant strains of *Staphylococcus aureus*.

Cephalosporins

As an alternative to penicillin, cephalosporins have many advantages. The most important advantage is their broad spectrum of activity against Gram-positive bacteria as well as many Gram-negative bacterial responsible for skin infections. This results in fewer failures of initial therapy. Less frequent dosing regimens such as once or twice daily dosing common among the new cephalosporins is another positive for the patient and greatly improves compliance. Cephalosporins are very safe and well-tolerated agents. Their major disadvantage is the higher cost. In many parts of Africa, cephalosporins are only slightly more expensive than penicillin and are available from the pharmacist without a prescription. This gives them an advantage in those markets where resistance is common. Cephalosporin usage is generally limited to industrialized countries and areas where penicillin-resistant *Staphyloccus aureus* predominate. The safety and tolerance of these agents plus their high efficacy have made them popular in communities where cost is only a minimal issue. The convenience of twice a day dosing has also played a role in their increased use.

Macrolides

The macrolides have some advantages over penicillins in treating skin and skin structure infections. The major advantage is that they act on a different site than penicillins and cephalosporins. They are not affected by beta-lactamase production and can be used to treat penicillin-resistant *Staphylococcus*. Macrolides are very safe drugs, and they have a much lower incidence of allergic reaction when compared to penicillins. Serious allergic reaction, such as anaphylaxis, occurs in 1 in 10,000 patients treated with penicillins[6] but less than 1 in 1 million patients treated with erythromycin. Erythromycin has a potent effect on the motilin receptors in the gastrointestinal tract, and the anhydrosis metabolite of erythromycin produced by the action of stomach acid on erythromycin is significantly more active.[7] This results in a significant number of patients who cannot tolerate erythromycin because of abdominal pain, cramping, nausea, and vomiting. The newer macrolides are much better tolerated and this is no longer a problem. Some strains of *Staphylococcus aureus* have inducible macrolide resistance, which can produce problems when they are overused.[8] Macrolides are not active against methicillin-resistant strains of staphylococci. Macrolides use is much more limited worldwide. One of the reasons for limited use has been the gastrointestinal intolerance seen in many patients given erythromycin. The countries with the highest consumption of macrolides are those where the newer generations of macrolides have been available for over 5 years.

Factors Affecting Antibiotic Usage

Economics

The cost of purchasing antibiotics can account for the use of the least expensive antibiotic for treating skin infections. In general, penicillin is the least expensive as long as the majority of infections treated are Group A *streptococcus* or penicillin-susceptible *Staphylococcus aureus*. If the predominant organism is *Staphylococcus aureus*, then penicillin failure will negate the savings. This tends to be true in more tropical climates and in industrial countries where penicillin resistance is the rule. In the United States and other developed countries, the more affluent portion of the population expects that initial treatment will be effective. Using an agent that results in failure can mean that the physician will lose his patient to other physicians who use more expensive but broader spectrum antibiotics. In Japan, the physician compensation for treatment is limited by the government but they are allowed to dispense medication. The cost of the medicine includes a percentage of profit for the physician. The cost of the drugs is also controlled, but the physican is not limited in his choice of agents. The newer agents are more expensive and the percentage of profit going to the physician is higher. This results in the newer, more expensive agents being used preferentially.

Regulatory

Every country has a regulatory agency that decides which drugs are approved for sale in its country. They have profound effects on which agents are available for treatment of skin infections. The Food and Drug Administration (FDA) regulates the use of drugs within the United States. The FDA requires extensive studies to prove both safety and efficacy. The cost of these studies, which must be done in most cases in the United States, limits the application to drugs that have some advantage over presently approved drugs.

Japan has led the world in the last 30 years in the development of new antimicrobial agents. Many of these agents are not available outside of Japan because of the lack of experience of the Japanese in obtaining approval in other markets. The Japanese are now becoming much more aggressive in the global development of their drugs.

The French are very nationalistic and agents developed by non-French companies with no marketing agreement with French companies are frequently delayed in their approval. France is the largest macrolide market in the world. It is of interest that oxacillin is the most common agent used to treat skin infections in this market. The Scandinavians have been very logical and concerned with cost and safety. They generally limit the number of agents from any drug class. They then select the agents that they feel are the most effective and safest. The physicians in Scandinavia tolerate the government control of their practice to an extent that would not be possible in other countries.

Australia was isolated from the other continents and developed unique flora and fauna. The susceptibility patterns of the skin pathogens in Australia would suggest a similar phenomena because the organisms are generally more susceptible than the organisms seen in other industrialized nations. This may be due to the very slow approval process in Australia and the lack of many of the newer agents as a result of the slow approval.

Resistance

The development of resistance can significantly alter the use of antimicrobial agents. In countries where the use of broad-spectrum antibiotics has been limited, such as Scandinavia and Australia, there has been little development of resistance in the skin pathogens. In the areas of the world where broad-spectrum antibiotics have been used inappropriately, there has been a gradual increase in resistant organisms and an ever-increasing need for new more potent anti-microbial agents. South Africa has produced some of the most resistant skin pathogens. The first isolates of penicillin-resistant *Streptococcus pneumoniae* were isolated in South Africa.[9] Recently, penicillin-resistant strains of Group A *streptococcus* have been seen. *Staphylococcus aureus* has always been a problem and penicillin resistance developed rapidly. With the use of beta-lactamase-stable penicillins and cephalosporins came the development of methicillin-resistant staphylococcus. The macrolides were of some use but inducible resistance meant that high usage would be followed by increasingly resistant strains.[8] The quinolones appeared to be an answer to this problem, but shortly after their introduction quinolone resistant strains of staphylococcus were found.[10-14] They are now becoming increasingly common and newer agents will be needed to combat development of resistance.

Future Trends

Third world countries will be ravaged by increasing populations, AIDS, and decreasing funds for health care. The use of even the least expensive agents to treat skin infection will become prohibitive. The former eastern block countries will have a rapid increase in the availability of newer agents. The common use of more potent agents is still relatively uncommon globally. As resistance patterns continue to change, the increase in foreign travel will result in a more rapid exchange of resistant strains of bacteria. The need for new antimicrobial agents with activity against these resistant strains will place a demand for agents with activity against mechanisms that the present agents do not address. Even with these changes there will still be a great amount of diversity between the agents used. The global diversity in the treatment of skin infections will continue to prove that there is always more than one way to treat a skin infection.

References

1. Galen W, Craft JC, Cohen I, et al: Bacterial disease. In: Schachner LA, Hansen RC, eds. Pediatric Dermatology, New York: Churchill Livingstone, 1988:1261–1369.
2. Swartz MN: Skin and soft tissue infections—cellulitis and superficial infections. In: Mandell GL, Douglas RG, Jr, Bennett JE, eds. Principles and Practices of Infectious Diseases, 2nd ed. New York: John Wiley & Sons, Inc. 1985:598–609.
3. Esposito AL, Adam D: Infection of skin and subcutaneous tissue. In: Eichenwald HF, Ströder J, eds. Current Therapy in Pediatrics—2. New York: B.C. Decker, 1989:698–704.
4. Parish LC, Witkowski JA: Systemic management of cutaneous bacterial infections. Am J Med 1991;91(6A):106S–110S.
5. Powers RD: Soft tissue infections in the emergency department: the case for the use of "simple" antibiotics. South Med J 1991;84(11):1313–1315.
6. Idsoe O, et al: Nature and extent of penicillin side reactions with particular reference to fatalities from anaphylactic shock. Bull WHO 1968;38:159.
7. Sarna SK, Soergel KH, Koch TR, et al: Gastrointestinal motor effects of erythromycin in humans. Gastroenterology 1991;101:1488–1496.
8. Westh H, Jensen BL, Rosdahl VT, Prag J: Development of erythromycin-resistance in Staphylococcus aureus as a consequence of high erythromycin consumption. J Hosp Infect 1989;14:107.
9. Appelbaum PC, Bhamjee A, Scragg JN, et al: Streptococcus pneumoniae resistant to penicillin and chloramphenicol. Lancet 1977;2:995–997.
10. Nakanishi N, Yoshida S, Wakebe H, et al: Mechanisms of clinical resistance to fluoroquinolones in Staphylococcus aureus. Antimicrob Agents Chemother 1991;35:2562–2567.
11. Thomson KS, Sanders CC, Hayden ME: In vitro studies with five quinolones: evidence for changes in relative potency as quinolone resistance rises. Antimicrob Agents Chemother 1991;35:2329–2334.
12. Harnett N, Brown S, Krishnan C: Emergence of quinolone resistance among clinical isolates of methicillin-resistant Staphylococcus aureus in Ontario, Canada. Antimicrob Agents Chemother 1991;35:1911–1913.
13. George RC, Ball LC, Norbury PB: Susceptibility to ciprofloxacin of nosocomial gram-negative bacteria and staphylococci isolated in the UK. J Antimicrob Chemother 1990;26(suppl F):145–156.
14. Kaatz GW, Seo SM, Ruble CA: Mechanisms of fluoroquinolone resistance in Staphylococcus aureus. J Infect Dis 1991;163:1080–1086.

46

Antifungal Therapy

G. Cauwenbergh

During the past 25 years, there has been a rapid evolution in the pharmacotherapy of mycoses. Together with the rapid evolution of pharmacotherapy of the mycoses, the world has also seen an increased importance of the economic aspects of antimycotic development and marketing. The world market for antimycotics in 1980 was valued at a total of 350 million US$. About 10% of this came from the sale of systemic (intravenous or oral) antifungals. In 1990, the antifungal world market was estimated at 1.5 billion US$ of which almost 400 million US$ was attributed to systemic antifungals. Obviously, this important increase in market value has induced more interest in research activities in the field of antifungals leading to more costly new treatment modalities.

The five most prescribed antifungals today are miconazole, clotrimazole, ketoconazole, nystatin, and econazole. This list gives some idea of the place taken by one group of antifungal drugs today: the azoles. Roughly, 70% of all antifungals used today belong to this chemical category. Although highly pathogenic fungi represent only a minority, the importance of opportunistic infections is increasing from year to year.

Human resistance to fungal infections is undermined by a number of factors, and both exogenous and endogenous factors are capable of increasing the pathogenicity of certain fungi. Fungal growth may be stimulated when the host is treated with antibiotics, oral contraceptives, or cytostatics. Exogenous factors such as protheses, catheters, and valves may give rise to an increased incidence of mycoses. In immunocompromized patients and diabetics, saprophytic fungi may become pathogenic due to disturbances in the internal environment. These patients may present chronic mucocutaneous candidosis (CMC) due to *Candida albicans*. *Aspergillus fumigatus* and *A. niger* may become moderately to highly pathogenic in the presence of previously mentioned predisposing factors.

To mycologists, each fungal infection has something specific, either in its symptomatology or its etiology; however, this is less obvious to practitioners. The incidence and the severity of the pathology are sometimes underestimated.

Should the physician opt for systemic or topical treatment? On the other hand, which arguments will convince the patient to use one or both forms for the minimum period recommended? It is typical for mycoses that the period of treatment generally exceeds 1 week and may even last a few months. There is still a strong tendency to treat the organ or the part of the organ affected by the pathogenic microorganism. This is justifiable in the case of localized unifocal mycoses of the skin caused by dermatophytes.

Oral treatment offers the advantage of bringing back all the lesions at all sites under control, in addition to the absence of unpleasant cosmetic effects. In certain cases, it may be preferable to use oral treatment for *C. albicans* vaginitis tinea and for extensive and persistent versicolor, caused by *Malassezia furfur*.

In the case of onychomycosis, combination treatment, topical plus systemic, is required. It

TABLE 46.1. Mycoses.

Superficial	Deep
Dermatophytosis	Aspergillosis
Trichophytosis	Blastomycosis
Microsporosis	Candidosis
Epidermophytosis	Chromomycosis
Tinea versicolor	Coccidioidomycosis
Candidosis	Cryptococcosis
	Histoplasmosis
	Maduromycosis
	Paracoccidioidomycosis
	Sporotrichosis

is preferable to use oral treatment for deep and systemic mycoses, although intravenous or intrathecal treatment is sometimes required.

The final choice of a suitable antimycotic and the route of administration are determined by many factors:

- safety of the antimycotic
- ease of administration
- broad-spectrum activity
- rapid clinical improvement associated with mycological cure.

Topical Antifungal Therapy

Older Compounds

Some antimycotics have been used for a long time; Whitfield's ointment is a typical example (1907). The ointment usually contains 6% benzoic acid and 3% salicylic acid. The action is attributed to the keratolytic effect of the salicylic acid and the direct effect of benzoic acid on the fungus. The main advantage of this ointment is its low price. This combination is now replaced by more active modern antimycotics.

Long ago, the antimycotic effect of aliphatic carboxylic acids with increasing number of C atoms was discovered. The optimum is 11 C atoms, undecylenic acid. This substrate is used in several ointments. Other drugs are a combination of a keratolytic agent (mesulfen) and the well-known antimycotic zinc un-

decylenate. This cream also contains zinc naphthenate, terpineol, chlorcresol, and methyl salicylate. The last substance has a deeply penetrative effect: It combines antimycotic and antibacterial properties and is used to treat swimmer's dermatitis. The cream must not be used on open skin areas infected by bacteria. Some foot powders are a combination of zinc undecylenate, boric acid, hexachlorophene, and salicylic acid.

Tolnaftate, which is active against dermatophytes, is the active component in another antifungal powder; it also contains cetylpyridinium chloride and talcum venetum. In addition to tolnaftate and cetylpyridinium chloride, the ointment also contains polyethylene glycol. This preparation is not active against *C. albicans*.

Specific Compounds

Nystatin

Together with amphotericin B, pimaricin (natamycin), trichomycin, candicidin, filipin, etruscomycin, and hamycin, nystatin belongs to the group of polyene-antimycotic antibiotics. During the past 30 years, approximately 200 polyenes have been isolated from different *Streptomyces* strains. Nystatin is obtained from *Streptomyces noursei*. The polyenes are characterized by a macrolide ring and differ from one another by the number of carbon atoms in the ring structure,[12-37] the number of hydroxyl groups,[6-14] and the presence or absence of carbohydrate.[1]

All of the polyenes alter the membranes permeability of sensitive cells by forming a complex with the sterol present in the membranes. Due to this binding to sterols, potassium ions are lost. Both nystatin and amphotericin B bind more strongly to ergosterol than to cholesterol. Ergosterol is the principal sterol in the membrane of yeasts and fungi, whereas the cell membrane in mammals contains mainly cholesterol. This difference in binding capacity is probably responsible for the selectivity.[1,2] Because bacteria, with the exception of *Mycoplasma* and *Acholeplasma*, contain no sterols, polyenes have no antibacterial activity.

Nystatin has a local fungicidal and fungistatic action against *C. albicans*. This polyene is not hydrosoluble. It is absorbed to a very limited extent from the digestive tract, which limits the field of indications after oral administration to candidoses of the oral cavity, the esophagus, and the intestines. It should be mentioned that oral administration of large doses may cause gastrointestinal disorders (nausea, vomiting, diarrhea). Nystatin is too toxic for parenteral administration. Nystatin is mainly used to treat vaginal and oral infections and localized skin lesions, including *Candida* intertrigo and *Candida* diaper dermatitis. It may also be used as prophylaxis during treatment with antibiotics.

Dosage: Cream or ointment (100,000 IU/g) to be applied twice daily. The cream used in gynecology contains 25,000 IU/g; oral suspension (100,000 IU/g) 4 times per day 1 ml; if necessary, the dosage may be increased; tablets (500,000 IU per tablet) 3 times per day 1 or 2 tablets.

Natamycin

Natamycin or pimaricin is a polyene with only four conjugated double bonds. This tetraene is obtained from *Streptomyces natalensis*. Like the other polyenes, pimaricin induces K^+ release from cells with membranes containing 20–40 mol% ergosterol (this is also the ergosterol concentration in the membrane of *Saccharomyces cerevisiae*).

Natamycin is not hydrosoluble or soluble in most organic solvents. It is not absorbed in the digestive tract.

Indications: Skin and nail infections with *C. albicans*; intertrigo and fissures at the corner of the mouth (perleche) caused by *C. albicans*; *Candida* vulvitis and vaginitis. Natamycin plays an important role in the treatment of mycotic keratitis. Natamycin also appears to be active against the protozoa *Trichomonas vaginalis*.

Side effects: Nausea or diarrhea may occur during oral treatment.

Dosage: Apply the cream several times per day. The eye ointment contains 10 mg natamycin per g ointment. This ointment should be applied 2 to 4 times per day. Vaginal tablets contain 25 mg natamycin per tablet. This tablet is inserted vaginally every evening for 20 days. 100 mg coated tablets can be used to treat intestinal candidosis. For adults, 1 coated tablet 4 times per day is prescribed during 1 week. Infants and children should receive 1/2 coated tablet 2 to 4 times per day.

Amphotericin B

Amphotericin B, an important polyene antibiotic, is administered almost exclusively via the intravenous route and is, therefore, discussed in more detail under the systemic antimycotics The vaginal suppositories contain 50 mg amphotericin B and 100 mg tetracycline base per tablet. The tablets for oral use contain 50 mg amphotericin B, 250 mg tetracycline base, and 125 mg sodium hexametaphosphate.

Synthetic Antimycotics

Because of their limited activity, small spectrum, and side effects, the older topical antimycotics have generally been surpassed by newer antimycotic chemotherapeutic agents. These newer antimycotics for topical use include the imidazole derivatives clotrimazole, miconazole, econazole, isoconazole, sulconazole, fetinconazole, oxiconazole, bifonazole, butoconazole, zinoconazole, tioconazole, and the triazole derivative, terconazole.

The introduction of the azole derivatives represents a milestone in the treatment of mycoses.

Clotrimazole

The imidazole derivative clotrimazole (Fig. 46.1) was introduced in 1969. Clotrimazole or

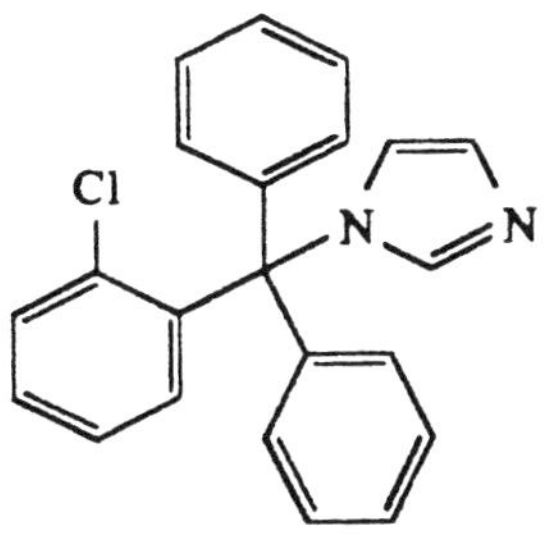

FIGURE 46.1. Chemical structure of clotrimazole.

chlordiphenyl benzylimidazole is a nonhydro-soluble antimycotic for topical application, with a broad-spectrum activity against mycoses of the skin and the vagina. This antimycotic, which was introduced for topical use, shows *in vitro* activity against dermatophytes, species of *Candida*, *Aspergillus*, *Coccidioides immitis*, *Histoplasma capsulatum*, *Cryptococcus neoformans*, and *Madurella* species. *Petriellidium* (*Allescheria*) *boydii* and *Phialophora* species are less sensitive.

As with the other azole derivatives, the antimycotic activity is based on inhibition of the cytochrome P-450-dependent ergosterol biosynthesis. This inhibition not only results in a reduction of ergosterol but also in an accumulation of C-14 methyl sterols. They disturb membrane permeability, inhibit cell replication, and are basically responsible, in combination with the reduction of ergosterol levels, for the antifungal action. Clotrimazole and other azole derivatives have a different mode of action than the polyenes, for example, amphotericin B. The latter bind to the ergosterol present in the membranes of yeasts and fungi, but azole derivatives inhibit the biosynthesis of ergosterol. (For further information concerning the mode of action of azole derivatives, see Refs. 8–11).

Clotrimazole is only partly absorbed in the digestive tract. It is a microsomal enzyme (cytochrome P-450) inductor and induces its own metabolism. This explains why it is not active in vivo against the etiologic agents of deep mycoses, including *H. capsulatum*, *C. immitis*, and *C. neoformans*. Enzyme induction also produces increased levels of other liver enzymes, such as transaminases. Because of this and possible side effects such as nausea, vomiting, and hallucinations at times (cerebral toxicity), the use of clotrimazole is limited to topical application.

Side effects: Topical application of clotrimazole is very well tolerated; local allergic reactions and generalized skin irritations may occur occasionally.

Dosage: cream (containing 10 mg clotrimazole/g) applied 2–3 times per day until 2 weeks after all symptoms have disappeared. Vaginal tablet (containing 100 mg clotrimazole); 1–2 tablets once per day (preferably in the evening) are inserted deeply into the vagina for 6–12 consecutive days.

Miconazole

Miconazole nitrate (Fig. 46.2), the 1-phenethyl-imidazole derivative first described in 1969, interferes at low doses with the cytochrome P-450-dependent ergosterol biosynthesis in yeasts and fungi. The result is an accumulation of C-14 methylated sterols on the one hand and reduction of the ergosterol levels in the membranes on the other hand.[12] In analogy to clotrimazole, this leads to a disturbance in the membranes; it results in inhibition of cell replication, mycelium development (in *C. albicans*), and finally, cell death. High concentrations of miconazole (which may be achieved with topical use) disturb the orientation of phospholipids in the membranes, which produces leaks.[13]

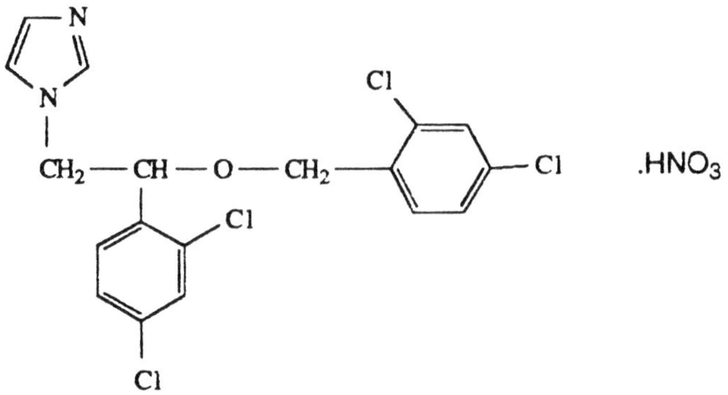

FIGURE 46.2. Chemical structure of miconazole.

Miconazole has a potent antifungal action against dermatophytes and *Candida* species. It is also active against Gram-positive bacilli and cocci. In vitro, it is effective against *Trichomonas, Leishmania,* and *Plasmodium.*

Miconazole is only moderately absorbed in the digestive tract. After intravenous administration, it is rapidly metabolized.

Indications: Infections of skin and nails due to dermatophytes or *Candida* species; vulvovaginal infections due to *Candida* species. Miconazole is used orally for prophylactic purposes in patients who have been treated with cytostatics or immunosuppressants (in particular, to prevent candidosis of the mouth and digestive tract).

Side effects: Nausea may occur during oral treatment. Miconazole tablets may increase the anticoagulant effect of coumarin derivatives. Topical treatment with cream or powder is well tolerated. Local irritation and allergic reactions of the skin and mucosa occur only rarely.

Dosage

- tablets (containing 250 mg miconazole base per tablet): children: 20 mg/kg/day, adults: 1 tablet 4 times per day;
- oral gel (20 mg miconazole per g); infants: 25 mg 4 times per day; older children and adults: 50 mg 4 times per day;
- cream (2% miconazole nitrate), powder, lotion, and tincture; skin infections: 1–2 times per day, usually 2–5 weeks; nail infections: 1–2 times per day (cure after 2 or more months); vulvovaginal infection: 5 g cream to

be applied vaginally once a day (before retiring) for at least 5 days;
- (200 mg miconazole nitrate per ovule): insert 1 ovule deeply into the vagina once per day (in the evening) for 7 days;
- 1200 mg: insert a single suppository deeply into the vagina;
- tincture (20 mg miconazole per ml): apply twice per day;
- lotion (20 mg per g): apply once or twice per day;
- tampon (100 mg miconazole nitrate per tampon): insert a tampon into the vagina twice per day for 5 days.

Econazole

Chemically, econazole (Fig. 46.3) is closely related to miconazole. The clinical indications are almost identical. Econazole is available as a vaginal cream and suppository containing respectively 1% and 150 mg econazole nitrate. For mycoses of the skin, several forms are available: cream, spray powder, spray solution, lotion. All these formulations contain 1% econazole nitrate. The dosages are practically identical to those of miconazole.

Isoconazole

Like econazole, both the chemical structure and the clinical indications of this imidazole derivative closely resemble those of miconazole. It is available as a vaginal tablet (300 mg isoconazole nitrate per tablet). In some countries, isoconazole (Fig. 46.4) is also available as a cream for dermatological use and as a cream and suppository for treatment of vaginal candidosis.

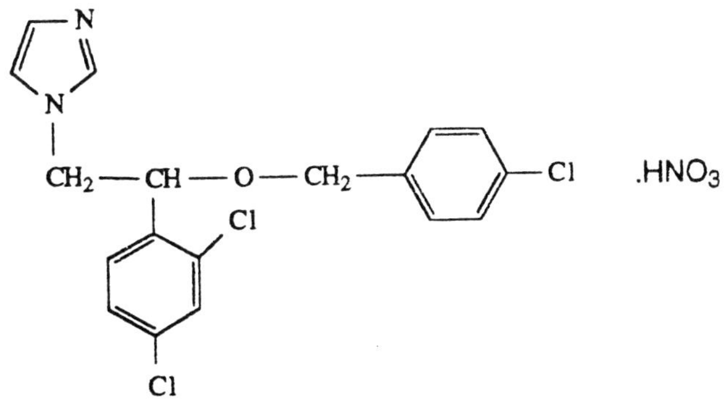

FIGURE 46.3. Chemical structure of econazole.

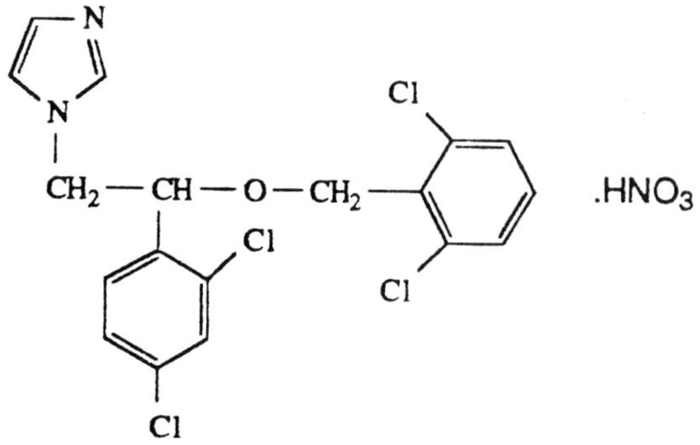

FIGURE 46.4. Chemical structure of isoconazole.

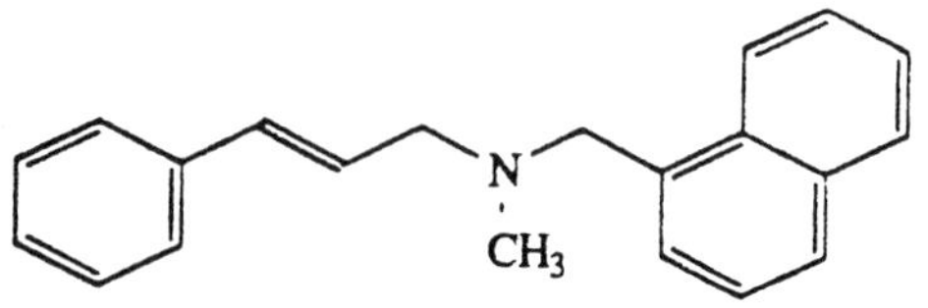

FIGURE 46.5. Chemical structure of naftifine.

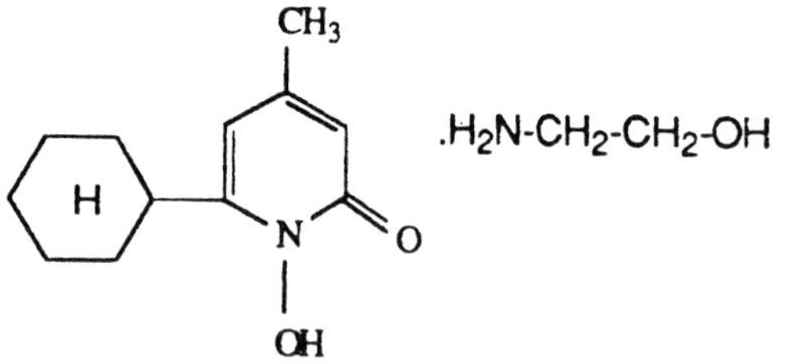

FIGURE 46.6. Chemical structure of cyclo-piroxolamine.

Naftifine

Naftifine (Fig. 46.5) belongs to the allylamines, a new class of antimycotics.[14] It is used to treat superficial mycoses and is particularly active against dermatophytes. Like the azole derivatives, it inhibits the biosynthesis of ergosterol, however, naftifine does not inhibit the cytochrome P-450-dependent C-14-demethylase, but inhibits the epoxydation of squalene. Squalene epoxydase catalyzes the first step in the conversion of squalene via lanosterol to ergosterol in yeasts and fungi or to cholesterol in mammalian cells. The squalene epoxydase in *C. albicans* is 150 times more sensitive to naftifine than the enzyme in rat liver.[15] Naftifine is available as a 1% cream.

Cyclopiroxolamine

Cyclopiroxolamine (Fig. 46.6) is a topically active antimycotic, available as a cream and powder.[16] The biochemical basis for its action in fungi has not been totally elucidated. This compound is used mainly in the treatment of mycoses of the skin and nails. A special formulation for topical treatment of nail mycoses has been developed. The initial clinical results have been encouraging but larger-scale studies were not able to confirm these initial good results.

Ketoconazole

Initial observations indicating that oral administration of ketoconazole (Fig. 46.7) produced good results in seborrheic dermatitis and

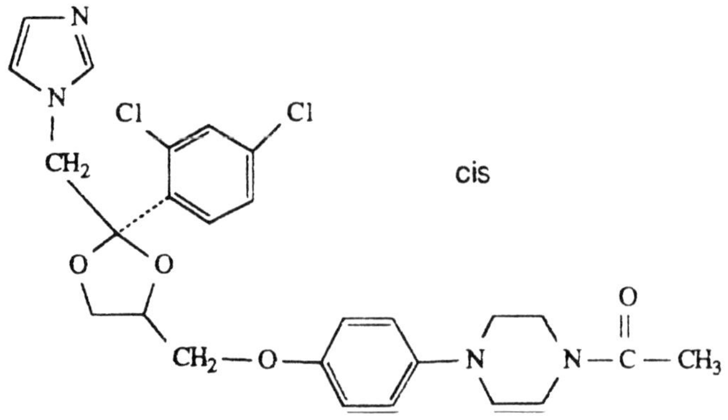

FIGURE 46.7. Chemical structure of ketoconazole.

seborrhea led to the development of a 2% cream and a 2% shampoo (scalp gel) of this antimycotic.[17,18] Naturally, these two topical forms of ketoconazole are highly active against superficial mycoses. The main application of these two topical forms is the treatment of seborrheic dermatitis and seborrhea. Ketoconazole's potent pityrosporicidal effect at concentrations of 100 ng/ml to 1 μg/ml forms the rationale of this activity. Recent work indicating an anti-inflammatory effect of ketoconazole may help to explain the apparent superiority of the drug in seborrheic dermatitis and dandruff.

Haloprogin

Haloprogin or 3-iodo-2-propynyl 2,4,5-trichlorophenyl ether is an almost insoluble antifungal for topical use, available in the United States. It was developed in 1963 and it is active against dermatophytes. The drug's effect against *Candida* spp. is rather limited. Its worldwide use is extremely limited to date.

Other Antimycotics

Most of the topical antimycotics still being developed or limited in availability are azole derivatives (mostly imidazole). The list includes butoconazole, oxiconazole, omoconazole, zinoconazole, and sulconazole (Fig. 46.8). Generally speaking, these newer azoles offer no additional therapeutic advantages compared to existing substances. These drugs are already available in certain countries, but are not yet commercialized on a worldwide scale.

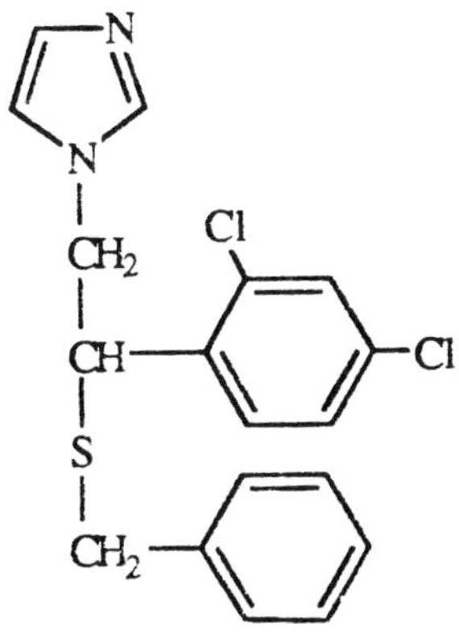

Amorolfine is a molecule that is totally different from this group; it is a morfoline derivative.[19] This substance has a broad-spectrum activity and a fungicide effect at fairly low concentrations. The development of a nail varnish for treatment of onychomycoses could be very interesting. For dermatologic use, a broad range of topical formulations has been developed. The mechanism of action of amorolfine is not P-450 related, although the end result is the same as that of allylamines and azole derivatives. Amorolfine disturbs the biosynthesis of ergosterol leading to disturbances in the fungal cell membranes.

Systemic Antimycotics

Potassium Iodide

When potassium iodide is administered orally for several weeks,[6-8] a therapeutic effect may be obtained in the subcutaneous form of sporotrichosis (amphotericin B is used IV to treat systemic sporotrichosis).

Dosage: Usually, a saturated solution in water is used (1 g/ml). The usual oral dose is 30 mg/kg/day. Children should receive 5 droplets, 3 times per day (after meals); the dose may be increased to 15–20 droplets.
Side effects: Digestive disorders, swelling of the salivary glands, and lacrimation. Thyroid function tests may be disturbed.

Griseofulvin

Although griseofulvin (Fig. 46.9) was first isolated in 1939 and was described as a metabolite of *Penicillium griseofulvum*,[20] its action against *Microsporum* and *Trichophyton*

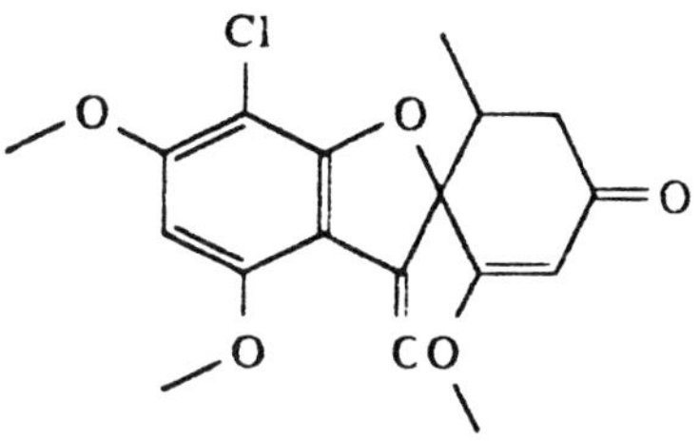

FIGURE 46.8. Chemical structure of sulconazole.

FIGURE 46.9. Chemical structure of griseofulvin.

was only discovered in 1958. Several modes of action were suggested for $(+)$ 7 chloro-4, 6-demethoxy-coumaran-3-one-2-1'-(2'-methoxy-6'-methylcyclohex-2'-en-4'-one($C_{17}H_{17}ClO_6$); this antibiotic derived from *P. griseofulvum*. It interferes with the synthesis of the hyphe walls, with the biosynthesis of nucleic acids and with the synthesis of chitine. The interaction with microtubules has also been described. The sensitivity of a cell seems to depend particularly on the ability to form griseofulvin nucleic acid complexes. (Further information concerning griseofulvin can be found in Ref. 21.)

After oral administration, griseofulvin is absorbed moderately. The absorption is increased when it is administered together with oil or fat. Micronization also increases the absorption greatly in the digestive tract. (Griseofulvin with a particle diameter of 3.7 μm reaches twice the plasma levels of griseofulvin with a particle diameter of 10 μm.)

Griseofulvin is found in the outer layers of the stratum corneum. Perspiration plays an important role in its distribution to the skin. Kinetic studies in the nail have indicated that griseofulvin is incorporated in the keratin via the nail matrix. The use of short-term high-dose pulse therapy in onychomycoses, however, has not resulted in adequate response rates.

Indications: Mycoses of the skin, hair, and nails due to species of *Trichophyton*, *Epidermophyton floccosum*, and *Microsporum*. Yeasts and bacterial are not sensitive. Griseofulvin has a very weak effect against *Aspergillus*.

Side effects: Headache and gastrointestinal disorders may occur, but are usually only temporary. Occasionally, urticaria, erythema, or photosensitivity are observed. Griseofulvin is a strong inducer of the mixed function oxidase in the liver. It, therefore, has a stimulating effect on the conversion of various other drugs, including oral anticoagulants for example. It also affects the biosynthesis of porphyrin; this may result in the accumulation of protoporphyrin in hepatocytes.

Dosage

- Children: 10 mg/kg/day or 2 tablets or 125 mg micronized griseofulvin per day;

- Adults: 4 tablets of 125 mg per day or 1 × 500 mg tablet.

tinea corporis, treatment may last longer than 6 weeks. Onychomycosis may last up to 6 months, certainly if the toenails are involved.

Precautions: Caution is required in patients with impaired kidney or liver function or hematological disorders.

Contraindication: Pregnancy.

Amphotericin B

This heptane macrolide antibiotic (Fig. 46.10) is produced by *Streptomyces nodosus*. It has fungistatic and fungicide properties and is effective against *Candida* species and the etiologic agents or systemic mycoses, including *Histoplasma capsulatum*, *Blastomyces dermatitidis*, *Coccidioides immitis*, and *Cryptococcus neoformans*. It is also active against *Sporothrix schenckii*. Like nystatin, this polyene has a greater affinity for ergosterol than cholesterol. Consequently, much lower levels of amphotericin B are required to induce potassium release in *C. albicans* than in mammalian cells. Potassium release is secondary to the increased flux of protons.[1] In yeasts, the proton gradient plays an important role in the function of the plasma membrane. The transport of amino acids and other nutrients depends on this proton gradient.[22]

Absorption is minimal after oral and topical administration. In order to obtain a systemic effect, the compound must be administered intravenously. Plasma levels are fairly stable during the first 24 h: Only a small fraction is eliminated via urine during this period. The polyene can be detected in urine up to 3 weeks after treatment. Diffusion of amphotericin B into cerebrospinal fluid is only moderate. (More information concerning polyene antibiotics can be found in Refs. 1–4 and 23.)

Side effects: during intravenous administration several side effects should be taken into account. The main side effects are noted in the glomeruli of the renal parenchyma and include thickening of the basal membrane with hyalinization and in the tubuli, where

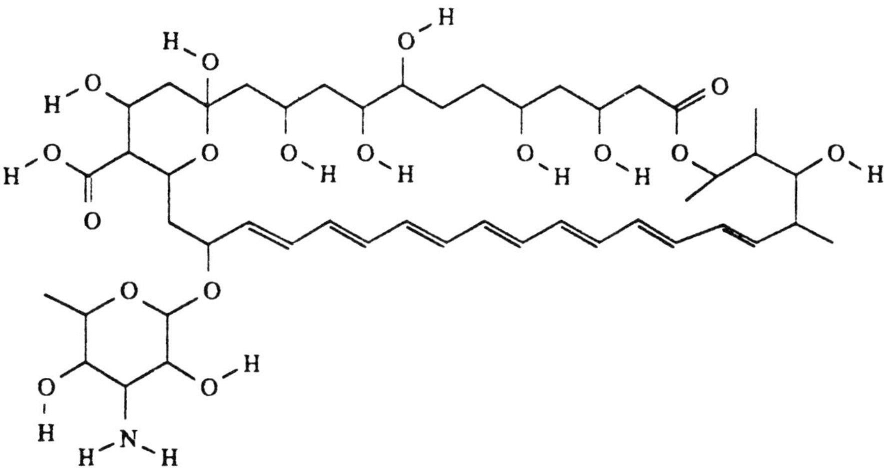

FIGURE 46.10. Chemical structure of amphotericin B.

focal or generalized degeneration and ne-phrocalcinosis may occur. Hypokalemia is an important consequence of nephrotoxicity. Headache, nausea, and vomiting are usually the first signs of toxicity. The dosage should be reduced until these side effects disappear. Vomiting, fever, and headache may be prevented by the administration of anti-histamines and corticosteroids.

Dosage: Amphotericin B is administered over a 6-h period via a slow intravenous infusion. The recommended concentration is 0.1 mg/ml. The initial dose is 0.1–0.2 mg/kg/day. The dose is then increased to 1 mg/kg/day. The daily dose must never exceed 1.5 mg/kg. The duration of the treatment depends on the nature and the extent of the infection.

A marked improvement is generally noted after 4–8 weeks of treatment. Treatment is often continued until a total dose of 3 g is reached. In the case of coccidioidomycosis, for example, treatment with 0.4–0.8 mg/kg/day may last months. The polyene is administered intrathecally to treat *Coccidioides* meningitis, however, the results are only moderate. It is very important to check renal and hepatic function during treatment with amphotericin B.

Flucytosine

Flucytosine (Fig. 46.11) or 5-fluorocytosine (4-amino-5-fluoro-2-pyrimidone, 5-FC) is a pyrimidine derivative that is very effective against *Candida albicans*, *Cryptococcus neofor-mans*, and *Torulopsis glabrata*. It is also active against *Aspergillus*, *Phialophora*, and *Clado-sporium*. The protozoa *Acanthamoeba culbert-soni* and *Leishmania* are sensitive to flucytosine. (See Refs. 1 and 24 for a general review.)

Flucytosine is very well absorbed in the digestive tract, which is why oral administration is preferable. Plasma levels of 30–40 mg/l were obtained after a dose of 30 mg/kg body weight. Approximately 90% of the pyrimidine derivative is found unaltered in urine, indicating that it is highly suitable for the treatment of renal candidosis. High concentrations were also noted in cerebrospinal fluid; the average concentration is approximately 75% of the plasma concentra-tion.

With the aid of cytosine permease, flucytosine reaches the fungal cell, where it is converted by cytosine deaminase into 5-fluorouracil. Cytosine

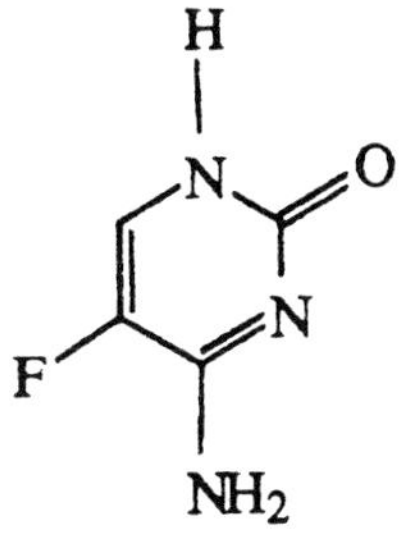

FIGURE 46.11. Chemical structure of flucytosine.

deaminase is not present in the host, which explains the low toxicity of 5-FC. 5-Fluorouracil is then phosphorylated and incorporated into RNA. 5-Fluorouracil may also be converted into 5-fluorodeoxyuridine monophosphate, which is a very potent and specific inhibitor of thymidylate synthetase. As a result, no more thymidine nucleotides are formed, which, in turn, leads to a disturbance of the DNA synthesis. These effects produce an inhibition of the protein synthesis and cell replication.[1,23,24]

5-Fluorouracil cannot be used as an antimycotic. It is poorly absorbed by the fungus to begin with and is also toxic for mammalian cells.

Flucytosine-resistant strains can develop very rapidly. These mutants may have a disturbed 5-FC metabolism, or a compensatory mechanism for the disturbed necleic acid functions. No cytosine permease was found in a resistant Cryptococcus neoformans strain, whereas cytosine deaminase was absent in resistant C. albicans strains. According to Kerridge and Whelan,[1] a deficiency of uridine monophosphate pyrophosphorylase occurred frequently in resistant C. albicans strains.

Dosage: Flucytosine 150–200 mg/kg orally in 4 portions every 6 h. A 1% flucytosine solution was developed for intravenous administration. In some countries, a 10% ointment is also available.

Side effects: In patients with normal renal function, flucytosine is seldom toxic. Occasionally, severe toxicity may be observed (leukopenia and thrombocytopenia). It is recommended to determine plasma levels and to check the dose in patients with impaired renal function. Liver function tests (transaminases and alkaline phosphatase) should be performed regularly. In some patients with high flucytosine plasma levels, hepatic disorders have been observed.[24]

Miconazole

Miconazole (Fig. 46.2) is also available as a sterile solution for intravenous infusion. Has a therapeutic effect on systemic mycoses due to C. albicans, Aspergillus fumigatus, Cryptococcus neoformans, Blastomyces dermatitidis, Histoplasma capsulatum, Coccidioides immitis, Paracoccidioides brasiliensis, and Petriellidium boydii.

The recommended dosage produces plasma levels that exceed the in vitro MIC values for the previously mentioned fungi. Doses >9 mg/kg generally produce plasma levels of ≥1 mg/L.

Side effects: Large doses may cause loss of appetite, nausea, and vomiting. Very rapid infusion may lead to transistory cardiac arrhythmia and tachycardia. During prolonged and repeated intravenous administration, liver function tests are recommended. Cremophor, the solvent, may induce hypertriglyceridemia.

Dosage: The daily dose is approximately 10 mg/kg (= 1 ml). Depending on individual tolerance, the dose may be increased to 30 mg/kg (= approx. 1800 mg). The infusion should last at least 30 min. In children, the dose administered via infusion should not exceed 15 mg/kg.

Ketoconazole

For treatment of systemic mycoses with amphotericin B or miconazole IV, the patient must be admitted to the hospital; this is not always possible (particularly in areas where systemic mycoses occur frequently) or desirable because of the expense. For these reasons, it was necessary to find an antimycotic that combined safety and broad-spectrum activity with oral administration.

Ketoconazole (Fig. 46.7), which is orally active, met most of these requirements. This inhibitor of the ergosterol biosynthesis is a N-substituted imidazole that differs from its precursors by the presence of a dioxolane ring. (See Refs. 6 and 7 for a general review.)

Ketoconazole is rapidly absorbed in the digestive system after oral administration. Sufficient gastric acid is required to dissolve the compound and for absorption. Therefore, medication that affects gastric acidity (for example, cimetidine and antacids) should not be combined with ketoconazole.

Plasma levels of 3–5 μg/ml are obtained 2 h after administration of 200 mg ketoconazole. No accumulation in the bloodstream was noted after a 30-week treatment with this dose. The half-life is approximately 8 h. When ketoconazole is taken with meals, higher plasma levels are obtained. Distribution studies using radioactive ketoconazole in rats show radioactivity mainly in the liver and the connective tissue. Radioactivity is also present in the subcutaneous tissue and the sebaceous glands. After 1 dose of 200 mg in humans, ketoconazole is found in urine, saliva, sebum, and cerumen.

Like miconazole, the mode of action is based on a selective inhibition of the cytochrome P-450-dependent biosynthesis of ergosterol. This results in disturbed membrane permeability and membrane-bound enzymes.[8,10,23,25]

Ketoconazole is active against dermatophytes (*Microsporum, Trichophyton, Epidermophyton*), yeasts (*Candida* species, *Cryptococcus*), and the dimorphous fungi (*Coccidioides, Histoplasma,* and *Paracoccidioides*). Activity was also demonstrated in patients with aspergillosis, and in a limited number of patients with chromomycosis and sporotrichosis, promising results were obtained. It should be noted that some *Leishmania* species are sensitive.

For the agent is indicated: Infections of the skin and nails due to dermatophytes and/or yeasts; yeast infection of the gastrointestinal tract; chronic recurring vaginal candidosis; systemic fungal infections.

Side effects: Ketoconazole is well tolerated by most patients. Gastrointestinal symptoms or pruritus were noted in 1–3% of the patients. Occasionally, liver enzymes may be increased temporarily. Normalization usually occurs during treatment. Three hundred of the estimated 4 million patients treated developed hepatitis, that is, 1 per 15,000 patients.[26]

Treatment with ketoconazole should be discontinued when clinical and/or laboratory indications of hepatitis are present.[7,27] In the case of prolonged treatment, it is advisable to check liver function twice a month during the first month of treatment, followed by monthly checks. With large doses (600 mg–1.2 g/day) a reversible inhibition of the testosterone synthesis is observed.[28]

Dosage: For all the indications, except vaginal candidosis, 1 tablet (= 200 mg) per day is normally prescribed. The treatment should be continued without interruption for at least 1 week after the symptoms have disappeared and until all the cultures are negative. If the clinical result is not satisfactory, 400 mg may be administered.

The period of treatment, with the exception of vaginal candidosis, depends on the clinical and mycological results. In the case of recurrent vaginal candidosis, 400 mg per day is prescribed for 5 days. Recent studies with *Pityriasis versicolor* have demonstrated that shorter treatments (1 tablet for 5–10 days) also produce good results. Children (≤ 20 kg) are given 50 mg per day. When they weigh between 20 and 40 kg, 100 mg/day is given. This is increased to 200 mg/day for children weighing > 40 kg.

Contraindications: pregnancy.

Itraconazole

Itraconazole (Fig. 46.12) is a highly lipophilic compound with a triazole structure. Compared to ketoconazole, itraconazole has a broader spectrum (including *Aspergillus* spp.)[29,30] and an in vitro activity that is a factor of 10 higher for most species other than ketoconazole. This in vitro superiority is also confirmed by animal experiments. Compared to ketoconazole, itraconazole is a much more selective inhibitor of the cytochrome P-450-dependent ergosterol biosynthesis in yeasts and fungi (see Refs. 29 and 30 for a review). Pharmacokinetically, itraconazole has a much longer bioavailability (± 24 h) and a greater tissue affinity. In general, itraconazole tissue levels are significantly higher than the corresponding plasma levels.

Pharmacokinetic studies in the skin and in the nails have shown that the itraconazole levels in the keratin are not only higher than the corresponding plasma levels but therapeutic levels persist for several weeks (skin) or months (nails) after discontinuation of therapy. This favorable cutaneous pharmacokinetic profile results in the possibility of treating skin infections for short-fixed treatment periods. It

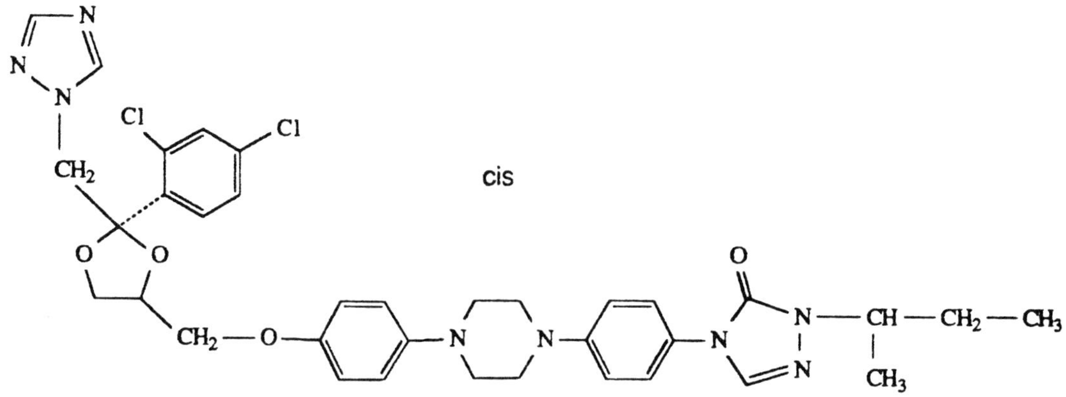

FIGURE 46.12. Chemical structure of itraconazole.

has been established toxicologically that therapeutic doses of itraconazole do not interfere with the steroid metabolism in humans. Itraconazole does not affect the liver as much as ketoconazole. There are few side effects: headache, nausea, vertigo, and intestinal disorders.

Itraconazole is used to treat vaginal candidosis (single-day treatment with 200 mg b.i.d.), tinea versicolor (200 mg o.d. for 1 week), tinea corporis/tinea cruris (100 mg o.d. for 2 weeks), and tinea pedis/tinea manus (100 mg o.d. for 4 weeks). Studies in onychomycoses show that 200 mg itraconazole for 3 months results in 80% mycological cure 6 months after stopping treatment. Itraconazole is contraindicated during pregnancy.[32]

Fluconazole

Fluconazole (Fig. 46.13) is a hydrosoluble bis-triazol tertiary alcohol.[33] The substance has a broad spectrum but has little activity in vitro, however, animal experiments reveal a broad spectrum and a potent effect. At the tested daily dose of 50 mg, fluconazole appears to be slightly less active against dermatophytes. The substance is used mainly to treat vaginal candidosis (a single capsule of 150 mg) and oral and esophageal candidosis (50 mg o.d. for 14 days). In a number of countries (e.g., England), the maximal period of treatment is 14 days. Although fluconazole has been used for treatment of skin mycoses, the results have not been superior than those of ketoconazole both in percent cure and treatment length.

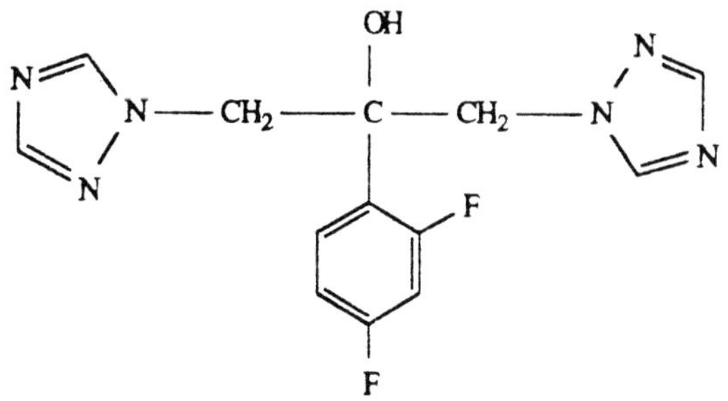

Toxicological studies have demonstrated that there are no important problems with fluconazole. Therapeutic doses of fluconazole may cause enzyme induction in the liver. This suggests that interactions with other drugs cannot be excluded.

The side effects are similar to those of itraconazole and include nausea, headache, and vertigo. Occasionally, increased liver enzymes may be noted. More recently, it has been demonstrated that long-term suppressive maintenance treatment with 50 or 100 mg fluconazole daily in AIDS patients may result in a selection of more therapy resistant strains of *C. albicans* and in a shift of pathogen toward the nonalbicans species of the genus *Candida*.

Like itraconazole, fluconazole is contraindicated during pregnancy.

Terbinafine

Terbinafine is an orally active allylamine derivative with a pronounced activity against

FIGURE 46.13. Chemical structure of fluconazole.

dermatophytes. Although in vitro antifungal activity against some strains of *C. albicans* and *Aspergillus fumigatus* could be demonstrated, the concentrations required for this effect were usually too high to have clinical relevance.[34] Terbinafine has a fungicidal effect on dermatophytes in vitro, but the presence of serum lowers this effect. Animal studies indicate no superiority over itraconazole in dermatophytosis.

The action of terbinafine is derived from the inhibition of the squalene epoxydase enzyme.[35] This inhibition results in a disturbed ergosterol biosynthesis and impaired cell membrane functions. Clinical studies have shown 80–90% response rates in dermatophytoses when terbinafine was given at a daily dose of 200 mg for 2–6 weeks. Studies in onychomycoses have shown that 250 mg for 6 months results in 75% cure. The same dose for 3 months appears to give similar results.

The side-effect profile of terbinafine is minor with only headache occurring as a relatively frequent complaint. Other side effects include nausea and gastrointestinal complaints. Thus far, biochemical monitoring has not shown consistent abnormalities in liver or renal function.

Acknowledgment. I would like to thank Ms. Hilde Dergent for typing the manuscript and adapting it completely after review.

References

1. Kerridge D, Whelan LE: In: Trinci APJ, Ryley JF, eds. Mode of Action of Antifungal Agents. British Mycological Society Symposium 9, Cambridge: Cambridge University Press, 1984: 343–375.
2. Gale EF, Cundliffe E, Reynolds PE, et al: The molecular Basis of Antibiotic Action, 2nd ed. London: John Wiley & Sons, 1981:201–219.
3. Medoff G, Kobayashi GA: In: Speller DCE, ed. Antifungal Chemotherapy. London: John Wiley & Sons, 1980:3–33.
4. Medoff G, Brajtburg J, Kobayashi GS: *Ann Rev Pharmacol Toxicol* 1983;**23**:303–330.
5. Holt RJ: In: Speller DCE, ed. Antifungal Chemotherapy. London: John Wiley & Sons, 1980:107–147.
6. Levine HB: Ketoconazole in the Management of Fungal Disease, Sydney: Adis Press, 1982.
7. Jones HE: In: Fleischmajer R, ed. Progress in Diseases of the Skin, Vol. 2. New York: Grune & Stratton, 1984:217–249.
8. Vanden Bossche H, Lauwers W, Willemsens G, et al: *Pesticide Sci* 1984;**15**:188–198.
9. Vanden Bossche H, Willemsens G, Marichal P, et al: In: Trinci APJ, Ryley JF, eds. Mode of Action of Antifungal Agents, British Mycological Society Symposium 9. Cambridge: Cambridge University Press, 1984:21–41.
10. Vanden Bossche H: In: McGinnes, ed. Current Topics in Medical Mycology, Vol. 1. New York: Springer-Verlag, 1985:313–351.
11. Vanden Bossche H, Marichal P, Gorrens J, et al: *Pesticide Sci* 1987;**21**:289–306.
12. Vanden Bossche H, Willemsens G, Cools W, et al: *Chem Biol Interact* 1978;**21**:59–78.
13. Vanden Bossche H, Ruysschaert JM, Defrise-Quertain F, et al: *Biochem Pharmacol* 1982: 2609–2617.
14. Petranyl G, Ryder NS, Stütz A: *Science* 1984;**224**:1239–1241.
15. Ryder NS: In: Nombela C, ed. Microbial Cell Wall Synthesis and Autolysis. Amsterdam: Elsevier Science Publishers, 1984:313–312.
16. Farkas B, Kemény L, Csato M: In Tümbay E, ed. The Efficacy of Cyclopyroxolamine in the Treatment of Mycosis and its Influence on the Keratinocyte Killing Activity. Turkish Microbiological Society, 1986:35.
17. Stratigos JD, Antoniou CHR, Katsambas A, et al: Mosby (St Louis), *J Am Acad Dermatol* 1987;**19**(5) (part 1):850–853.
18. Cauwenbergh G, De Doncker P, Schrooten P, Degreef H: *Int J Dermatol* 1986;**25**(8):541.
19. Polak A, Dixon DM: In: Fromtling RA, ed. Recent Trends in the Discovery, Development and Evaluation of Antifungal Agents. JR Prous Science Publishers, S.A., 1987:555–573.
20. Oxford AE, Raistrick H, Simonart P: *Biochem J* 1939;**33**:240–248.
21. Davies RR: In: Speller DCE, ed. Antifungal Chemotherapy. London: John Wiley & Sons, 1980:49–82.
22. Foury F, Goffeau A: *J Biol Chem* 1974;**250**:2354–2362.
23. Vanden Bossche H, Willemsens G, Marichal P: *CRC Crit Rev Microbiol* 1987;**15**:57–72.
24. Scholer HJ: In: Speller DCE, ed. Antifungal Chemotherapy. London: John Wiley & Sons, 1980:35–106.
25. Vanden Bossche H, Willemsens G, Cools W, et

al: *Antimicrob Agents Chemother* 1980;**17**:922–928.

26. Lewis JH, Zimmerman HJ, Benson GD, Ishak KG: *Gastroenterology* 1986;**86**:503–513.

27. Janssen PAJ, Symoens JE: *Am J Med* 1983:80–85.

28. Varden Bossche H, Lauwers W, Willemsens G, Cools W: In: Schroeder F, eds: European Organization for Research on Treatment of Cancer. New York: Alan E Liss Inc., 1985:187–196.

29. Van Cutsem J, Van Gerven F, Van De Ven M-A, et al: *Antimicrob Agents Chemother* 1984;**26**:527–534.

30. Vanden Bossche H, Mackenzie DWR, Cauwenbergh G, eds: Aspergillus and Aspergillosis. New York: Plenum Press; 1988.

31. H. Vanden Bossche: In: Fromtling RA, ed. Recent Trends in the Discovery, Development and Evaluation of Antifungal Agents, J.R. Prous Science Publishers, S.A., 1987:207–221.

32. Cauwenbergh G, De Doncker P: *Drug Dev Res* 1986;**8**:317–323.

33. Troke PF: In: Fromtling RA, ed: Recent Trends in the Discovery, Development and Evaluation of Antifungal Agents. JR Prous Science Publishers, S.A., 1987:103–112.

34. Van Cutsem J, Janssen PAJ: 28th Interscience Conference on Antimicrobial Agents and Chemotherapy, Los Angeles, CA, 1988:141.

35. Ryder NS, Fromtling RA, ed. Recent Trends in the Discovery, Development and Evaluation of Antifungal Agents. JR Prous Science Publishers, S.A., 1987:451–459.

47

Antiparasitic Therapy

Mohamed Amer

Animal parasites are divided into two groups:

1. Protozoa (unicellular).
2. Metazoa (multicellular), which are characterized by segmentation of the ovum.

Both are divided into phyla, the most important of which are:

1. protozoa,
2. nemathelminthes, parasitic worms,
3. arthropoda.

Each phylum is divided into classes, and further into orders, families, genera, and species.

In this chapter, the treatment of the most common diseases caused by each phylum is discussed. The prevention of these diseases, when feasible, will be mentioned.

Protozoa

Cutaneous Amoebiasis

Cutaneous amoebiasis is caused by *Entamoeba histolytica*; in patients with AIDS, it may be caused by *Acanthamoeba castllani*.

The disease usually presented by deeply invading ulcer or ulcerative granuloma (Amoeboma) which is usually very painful. The common sites are the perianal region and in or around a surgical wound in the abdomen. This may be the only manifestation of the disease or it may be associated with the involvement of other organs;[1] treatment varies accordingly.

Treatment

Combinations of drugs may be necessary because some are more effective in the gut lumen (e.g., metronidazole, emetine, and dehydroemetine) and others are active systemically[2] (e.g., diloxanide and tetracyclines). Chloroquine is often given as a supportive treatment for liver abscesses.

1. Metronidazole: given in a dosage of 800 mg 3 times daily for up to 10 days (35–50 mg/day for children) is probably the safest in treating cutaneous infection.
2. Tinidazole: given as a single daily dose of 2 g for 3–5 days (50–60 mg body weight for children) may be more effective.
3. Local cleansing of cutaneous ulcer with antiseptic solutions may be necessary.

Cutaneous lesions usually respond rapidly with improvement occurring in 4–5 days.

Trypanosomiasis

Two distinct types of infection by protozoan of the genus *Trypanosoma* exist, the African and the American forms. The African form is subdivided into two clinical varieties, gambiense and rhodesiense trypanosomiasis, both transmitted by tsetse flies.

Cutaneous lesions are usually limited to the site of initial fly bite. A chancre develops at the entry site 5–10 days after the bite. It is a painful red nodule usually on the exposed parts and associated with regional lymphadenopathy. Scratching may lead to secondary infection and ulceration. The secondary or invasive stage usually develops 1–3 weeks after the initial bite and is manifested as fever accompanied or shortly followed by a characteristic eruption.[3] The eruption consists of transient erythematous of annular or serpiginous plaques. Painful transient edema of the hands, feet, and eyelids usually occurs.

Treatment

Treatment of African trypanosomiasis depends on the stage of the disease.[3]

In the early stages, suramin is the drug of choice administered intravenously in a freshly prepared solution. The first test dose of 0.1 g is followed by 1 g weekly for 6 weeks if no renal toxicity develops.

Pentamidine may be given in cases of gambiense infection intramuscularly in a freshly prepared solution of 4 mg/kg every other day for a total of 10 injections.

Arsenkal preparations such as melasoprol and suramin may be given in late stages when CNS involvement occurs.

The American Trypanosomiasis

American trypanosomiasis also called Chaga's disease is caused by *Trypanosoma cruzi*. The acute stage of the disease (1–4 months) is the only form associated with cutaneous manifestations.

Chagoma, the most distinctive feature of this stage, is a boardlike tender induration associated with regional lymphadenopathy. Unilateral eyelid edema, conjunctivitis, and periauricular adenopathy is known as Romana's sign.

Treatment

The treatment of choice in the acute stage depends mainly on two effective specific parasiticidal drugs. Nifurtimox, administered in 3 divided doses of 8–10 mg/kg body weight for 2–3 months. Children under 2 years of age receive 20 mg/kg body weight; those over 2 years received 15 mg/kg/day in four divided doses. Side effects such as anorexia, insomnia, and polyneuritis are dose related and often

disappear after dose reduction. The second drug of choice, benznidazole (Rochagan), is administered in 5 mg/kg body weight doses for 2–3 months. Photosensitivity, erythema multiforme, and erythroderma are common side effects.

There is no specific effective therapy for the chronic form of the disease and the treatment is usually symptomatic.

Prevention depends chiefly on avoidance and/or irradication of the insect vector. Community public health measures are mandatory to eliminate breeding places.

Leishmaniasis

Leishmania is a genus of protozoan parasite that infects a broad range of hosts including insects, amphibians, and mammals including humans. In the human host, *Leishmania* is an obligate intracellular parasite, transmitted by the bites of the infected female sandflies. Transmission to humans is usually from infected nonmammalians reservoirs and, depending on the parasite species, can result in cutaneous, mucocutaneous, or visceral disease.

Classification

A. Old World cutaneous leishmaniasis is caused by the following:
1. *L. tropica minor*. This organism causes the urban, usually anthroponotic, cutaneous leishmaniasis. It is found in the Near East from Turkey to India, North and West Africa, and Mediterranean Europe.
2. *L. tropica major*. This form causes the zoonotic rural cutaneous leishmaniasis in Iran, Pakistan, the Middle East, and North and West Africa. Rodents are the main reservoirs.
3. *L. aethiopica*. This species commonly causes diffuse cutaneous leishmaniasis in the highlands of Ethiopia and Kenya. The hydrax is the reservoir.
B. New World cutaneous leishmaniasis is found in Central and South America.

It is caused by species of *L. mexicana* complex (e.g., *L. mexicana mexicana*) and the *L. braziliensis* complex (e.g., *L. braziliensis panamenesis*).

Mucocutaneous leishmaniasis, found in South America, is caused by *L. braziliensis*. It is a life-threatening disease.

When considering the treatment of cutaneous leishmaniasis, one must keep in mind the wide variety of species/subspecies of the parasite involved. The clinical form taken by the infection depends on the immunologic response of the host. The host's defense to these intracellular pathogens largely depends on the cell-mediated immune response.

The most common form of cutaneous leishmaniasis is acute cutaneous leishmaniasis (ACL), also known as Oriental sore or Baghdad boil. This lesion is at the center of the spectrum. The initial nodular erythematous lesion usually breaks down to form an ulcer. Such lesions heal spontaneously in weeks or months but usually leave a scar.[4]

At the anergic end of the spectrum is diffuse cutaneous leishmaniasis (DCL). The primary lesion spreads and the parasite is disseminated throughout the whole body surface. The infection is usually very chronic.

The hypernergic end of the spectrum includes: (1) chronic cutaneous leishmaniasis (CCL), which follows from ACL that does not heal. There may be erythematous papules at the edge of the lesion. (2) Recurrent cutaneous leishmaniasis (RCL), also known as leishmaniasis recidivans. It occurs at or near the acute lesions that have completely or partly healed. These lesions can appear months or years after the healing of the primary lesion.[5]

Treatment

The leishmaniases, like the trypanosomiases and microfilariases, have not seen major advances in their treatment in the last decades. The detection and treatment of human cases are considered very important for controlling cutaneous leishmaniasis. Control of the vector sandfly and the animal reservoir, for example, the rodents and wild hydraxes, is also needed.

Spontaneous healing also occurs. For the first 2 or 3 months the lesions continue to become progressively worse, then healing begins and is complete within 12–15 months. Considering this fact and that recovery is supposed to confer lifelong immunity a pertinent question could be asked:[4] *Why* treat leishmaniasis?

In New World cases, there is, of course, the fear of the consequences of *L. braziliensis* infections. *L. braziliensis* infections are already treated. In the Old World, ACL treatment is desired where there are lesions on exposed parts of the body, especially the face. The healed scars and areas of depigmentation are ugly. Another reason to treat is to prevent secondary bacterial infection of the lesions.

Infections with *L. aethiopica* should receive special attention because they involve large areas of the body surface and tend to have a long course. Healing of these lesions gives rise to severe fibrosis that, for example, may restrict the use of fingers.

Another reason for the need to treat is that treatment is one of the most important methods of controlling the disease in the population.[6]

Traditional Therapies

1. **Pentavalent antimonials**, such as glucantime (methyl glucamine antimoniate) and pentostam (sodium stiboglycate), are the most commonly used in a dose of 10 mg antimony/kg body weight for adults, 20 mg/kg body weight for children by intravenous or intramuscular injection daily, plus local infiltration with either of the drugs. In chronic leishmaniasis (the hypernergic spectrum), intralesional steroid should be tried in conjunction with antimonial to shift the hypernergic activity toward a normogenic response.

   Toxicity includes headache, fainting, muscle and joint pain, ECG changes, and seizures. Antimonials should be avoided in patients with myocarditis, hepatitis, or nephritis. The mechanism of action of antimonials is unclear. Numerous enzymes of the parasites are inhibited selectively. Of significance, phosphofructokinase, which catalyzes a rate-limiting step of glycolysis, is inhibited.[7]

2. **Amphotericin B** has been used and found effective in the mucocutaneous form. The drug should be diluted in 5% dextrose solution and given 1 mg/kg over 6 h on

alternate days. Amphotericin B is very toxic to the kidney. Urea and urine protein levels should be carefully monitored. Decreased serum potassium levels are found in 25% of patients receiving the drug. Infusions of amphotericin B are associated with thrombophlebitis. This can be prevented by adding small amounts of heparin to the infusion.

Details of the mechanism of action of amphotericin B are not clear. In fungal infections, its action is likely to occur through interaction with ergosterol in fungal membranes.

Other Drugs

1. **Metronidazoles**: used in protozoal infections amoebiasis and trichomoniasis. Its selective toxicity is probably due to the reduction of a nitro group on the drug inside the parasite. It now appears that metronidazole is unlikely to play a primary role in the therapy of leishmaniasis.
2. **Nifurtimox**: this is the drug of choice in American trypanosomiasis (Chaga's disease), where it is active against the amastigote phases of the parasite. The dose is 8–10 mg/kg/day for 3–120 days. However, the dose takes too long to administer.
3. **Rifampicin**: in one trial using 1200 mg/day, clinical cure occurred in 3–8 weeks in 41 of 46 cases of cutaneous leishmaniasis.

   Rifampicin has been tried with other drugs, for example, with isoniazid, pentamidine, sodium stibogluconate, or amphotericin B.
4. **Antimalarials**: for example, 8-aminoquinoline (Quinacrine) 5–10% solution may be administered intralesionally with good anticipated results.
5. **Levamisol**: has an immunopotentiating effect on T-cells. Butler[8] observed that even in an endemic area the prevalence of cutaneous leishmaniasis is low. He believes that most local inhabitants are inoculated in early life with the parasite by sandflies and have subclinical infections. This gives long-term immunity. Butler proposes that clinical cutaneous leishmaniasis infections in later life are due to a declining cell-mediated immunity, which can be potentiated by levamisol. In this trial, 28 patients were cured with levamisol

without other medication. This interesting proposal requires further investigation.
6. **Phenothiazines**: include chlorpromazine and are psychoactive drugs.

   Henriksen and Lenden[9] treated 3 patients with *L. aethiopica* diffuse cutaneous leishmaniasis with topical chlorpromazine. Inflammation improved, and parasite smears were negative after 1 month of treatment.
7. **Allopurinol**: used in hyperuricemia. Oral allopurinol (15 mg/kg/day) produced questionable cure in two of five patients with mucocutaneous leishmaniasis. There was clinical cure in the two patients after 2 months from start of treatment, but there was still a significant fluoresence antibody titre at 1 year.[10]
8. **Ketoconazole**: Urcayo and Zaias[11] report on oral ketoconazole (400 mg/day for 3 months) being effective on six Nicaraguan patients with early skin lesions.

Experimental Agents

1. **Difluoromethylornithine** (DFMO) blocks polyamine synthesis (have important functions in the growth of *Leishmania*) by inhibiting ornithine decarboxylase (ODC) essential for polyamine synthesis.[12]
2. **Antipain and leupeptin**, the peptide analogues, lead to inhibition of cysteine proteinases and stop the in vitro multiplication of the parasite.[13]
3. **Transfer factor** is a dialyzable extract of leukocytes obtained from healthy donors who have recovered from cutaneous leishmaniasis. This factor is injected subcutaneously near the skin lesion of the patient.

Nonmedical Treatment of Leishmaniasis

1. **Plastic surgery** has an important role in treating disfiguring scars, especially scars of *Leishmania recidivans*.
2. **Heat therapy** has been used quite often in the past. Leishmania organisms are very thermosensitive to both heat and cold.
3. **Cryotherapy** with a carbon dioxide cryomachine is short and quick and gives little discomfort. Cryotherapy also spares pregnant and weak patients from toxic drug effects.

Parasitic Worms

Parasitic worms infect humans worldwide and are particularly common in tropical countries. There are two main groups, roundworms (Nemathelminthes) and flatworms (Platyhelminthes). A single class of Nemathelminthes causes disease, Nematodes. There are two important classes of Platyhelminthes, Trematoda (flukes) and Cestoda (tapeworms).

Nematodes

Nematodes that are parasitic in humans may be intestinal or tissue roundworms.

Enterobiasis

Anal and perineal pruritus at night especially in children are the leading symptoms.[14] Synonyms are pinworm, oxyuriasis, and threadworm.

Treatment

1. **Mebendazole**, given as a single oral dose of 100 mg for all ages, has cure rate of 90–100%. There is a minimal absorption of this drug which seems to be free of side effects.
2. **Levamizole** in a single oral dose of 3–5 mg/kg body weight may be another alternative.

Either mebendazole or levamizole should be given a second time after 2 weeks.

Human Hookworm Disease

The disease occurs in nearly all subtropics and tropics and is caused by two intestinal hookworms, *Necator americanus*, the New World hookworms, and *Ancylostoma duodenale*, the Old World hookworms.

Larvae penetrating the skin cause ground itch: severe pruritus, erythema, edema, papular, and vesicular or bullous eruptions developed, usually on the feet. It is transient, subsiding spontaneously in 2 weeks unless complicated by secondary bacterial infection. The rash is more common with *Necator* sp. infections.[15]

Treatment

1. Topical application of thiabendazole may be helpful.
2. If secondary infection occurs, antibacterials should be administered.
3. The treatment of intestinal disease depends mainly on tetrachloroethylene in cases of *Necator* sp. infections given in a gelatinous capsule on an empty stomach preceded by a saline purge the day before. The dose is 5 capsules (1 ml each) for adults and 0.1 mg/kg body weight for children. Another saline purgative is given a few hours later. Treatment should be repeated 2 weeks later if 3 successive stool examinations show eggs still present.
4. For *A. duodenale* infections, pephenium hydroxy naphthoate (Alcopara) is preferable. Two packets of 2.5 g on an empty stomach is given to adults; half of this dose may be given to children. In heavy infections, this may be repeated in 15 days.
5. Thiabendazole is also effective.
6. In case of mixed infections with *Ascaris*, piperazine may be used before the treatment of hookworms.
7. Anemia should be corrected.

Strongyloidiasis

Strongyloides stercoralis is a roundworm with a life cycle similar to that of the hookworm but with a heterogenic nature yielding alternating parasite and free living generations.

The skin changes are pronounced and occasionally characteristic. They are caused by penetration of the larvae or allergic reaction. The dermatitis that develops due to penetration of the skin by the larvae is similar to the ground itch but less intensive. Later in the disease, urticarial eruption associated with erythema lasting for several days may occur. This may be associated with a peculiar type of creeping eruption. This migrates at a rate of several centimeters per hour in a serpiginous manner. This is called larvae currens to differentiate it from larva migrans caused by

Ancyclostoma braziliensis (the dog hookworms).[16]

Treatment

1. **Thiabendazole**, 25 mg/kg body weight, orally for 3 days may be effective.
2. **Ivermectin** is an antiparasitic agent used extensively in veterinary practice and has shown promise for the treatment of strongyloidiasis.[17]

The control of the disease depends mainly on improvement of waste disposable facilities.

Trichiniasis (Whipe worms)

Trichouris trichura infection is more prevalent in moist and warm tropical regions, especially in rural areas. The infection occurs by ingestion of infective ova that originated directly or indirectly from the soil.

The only important skin eruption is urticaria and may be due to systemic hypersensitivity.

Treatment

Mebendazole and thiabendazole may be used.

Gnathostomiasis

The characteristic of the infection caused by *Gnathostoma spinigerum* is that it combines features of creeping eruption and myasis. Human is a dead end host; the parasite fails to mature and wanders in human tissue as long as 10 years. The usual route for migration leads from stomach to liver, skeletal muscles, and subcutaneous tissues. Intermittent erythematous, edematous migratory plaques of different sizes appear suddenly. They are piuritis and may be associated with abscess formation or small haemorrhagic spots. Rarely the worm emerges spontaneously from the lesion.[18]

Treatment

1. **Surgical removal** of the parasite is the treatment of choice.
2. **Freezing,** with ethylchloride or dry ice, the advancing end of the lesion where the parasite is located has been reported effective.

Creeping Eruption

There is considerable confusion about the disorders included under this title. Several different parasites produce similar clinical pictures. *Ancylostoma brazieliense*, *A. caninum*, *A. duodenale*, *Necator A.*, *Uncinaria stenocephala*, and *Capillaria philippinensis* are some of these. The lesion arises as a result of tunneling of the larvae in the epidermis.

Treatment

The treatment depends on severity of infection:

1. Orally, **albendazole** is now replacing all other lines of treatment that have been of choice. It is given 400 mg b.i.d. for 1–2 weeks. Side effects are absent or minimal.
2. Topical and oral **thiabendazole** may also be effective.

Tissue Roundworms

Extraintestinal human nematodes include filarial worms, guinea worm, *Dracunculus medinensis*, and *Trichinella* species.

Filariasis

Wuchereria bancrofti and *Brugia malayi* cause bancroftian and malayian filariasis, respectively. The latter is more prevalent in Southeast Asia, whereas bancroftian filariasis is endemic in extensive tropicals and subtropicals. It has been reported in almost every country of these zones. Humans are only host for *W. bancrofti*, whereas *B. malayi* has been found in primates and felines. The bite of a mosquito of the genera *Culex*, *Aedes*, *Mansonia*, and *Anopheles* injects larvae of the parasite, which migrate to the lymphatics and lymph nodes and develop within about 1 year into mature worms.[19]

Clinical manifestations range from asymptomatic infection to severe elephantiasis.

Treatment

1. **Diethylcarbamazine** has been known as the drug of choice. It rapidly reduces the circulating microfilariae and may affect the

adult worm. The drug is given in tablet form starting with smaller doses:

50 mg for the first day,

50 mg t.d.s. for the second day,

100 mg t.d.s. for the third day

2 mg/kg body weight daily to complete a course of 3 weeks.

This course is advocated to minimize the Jarisch-Herxheimer reaction, which develops within 6 h after the first dose and reaches its maximum in 24–48 h. It usually subsides in 3–6 days even with the continuation of treatment. The reaction usually manifests itself with fever, orchitis, abdominal pain, bone aches, and arthritis. Antihistamines given at the beginning of treatment may help to control the reaction.

If clinical response is unsatisfactory, a second course after 3 months may be given. Treatment will not reverse elephantiasis.

2. Recently, **ivermectin** is suggested as an effective line of treatment of lymphatic filariasis. A single dose of 100–200 μg/kg ivermectin is given. Side effects are similar to those of diethylcarbamazine. The drug is suitable for mass treatment. The mechanism of action is not well understood.[17]

3. **Surgical treatment** may be needed to correct massive scrotal involvement, hydrocele, and elephantiasis.

Loiasis (LoaLoa)

This is a chronic infection limited to rain forests. It is caused by the filarial worm loaloa. It is transmitted by *Chrysops* flies. The adult, a wide threadlike worm measuring between 25 and 75 mm, migrates continuously through the subcutaneous tissue at a maximum rate of 0.5–1 cm. The adult worms appear in the eye, occasionally beneath the skin, and produce Calabar swellings.[19]

Treatment

1. **Diethylcarbamazine** is very effective in treatment of loiasis; it kills the adults and microfilariae. The dose is similar to that used for the treatment of bancroftian filariasis.

2. Low-dose **mebendazole** has also been used in a dosage of 100 mg t.d.s. for 45 days.

Onchocerciasis

Onchocerciasis is a filarial disease caused by *Onchocerca volvulus* and is transmitted by flies of genus *Simulium*. Twenty to forty million persons worldwide are victims of this disease. The disease may cause blindness and has a negative impact on economic development all over tropical Africa and in some countries of Asia. There are also foci in Central and South America. The most characteristic lesion is subcutaneous nodules that contain the worms and may be acute or chronic. Regional lymph node inflammation and ocular damage may also occur.

Treatment

Between 1982 and 1984 several reports from Aziz et al.,[20] Coulaud et al.,[21] and Awadzi et al.,[22] appeared about the effect of ivermectin in treating lightly infected individuals with single oral doses of ivermectin ranging from 5 to 200 μg/kg body weight. The drug appeared to be effective, safe, and well tolerated. It was also shown that ivermectin was as effective as diethylcarbamazine in its microfilaricidal effect and was associated with less significant skin reaction.

Ivermectin is now the drug of choice for treatment of *O. volvulus* infection in humans. It is administered as a single oral dose of about 150 μg/kg body weight. It is an effective microfilaricidal agent suppressing count in the skin and eyes and prevents progression of ocular disease. It is recommended to be given every 6 months.

The mechanism of action of ivermectin is not well understood. It is thought to block the action of the neurotransmitter GABA, as evident by its paralytic action on intestinal nematodes. In mammals, GABA-dependent neuronal transmission is only in the CNS, and ivermectin does not enter the CNS. In patients with onchocerciasis, ivermectin was found to decrease the motility of microfilaria and promote cell-mediated cytotoxicity. It also has been shown to inhibit release of microfilaria from the uterus of adult worms, which may affect transmission.

1. **Diethylcarbamazine** is given in cases of mild to moderate onchocercal dermatitis without

eye involvement. Several repeated courses of a long period may be needed to destroy the new load of microfilariae. The dosage is the same as for the treatment of filariasis.

2. **Suramin,** which is a urea derivative, may be used especially in treatment of cases with eye involvement. It is a microfilaricidal and it also kills the adult worms. The dosage is the same as for the treatment of trypanosomiasis. Urine examination should be performed before starting treatment and before each weekly injection to detect the possible presence of albumin. Arterial blood pressure should also be checked because the drug is very slowly eliminated through the kidneys. Renal dysfunction, pregnancy, hypertension, and severe anemia are absolute containdications. Side effects such as urticaria, edema especially of the palms and soles, arthritis, and erythroderma may be controlled by antihistamines or even corticosteroids, and there may be a need to interrupt treatment.

Platyhelminthes

Among platyhelminthes two types are of medical importance: *Trematoda* and *Cestoda*. The *Trematodes* of cutaneous importance are *Schistosomes* or blood flukes.

Cutaneous manifestations of *Schistosomes* can be divided into four types depending on the state of development of the parasite and the chronicity of systemic disease.[23]

1. Dermatitis schistosomica (swimmer's itch) caused by the penetration of the human or nonhuman cercariae through the skin.
2. Bilharzida or schistosomid (Katayama disease) is an allergic anaphylactoid reaction that occurs when large number of eggs (new antigenic materials) are released, and antibodies produced in response to the presence of developing worm cross react with them.
3. Bilharziasis cutna tarda is a specific schistosomal skin lesion caused by deposition of eggs in the dermis.
4. Lesions related to complications of schistosomiasis spider nevi, vulval leukoplakia, and rarely carcinoma of the vulva.

Treatment

Cercarial dermatitis may be prevented by thorough drying of skin immediately after leaving water; repellents such as citronella oil or protective clothes are also helpful. Antipruritic lotions and antihistamines may reduce the itching and, thus, prevent scratching from causing secondary infection, which may need a course of oral antibiotic. Norfloxacin may be given 400 mg twice daily for 5–10 days.

Oral preparations include lucanthone and niridazole (25 mg/kg body weight daily for 10 days). Hycanthone is available also in the form of intramuscular injections. Treatment of *S. mansoni* must be repeated several times. Anti-schistosomal treatment must start as early as possible before tissue reactions and fibrosis have become irreversible.[23]

Praziquantel is the drug of choice for the treatment of infections due to all species of *Schistosoma*. It is given as a single oral dose of 40 mg/kg. Side effects are few and include abdominal distress with or without nausea, headache, slight drowsiness, and, very rarely, itching of the skin and a rise in temperature.[24]

For schistosomal skin granuloma, the anti-schistosomal drugs will lead to involution of the lesions usually in 4–6 weeks, but larger lesions will respond better to intralesion triamcinalone (4 mg/ml) weekly for 1 month. Surgical excision of large lesions may be necessary.

References

1. Fujita WH, Barr RJ, Gottschalk WR: Cutaneous amoebiasis. *Arch Dermatol* 1981;**117**:309–310.
2. Knight R: The chemotherapy of amoebiasis. *J Antimicrob Chemother* 1980;**6**:577–593.
3. Foulkes JR: Human trypenosomiasis in Africa. *Br Med J* 1981;**283**:1172–1174.
4. Chong H: Oriental sore. A look at trends in and approaches to the treatment of leishmaniasis. *Int J Dermatol* 1986;**25**:615–623.
5. Farah F, Malak J: Cutaneous leishmaniasis. *Arch Dermatol* 1971;**103**:467–474.
6. Strick R, Barok M, Gasiorowski H: Recurrent cutaneous leishmaniasis. *J Am Acad Dermatol* 1983;**9**:437–443.

7. Gutteridge W, Coombs G: Biochemistry of parasitic protozoa. London: Macmillan, 1977.

8. Butler P: Levamisole and immune response phenomena in cutaneous leishmaniasis. *J Am Acad Dermatol* 1982;**6**:1070–1077.

9. Henriksen T, Lenden S: Treatment of diffuse cutaneous leishmaniasis with chlorpromazine ointment. *Lancet* 1983;**1**:126.

10. Marsden P, Cuba C, Barretta A: Allopurinol treatment in human leishmania braziliensis infections. *Trans Roy Soc Trop Med Hyg* 1984;**78**:419–420.

11. Urcayo F, Zaias N: Oral ketoconazole in the treatment of leishmaniasis. *Int J Dermatol* 1982;**21**:414–416.

12. McCann P, Bacchi C, Clarkson A: Further studies on difluoromethylornithine in African trypanosomiasis. *Med Biol* 1981;**59**:434–440.

13. Coombs G, Hart D, Capaldo J: Proteinase inhibitors as antileishmenial agents. *Trans Roy Soc Trop Med Hyg* 1982;**76**:660–663.

14. Broadbent V: Children's worms. *Br Med J* 1975:89.

15. Gilles HM, Williams EJW, Ball PAJ: Hookworm infection and anemia. *Quart Rev Med* 1964;**33**:1–24.

16. Stone OJ, Newell GB, Mullins JF: Cutaneous strongyloidiasis: larva current. *Arch Dermatol* 1972;**106**:734.

17. Campbell WC: Ivermectin: An update. *Parasitol Today* 1985;(1):10–16.

18. Radomyos P, Daengsvang S: A brief report on Gnathostoma spinigerum specimens obtained from human cases. *Southeast Asian J Trop Med Pub Hlth* 1987;**18**:215.

19. Davis BR: Filariasis. *Dermatol Clin* 1989;**7**:313–321.

20. Aziz MA, Diallo S, Diop IM, et al: Efficacy and tolerance of ivermectin in human onchocerciasis. *Lancet* 1982;**2**:171–173.

21. Couland JP, Lariviere M, Gervais MC, et al: Treatment of human onchocerciasis with ivermectin. *Bull Soc Pathol Exot Filiales* 1983;**76**:681–688.

22. Awadzi K, Dadzie KY, Schulz-Key H, et al: Ivermectin in onchocerciasis [letter]. *Lancet* 1984;ii:2921.

23. Amer M: Cutaneous schistosomiasis. *Int J Dermatol* 1982;**21**:44–46.

24. Mamoud AAF: Praziquantel for the treatment of helminthic infections. In: Stollerman GH, ed. Advances in Internal Medicine. Chicago: Year Book Medical Publishers, 1987:419–434.

Index

2,3-Dimercaptopropanol (BAL) for
    treatment of arsenic poisoning,
    184
Diphtheria, cutaneous, among
    Australian aborigines, 129–30
Dithranol for psoriasis, 240
DNA repair mechanism, inhibition by
    heat, 90
Dolphins, infection with *loboa loboi*,
    176
Dominican Republic, immigration to
    the United States from, 45
Donovanosis, among Australian
    aborigines,
    123, 130
Down's syndrome, 157
Doxycycline, cutaneous adverse
    reactions to, 73
Dracontiasis in Nigeria, 254–56
Dracunculosis, 3
    in the Caribbean, 177
Dracunculus medinensis, 177
    Guinea worm disease caused by,
    119, 254–56
Drugs
    contact dermatitis from, 271
    cost of, 316
        in Nigeria, 246
        in Rwanda, 267–68
        in South India, 292
    effect of, in porphyria variegata,
        281
    multidrug therapy, for leprosy,
        228, 293
    nephrotoxic, suramin, 251
    photoallergic dermatitis associated
        with, 72
    phototoxic dermatitis associated
        with, 72, 201
    prophylactic and therapeutic,
        interactions, 73
    reactions to, 230
    shortage of, in Malawi, 239
Dubin-Johnson syndrome, 159–60
Duhring's disease. *See* Dermatitis
    herpetiformis
Dum-Dum fever, 119
Dysautonomia, familial type II, among
    Ashkenazi Jews, 158
Dyshidrosis, 53
Dystrophy, cone-rod, 161

Ebola virus disease, 119
Econazole, 323
Economics
    of antibiotic usage, 316–17
    of antimycotic usage, 319
    See also Drugs, cost of;
        Socioeconomic factors
Ectodermal dysplasia, congenital, in
    Lebanon, 300
Ectoparasitic disease
    in large animals, 104, 106–7
    skin, in immigrants to western
        Europe, 54

Eczematides, among Afro-Caribbean
    immigrants to the United
    Kingdom, 59
Education
    Centre for the Investigation of
        Tropical Disease (CIET), 8
    in China, 37
    in Colombia, 188–89
    core curriculum, in dermatology,
        37
    in Germany, 218
    Institute of Dermatology, Thailand,
        11
    medical
        and the global village, 35–36
        international aspects of, 37–39
    of patients, in preventive
        dermatology, 67
    in Poland, 232
    in tropical medicine, 6
    in Venezuela, 208
Educational Commission for Foreign
    Medical Graduates (ECFMG),
    36–39
Egypt
    scabies in, 118
    survey of skin diseases in Sharkia,
        116
    tinea capitis in, 17
Ehlers-Danlos syndrome (EDS)
    among Afrikaners, 284
    effect of heat in, 89
    in Lebanon, 300
Ehrlich, Paul, 217
Eicosapentaenoic acid, for psoriasis,
    287
Elastosis, effect of radiation (UV and
    IR), 90
Elephantiasis, filarial, 3, 252–53,
    339
El Salvador
    immigration to the United States
        from, 45
    seasonal cycles of infections in,
        17
Emic point of view, defined, 28
Emporiatrics. *See* Travel medicine
Encephalitis
    in Chagas' disease among children,
        48
    propagation by mosquitoes, 101
Endocrine-related skin disease in
    animals, 104–5
Entamoeba histolytica, cutaneous
    amoebiasis caused by, 333
Enterobiasis, therapy for, 337
Entomophtharomycoses in South
    India, 294
Environment
    of Australian aborigines, 125, 127
    degradation of
        as a public health problem, 8
        from byproducts of copper
            smelting, 181–83
    and expression of disease, 3
    in Germany, 214–16

role in incidence of infections, 17
    dams building, 67
    role of, in disease, Nigeria, 247
    tropical, role in incidence of
        infections, 117–20
    See also Climate; Climatology;
        Culture
Eosin, phototoxic contact reactions
    associated with, 72
Epidemiology, 10–14
    of ashy dermatosis, 201–2
    and travel, 70
    of veterinary skin diseases, 104–5
Epidermolysis bullosa
    in Africa, 67
    among black people, in South
        Africa, 284
Epidermophyton floccosum, 117, 176,
    294, 306
    associated with tinea, in Colombia,
        192
    associated with tinea cruris, in
        Lebanon, 300
    infection among non-Aborigines in
        Australia, 135
Epilepsy as a stereotypically Jewish
    condition, 21
Epinephrine for erythermalgia, 88
Ergosterol
    in cell membranes, yeast and fungi,
        320, 324
    inhibition of synthesis of
        by azoles, 322
        by ketoconazole, 329
        by terbinafine, 331
Erythema
    keratolytic winter, 13C
        among Afrikaners, 282
    toxic, of the newborn, 89
Erythema ab igne, 87, 88–89
    in Nigeria, 259–60
Erythema chronica migrans, 174
Erythema dyschromicum perstans, 201–3
Erythema induratum in Korea, 103
Erythema multiforme
    from benznidazole, 334
    among blacks in South Africa, 275
    in Malawi, 242
    among non-Aborigines in Australia,
        135
    photosensitivity in, 71
    sulfadoxine/pyrimethamine
        associated with, 73
Erythema nodosum
    association with sarcoidosis, in
        Caucasians, 179
    association with tuberculosis, in
        South India, 294
Erythema nodosum leprosum, 197
Erythermalgia, 87–88
Erythrocyanosis crurum, effect of cold
    on, 71
Erythroderma
    from benznidazole, 334
    in graft-versus-host disease,
        transfusion, 288–90